SOCIAL WORK PRACTICE IN HEALTH CARE SETTINGS

Second Edition

Edited by

Dr. M. J. Holosko
Professor
School of Social Work
University of Windsor

Prof. P.A. Taylor
Associate Professor
School of Social Work
University of Windsor

Canadian Scholars' Press Inc.　　　Toronto　　　1994

Social Work Practice in Health Care Settings
Second Edition

Published in 1992 and reprinted in 1994 by
Canadian Scholars' Press Inc.
180 Bloor St. W., Ste. 402,
Toronto, Ontario   M5S 2V6
First edition published in 1989.

Canadian Cataloguing in Publication Data

Main entry under title:
Social work practice in health care settings
Includes bibliographical references.

ISBN   0-921627-99-8

1. Medical social work. I. Holosko, Michael H.
II. Taylor, P.A. (Patricia A.), 1936-.

HV687.S63   1992   362.1'0425   C92-093745-4

Printed and bound in Canada

TABLE OF CONTENTS

Dedication   v
Acknowledgement   vi
Preface   vii
Contributors   ix
About the Editors   xii

Section I
An Overview of Social Work Roles in Health Care:
A Case for Generalist Practice

Chapter 1. An Overview of Social Work Practice
            in Health Care Settings 3
            Rebecca Erickson and Gerald Erickson

        2. Social Work Practice Roles in Health Care:
            Daring to be Different..21
            Michael J. Holosko

        3. Insights About Social Work Field
            Placements in a Teaching Hospital:
            Preparation for Generalist Practice.....................................33
            Sonia Busca

Section II
Hospital-Based Practice

Chapter 4. Social Work Practice
            with Myocardial Infarction
            Patients and Families in an Acute Care Hospital 45
            Joanne Sulman and Godelieve Verhaeghe

        5. Social Work Practice with Infertility
            Patients in an In Vitro Fertilization Program....................63
            Sima K. Needleman

        6. The Role of the Social Worker in the Realm of
            HIV Disease...83
            Peter Quick

7. Perinatal Social Work Practice 101
   Catherine J. Cameron, Randee J. Moir and
   Marlene L. Rees-Newton

8. Social Work Practice with Childhood Cancer 121
   David W. Adams

9. Social Work Practice
   with Paediatric Bereavement Patients.............................141
   Michael Bull

10. Social Work Practice in Family
    Centred Airway Management..161
    Jean M. Lawrence

11. Social Work Practice
    with Ventilator-Assisted Patients...................................179
    Linda B. Fischer

12. Social Work Practice
    in a Women's Health Care Centre...................................193
    Deborah MacLean-Brine

13. Social Work Practice
    with Domestic Violence in Hospital Settings 215
    Don Ebert and Shan Landry

14. Social Work Practice in a Black
    Community-Based Teaching Hospital............................237
    Marvin D. Feit and Sheila D. Miller

15. Social Work Practice in Hospital-
    Based Crisis Intervention 253
    Robert J. Todd and Mary Webb

16. Social Work Practice in Critical Care
    and Trauma Units...273
    Irene Tiegs

17. Social Work Practice
    with Plastic Surgery/Burn Patients................................293
    Clifford N. Levy

18. Social Work Practice in a Psychiatric
    Ambulatory Care Setting...307
    Sherrill Hershberg and Craig M. Posner

19. Social Work Practice
    with Institutionalized Frail Elderly...................................323
    Len Fabiano and Ron Martyn

20. Social Work Practice on a Geriatric Consultation Team 353
    Bernice Wilson

21. Social Work Practice
    in Geriatric Assessment Units 373
    Patricia MacKenzie

22. Social Work Practice in Hospice Care.............................403
    Nina Millett Fish

23. Social Work Practice in Palliative Care............................419
    Margaret R. Rodway and Judith Blythe

24. Social Work Practice
    with Organ Transplant Patients..439
    M. Jane Bright

25. Social Work Practice
    with Chronic Pain Management 453
    Mario Spiler

26. Social Work Practice in a Multi-
    disciplinary Physical Rehabilitation Setting....................467
    Carolynn Campbell, Zora Jackson and Libusa Jeglic

27. Discharge Planning
    and the Role of the Social Worker 489
    Mary Ciotti and Susan Watt

28. Discharging Patients
    from an Acute Care Hospital...509
    Margaret A. Dimond and Theresa Jansen-Santos

Section III
Community-Based Practice

Chapter 29. Social Work Practice
with Family Caregivers of Frail Older Persons...............529
Ronald W. Toseland and Charles M. Rossiter

30. Social Work Practice
with Head Injured Persons 553
Sabine Huege and Michael J. Holosko

31. Social Work Practice
with Military Personnel
in a Health Care Setting......................................567
Marvin D. Feit and Raymond D. McCoy

32. Social Work Practice
with Community-Based Dementia Care........................587
Roberta Krakoff and Lucy Esralew

33. Social Work Practice in a Community-
Based Substance Abuse Program 601
Marvin D. Feit and Terence Mayes

34. Social Work Practice
in a Therapeutic Community Context.............................613
Neal Ruton and Tracey Foreman

35. Community Social Work Practice:
Health Promotion in Action....................................643
Judith Dunlop and Michael J. Holosko

Section IV
Postscript

Chapter 36. New Wave Social Work: Practice Roles
for the 1990s and Beyond 659
Patricia A. Taylor

DEDICATION

The editors dedicate this text to the memory of Dr. Gerald Erickson, Director of the School of Social Work, University of Windsor, whose deep involvement in social work was expressed in his lifelong concern for enhancing the profession's body of theoretical and clinical knowledge. In this pursuit, he was a supportive colleague and an inspiration always. His sudden death in the midst of this project was a loss to all who knew and respected him. "Lambs Forever," Gerry.

ACKNOWLEDGEMENTS

While the editors worked diligently on organizing and developing this text, many others contributed along the way. In particular, we are grateful for the support of President Ianni and the University of Windsor. We also acknowledge the contributions of Jennifer Erickson, Ingrid Sands, Todd Sands and Andrew Taylor (who designed the book's cover). Without such able assistance we would have been seriously restricted in this endeavour. We wish also to acknowledge the sacrifices of our most astute and supportive critics, Maurice Taylor and Ann Holosko. Their love, patience and assistance were invaluable. A sincere thank you to all the supporting cast.

PREFACE

In selecting articles for this book, the editors kept in mind two main points:

1) the rapidly changing nature of the delivery of health care services in North America characterized by:
   a) unique illnesses;
   b) complex social values and ethical issues and
   c) financial resources versus increasing health care costs and

2) the need for social work practice in health care systems to relate to these changes and respond in new, creative and meaningful ways.

Consequently, we selected articles in both Canadian and American health care systems that reflect social work practice into the 1990s. We asked authors to respond not only to a discussion of roles and responsibilities in terms of today's practice, but how they plan to assume new roles and responsibilities as practice demands change to meet the challenges of the 21st century.

The concentration on certain patient groups, such as the elderly, indicates what we believe is not only a trend but will constitute a new frontier for social workers practising in health care. For instance, the social and emotional needs of older people are integrated into their physical problems in a way that tests the limits of medical intervention but also challenges the expansiveness of social work intervention.

The contribution of social work practice to health care delivery is embedded in the present trend toward holistic medicine. Teaching social workers how to adapt and expand their skills to meet the demands of tomorrow is a responsibility of both practitioners and educators.

This text brings together, for the first time, original descriptive accounts of social work practice roles in health care settings. It is intended to inform practitioners and students alike about the practice roles and responsibilities social workers undertake in a variety of settings and health care systems. Implicit in each chapter is the notion that social work holds a unique and meaningful contribution to health care service delivery. It is our decided opinion that for too long, social work has been assumed to be under the aegis of medicine and it appears timely for the profession to better define its roles and responsibilities in more autonomous, non-medical ways. The organizational context of health care settings certainly lends itself to such delineations, as such settings are characterized by a need for high levels of accountability, inter-disciplinary collaboration, timely invention and effective decision making.

The text is organized according to three main sub-sections. **Section I**, entitled "An Overview of Social Work Practice in Health Care Settings," contains three chapters that form the framework for understanding social work practice roles in a variety of health care settings. Implicit in these chapters is the notion that social work should maintain its generalist orientation, and that it holds a unique position in health care systems. The remaining chapters in the text serve as testimony to these considerations.

The health care system *per se* is then dichotomized into either hospital-based practice or community-based practice. These represent the main organizational domains in which social work practice activities occur, although inevitably there is some overlap. **Section II**, "Hospital Based Practice," contains twenty-four chapters that cut across various ages, diseases, specialty groups and practice activities. **Section III**, "Community-Based Practice," contains seven chapters that emphasize the importance of practice activities that are tied to the community. Each chapter in sections II and III is blueprinted with the same sub-headings to ensure continuity of style and content. These are:

1) the clientele;
2) practice roles and responsibilities;
3) the potential for role development;
4) concluding remarks;
5) a case example and
6) references.

The final section (IV) provides a postscript of where practice roles seem to be evolving in the 1990s and beyond. This is based on identifying threads of commonality that emerged throughout the text and a projection of social work into the future. The cumulative experience and wisdom of these contributors prescribes an important message to students and practitioners alike. Social work is not only alive and well in health care systems, it is becoming integral to them, and, in our opinion, the sooner the profession recognizes this, the better.

P.A.T.
M.J.H.

CONTRIBUTORS

ADAMS, DAVID, W., CSW, MSW, Director, Social Work Services, McMaster University Medical Centre; Professor, Department of Psychiatry, McMaster University, Hamilton, Ontario, Canada.

BLYTHE, JUDITH, MSW, Palliative Care Coordinator, Bethany Care Centre, Calgary, Alberta, Canada.

BRIGHT, M. JANE, MSW, Social Worker, Lung and Liver Transplant Programs, Toronto General Hospital, Toronto, Ontario, Canada.

BULL, MICHAEL, MSW, CSW, Associate Director, Social Work Department, Victoria Hospital, London, Ontario, Canada.

BUSCA, SONIA, RSW, Social Worker, Children's Hospital, Winnipeg, Manitoba, Canada.

CAMERON, CATHERINE J., MSW, Social Worker, St. Joseph's Health Centre, London, Ontario, Canada.

CAMPBELL, CAROLYNN, MSW, Social Worker, The Rehabilitation Centre, Ottawa, Ontario, Canada.

CIOTTI, MARY, MSW, CSW, Assistant Clinical Professor, Department of Psychiatry, McMaster University; Department of Social Work, Chedoke McMaster Hospitals, Hamilton, Ontario, Canada.

DIMOND, MARGARET A., MSW, ACSW, Director, Department of Social Work and Discharge Planning, Henry Ford Hospital, Detroit, Michigan.

DUNLOP, JUDITH, MSW, Organizational Consultant, Windsor, Ontario.

EBERT, DON, MSW, Director of Social Work, University Hospital, Saskatoon, Saskatchewan, Canada.

ERICKSON, GERALD, D. Phil., Professor and Director, School of Social Work, University of Windsor, Windsor, Ontario, Canada.

ERICKSON, REBECCA, MSW, Researcher, Kidney Foundation of Canada, Toronto, Ontario, Canada.

ESRALEW, LUCY, MS, Consultant, Washington Heights-Inwood, Council on the Aging, New York, New York.

FABIANO, LEN, BA, RN, President, ECS Publications and Consulting Service, Seagrave, Ontario, Canada.

FEIT, MARVIN D., Ph.D., Associate Professor, Norfolk State University School of Social Work, Norfolk, Virginia.

FISCHER, LINDA B., MSW, Social Worker, Department of Social Work, St. Joseph's Health Centre, London, Ontario, Canada.

FOREMAN, TRACEY, MSW, Social Worker, Stonehenge Therapeutic Community, Guelph, Ontario, Canada

HERSHBERG, SHERRILL, MSW, RSW, Social Worker, Adult Partial Hospitalization Day Treatment Program, Winnipeg Health Sciences Centre, Winnipeg, Manitoba, Canada.

HOLOSKO, MICHAEL J., Ph.D., Interim Director, Associate Professor, School of Social Work, University of Windsor, Windsor, Ontario, Canada.

HUEGE, SABINE, MSW, CSW, Vocational Rehabilitation Counsellor, Ministry of Community and Social Services, Chatham, Ontario, Canada.

JANSEN-SANTOS, THERESA, MSN, MA, RN, Supervisor, Department of Social Work and Discharge Planning, Henry Ford Hospital, Detroit, Michigan.

JACKSON, ZORA, MSW, Director of Social Work, The Rehabilitation Centre, Ottawa, Ontario, Canada.

JEGLIC, LIBUSA, MSW, CSW, Social Worker, The Rehabilitation Centre, Ottawa, Ontario, Canada.

KRAKOFF, ROBERTA, ACSW, Associate Director, Social Work Services, Presbyterian Hospital, New York, New York.

LANDRY, SHAN, MSW, Home Care—Saskatoon, Saskatoon, Saskatchewan, Canada.

LAWRENCE, JEAN M., MSSA, ACSW, Social Worker, Neonatal Intensive Care Unit, William Beaumont Hospital, Royal Oak, Michigan.

MacKENZIE, PATRICIA, MSW, Assistant Professor, Faculty of Social Work, University of Regina, Regina, Saskatchewan.

MacLEAN-BRINE, DEBORAH, BSW, RN, Social Worker, Women's Health Care Centre, Victoria Hospital, London, Ontario, Canada.

MARTYN, RON, Master of Gerontology, Associate, ECS Publications and Consulting Services, Seagrave, Ontario, Canada.

MAYES, TERENCE, MSW, Substance Abuse Counsellor, Norfolk Substance Abuse Outpatient Services, Norfolk, Virginia.

LEVY, CLIFFORD H., BA, MSW, Social Work, Department of Social Work, Victoria Hospital, London, Ontario, Canada.

McCOY, Lt. RAYMOND D., MSW, ACSW, Head, Social Work Department, Naval Medical Clinic, Norfolk, Virginia.

MILLER, SHEILA D., DSW, Associate Professor, Norfolk State University, School of Social Work and Field/Research

Coordinator, Norfolk Commmunity Hospital, Norfolk, Virginia.

MILLETT FISH, NINA, BS, MSW, RN, President, PASSAGES, St. Louis, Missouri.

MOIR, RANDEE J., SSW, Social Worker, Department of Social Work, St. Joseph's Health Centre, London, Ontario, Canada.

NEEDLEMAN, SIMA K., MSW, ACSW, Social Worker, Jewish Hospital of St. Louis, St. Louis, Missouri.

POSNER, CRAIG M., MSW, RSW, Social Worker, Outpatient Department, Department of Psychiatry, Winnipeg Health Sciences Centre, Winnipeg, Manitoba, Canada.

REES-NEWTON, MARLENE L., MSW, Social Worker, Department of Social Work, St. Joseph's Health Centre, London, Ontario, Canada.

RODWAY, MARGARET R., Ph.D., Professor, Faculty of Social Welfare, University of Calgary, Calgary, Alberta, Canada.

ROSSITER, CHARLES M., Ph.D., Project Director, Caregiver Support Project, School of Social Welfare, and the Ringel Institute of Gerontology, University at Albany, State University of New York, Albany, New York.

RUTON, NEAL, MSW, Executive Director, Stonehenge Therapeutic Community, Guelph, Ontario, Canada.

SPILER, MARIO, MSW, CSW, Social Worker, St. Joseph's Health Centre, London, Ontario, Canada.

SULMAN, JOANNE, MSW, CSW, Social Work Supervisor, Mount Sinai Hospital, Toronto, Ontario, Canada.

TAYLOR, PATRICIA, BA, MSW, Associate Professor, School of Social Work, University of Windsor, Windsor, Ontario, Canada.

TIEGS, IRENE, BSc, MSW, Social Worker, Critical Care Trauma Centre, Victoria Hospital, London, Ontario, Canada.

TODD, ROBERT J., RN, Manager, Crisis and Aftercare Services, Grey Bruce Regional Health Centre, Ontario, Canada.

TOSELAND, RONALD W., Ph.D., Associate Professor of Social Work and Principal Investigator, Caregiver Support Project, School of Social Welfare, and the Ringel Institute of Gerontology, University at Albany, State University of New York, Albany, New York.

VERHAEGHE, GODELIEVE, MSW, CSW, Social Worker, Mount Sinai Hospital, Toronto, Ontario, Canada.

WATT, SUSAN, DSW, CSW, Associate Professor and Director, School of Social Work, McMaster University, Hamilton, Ontario, Canada.

WEBB, MARY, BSW, CSW, Crisis Worker, Grey Bruce Regional Health Centre, Ontario, Canada.

WILSON, BERNICE, BSW, Ed.D., Social Worker, Toronto General Hospital, Toronto, Ontario, Canada.

ABOUT THE EDITORS

MICHAEL J. HOLOSKO is Professor at the School of Social Work, University of Windsor. He has taught social work and nursing and been a consultant in the human service and health field for the past twelve years in Canada, the United States and Europe. His specialty areas are clinical and program evaluation, administrative skills and stress management. He has published numerous monographs, chapters and articles and conducted research studies in the areas of health care, social policy and evaluation. His recent text, co-edited with Dr. M. D. Feit, was *Evaluation of Employee Assistance Programs* published by the Haworth Press, in 1988. He also serves on the editorial board for the *Journal of Health and Social Policy*. He has served on numerous boards of directors for a variety of human service agencies including Health and Welfare Canada's Research Advisory Committee.

PATRICIA A. TAYLOR is an Associate Professor at the School of Social Work, University of Windsor. For the past twenty-four years she has taught courses in both the historical development and intervention of social work in health care. In addition, Professor Taylor has been the Director of Social Work in two general hospital settings and was responsible for the initiation of social work departments in four other hospital settings. Professor Taylor has been an active member of the executive of the Ontario Hospital Association Social Work Section and frequently acts as a consultant in the health care area. She has published articles and delivered papers in Canada, the United States and Great Britain on various aspects of health care. Most recently, she was elected to the Board of Directors of Family Service America and is a member of the editorial review committee of the *Journal of Social Casework*.

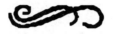

SECTION I
An Overview of Social Work
Roles in Health Care:
A Case for Generalist Practice

Chapter 1

AN OVERVIEW OF SOCIAL WORK PRACTICE IN HEALTH CARE SETTINGS[1]

Rebecca Erickson, MSW
Gerald Erickson, PhD

Abstract

Social Work in health care settings is the largest single field of practice for social workers in North America. Thus it is difficult to provide a comprehensive overview of the area in this limited space. This chapter assesses the health care field and makes nine observations useful for new social work practitioners and social work students: the medical world; a field of rapid change; site specificity; interdisciplinary teams; social work autonomy; patients' rights and advocacy; historical aspects; education and health services; and social work roles in health care settings.

AN OVERVIEW OF SOCIAL WORK PRACTICE IN HEALTH CARE SETTINGS

Any overview of social work practice in health care settings is necessarily a partial and incomplete review. The field is too vast for it to be otherwise. Indeed, it is the largest single field of practice for social workers. This overview will attempt, rather, to attend to those aspects of practice that cut across a variety of settings and organizations, and that may be applied to multiple populations in differing contexts. Given the extreme malleability of social work, sometimes seen as a weakness and sometimes as a great strength, the chapter in its presentation will also attempt to hold fast to the social work anchor in all practice settings — it is the social orientation, the social perspective itself, that is at the base of whatever domain can be claimed by social work as a "field of action." As Bracht (1978) noted, "...social work's uniqueness comes from its persistent focus on the physical, social-psychological and environmental health needs of clients" (p. 13).

The authors recognize that this uniqueness is also shaped in Canada and the United States by quite different health care policies governing health insurance, access to care and the health care organizations themselves. The United States, for example, remains the only country in the industrialized western world without a universal health care plan; however, for purposes of examining social work practice, many of these policy differences, as long as one is aware of them, can be taken as given. Certainly, one of the strengths of this book is that practice material has been gathered from sources in both countries representative of the leading edges of practice in two distinct systems.

SOME INITIAL OBSERVATIONS BY BEGINNING SOCIAL WORKERS IN HEALTH CARE

Both authors well remember their first days at a general hospital social work department and what seemed to be a great buzzing confusion. Newly graduated BSWs or MSWs entering employment in the health care field, trained as they are to survey the pertinent systems that surround them, are apt to make a number of early observations about both the settings and the various social work roles within them. Some of these likely observations are summarized below; i.e., what will recent graduates (or students) find when they enter a health care service?

I. The Medical World

Entry to health care settings may come as something of a culture shock for many beginning social workers. The medical world is populated by experts and the emphasis is on rapid and accurate assessment and treatment. There is little time for a leisured approach to relationship building with clients, and even less for a lengthy diagnostic formulation as preparation for treatment. There is, rather, a premium on rapid decision making about and with people in crisis; thus, the questions for the social worker are always: What needs to be done? What can I do? How can I do it? With whom can I do it?

Tiptoeing through the first few weeks of hospital practice can be an eye-opening experience for the student or new graduate. Faced with an array of professional groups, the new social worker quickly learns that the social work orientation to health care is unique in its holistic focus; however, in interdisciplinary settings, each professional may have differing views of what the others do, or should do, in relation to each other. This is particularly true in health care settings that have been dominated by the medical profession. Historically, social work in health care has been subordinate to the medical profession and thus the physicians' view of the patient has taken precedence. The primary difference between a social work perspective of health care and the medical model is that the latter views health, in negative terms, as the absence of disease. The medical profession focusses on the bio-medical aspects of care and is less interested in the social impact of health.

One consequence of this bio-medical focus is that there has been, in part, an emphasis in social work on helping people adapt to the demands of illness and hospitalization.

However, in recent years, the emphasis on developing autonomous social work practice in health care settings has led several authors to suggest that the time has arrived for social workers to expand their roles and promote a bio-psycho-social approach to health care practice (Caputi, 1978; Germain, 1984; Bywaters, 1986; Weick, 1986).

II. A Field of Rapid Change

The new social worker will observe a field undergoing rapid and continuous change. Advances in medical information and technology create new high risk populations (e.g., AIDS patients, organ transplant patients, family violence issues, etc.); further, changing demographics dictate an increasing concern with the elderly, single-parent families and lifestyle issues. The increasing proportion of elderly in the population will inevitably result in a concomitant emphasis on chronic health problems rather than acute illness. Health promotion and an emphasis on wellness, self-care and mutual aid and assistance are increasingly noted to be found in the forefront of health policy concerns (Germain, 1984; Rehr, 1984).

It is no accident that social work in health care settings is often characterized as a "struggle" (Weick, 1986; Germain 1984; Bywaters, 1986). Having a place to stand within the field, with a defined area of competence, a shared and recognized domain of autonomy, are all matters that are never finally settled (other than perhaps in specific sites) in the field, but rather are continuously subject to redefinition.

III. Site Specificity

Social work practice in health settings is markedly site specific; that is, social work activities and tasks may take quite different forms varying among, for example, practice in an acute care or teaching hospital, a small general hospital, an HMO, a community clinic, a medical group practice, a nursing home, a children's unit and so forth; further, there may be a sub-level of specificity between the type of site and among sites in the same category; for example, there may be distinctive differences between a general hospital that is a teaching centre versus one that is not, or between smaller and larger settings or urban and rural settings. The population served will vary depending on location and there may also be significant differences in social work functions and roles within the same category of health care organizations; for example, from one HMO to another.

Little can be taken for granted about social work practice in health care settings. Miller and Rehr (1983) stress the importance of understanding the particular organization and all its arrangements related to funding, accountability procedures, the structure and relationships among and between various services in the organization and the means by which new services may be introduced or current programmes changed. As they conclude, the social worker "...who appreciates the need to understand the structural and organizational arrangements of the setting will be more attuned to the patient's need and, therefore, will be a better practitioner" (Miller and Rehr, 1983, p. 18). As a corollary to this, we can add that an active stance is essential to the beginning social worker, a willingness to reach beyond what might otherwise be barriers, to have an inquiring attitude, to reach out and connect with others. Each setting is a unique organization and requires study and comprehension on the part of the new staff member or students.

IV. Interdisciplinary Team Collaboration

There are ample references in the literature on the importance of interprofessional collaboration of social workers with other health care professionals, including, for example, physicians, nurses, physiotherapists and occupational therapists. Some underlying assumptions of interdisciplinary teams are that the contribution and expertise of each professional are a vital and necessary part of the overall health treatment plan and that today's health care system is so complex and large that it requires the combined knowledge and presence of a range of professionals to navigate the system.

For the beginning social worker, it may seem difficult to initially understand the role differentiation in health care teams, as frequently there is an overlap of tasks and functions. Role blurring, interprofessional rivalry or "turf wars" may develop as each professional group tries to maintain some autonomy over their domain of expertise. The role of the social worker on health care teams is tremendously important as they are the only professional group that takes a central premise that a holistic perspective of a client (which considers the individual, social, familial, cultural and environmental dimensions of social functioning) is of utmost importance (Carlton, 1984).

In the same way that social work practice in health care will vary from setting to setting, it will also vary from team to team; for example, Lowe and Herranen (1981) distinguish between teams in acute care settings, which tend to emphasize crisis oriented work and have a strong co-ordinating function in patient care, and chronic care teams, which may focus more on patient maintenance issues.

Health care social workers function in a host or secondary setting; that is, the primary function of health care services has usually been directed to biomedical concerns, and other services (including social work) exist as a supplement to medical care. There has been increasing pressure to develop truly collaborative teams where the physician would be the "bio-medical specialist as part of (a) primary care team, appreciative of the psychosocial and social dimensions but not inexpertly attempting to provide them" (Wallace, Goldberg & Slaby, 1984, p. 65). The notion of a collaborative, rather than co-operative, health care team is appealing to those professional groups whose expertise seems often neglected by physicians; however, Abramson and Mizrahi (1986) believe that the strains and differences that exist between medicine and social work will continue due to inherent differences in their values, socialization and training. Similarly, Bywaters (1986) notes that running parallel to the public face of the development of collaborative teams, there has been another less visible development, a "history of interprofessional conflict...resistance, opposed to medical domination" (p. 663).

Inherent in the concern for providing good health care through collaborative rather than co-operative interdisciplinary teams is the necessity for social work to function as an autonomous profession. The need for professional autonomy has been a recurrent theme throughout the history of social work in health care, and will be developed further in the next section.

V. Autonomy

Individuals entering the field of social work will often hear reference to the need for professional autonomy. In health care, and other secondary social work settings, the emphasis becomes even more marked on defining social work as distinct from other professions.

In the early history of health care practice, social workers were dependent on referrals from physicians and were not encouraged, or allowed, to actively seek out cases on their own. In effect, the medical profession acted as an "intermediary gatekeeper for social work, by allowing only some people access to social work services" (Bywaters, 1986, p. 673); consequently, the roles and responsibilities of social work in health settings were determined by physicians and not social workers. The message to social workers was that they did not have the authority to make autonomous decisions (Ben-Sira, 1987). Abramson and Mizrahi (1986) suggested that if social work fashioned itself as a resource for physicians rather than the traditional handmaiden role, then it would be more likely to extend its sphere of influence in health care settings. They propose that if social work provides the instrumental services physicians expect from social work departments, it would be in a better bargaining position to "actively communicate" the need for other, less concrete, services.

The profession's ability to accurately gather data, to assess the psychosocial-environmental needs of health care consumers and to provide and develop resources to satisfy client needs is, paradoxically, contingent on its level of autonomy. In order for social work to achieve professional autonomy it must be able to describe what it does as distinct from other professions, how it does it and why it is important to do it. It must promote a psychosocial-environmental perspective that will encompass all aspects of good client care and aftercare.

VI. Clients' Rights and Advocacy

Historically, advocacy has been a primary social work function. In health care settings, social workers may act as advocates on their clients' behalf to obtain access to financial or other assistance, to develop resources and to improve policies affecting health care clients (Lurie, 1982).

Consumers of the health care system are frequently faced with a bewildering and complicated array of physicians, nurses, technicians and tests. If they are in a teaching hospital, they may find themselves explaining to each new group of interns their medical history and symptoms. It is important for hospitalized people to have an understanding of the procedures and tests to be performed upon them, and of the possible outcomes if they accept or refuse any treatment. The freedom to give fully informed consent is an important and basic right for every patient (Germain, 1984).

In long term care facilities, the issues and concerns of clients will be very different from those in acute care settings. Social workers may have to advocate on behalf of people for the provision of material goods and services; for example, in one hospital the dialysis unit television set had broken and the hospital administration could not stretch their budget to purchase a new television. For the people who were on dialysis three to six hours a day, and up to three days a week, the loss of the television was an important issue. They had individually approached the physician in charge of the unit but he was unable to help. When the situation was brought to the attention of the renal social worker, she was able to represent the patients' interests and obtain a new donated television set.

Some health care settings have "patient representatives" to advocate for patients. These are relatively new positions that are funded by hospitals. Generally, the patient representative is responsible for acting as a mediator between the patient and the health care system, and selectively interprets the patients' needs to other medical personnel and provides social support to patients and families (Miller & Rehr, 1983). One author recalls a situation where a person with AIDS was admitted to hospital on Monday for surgery three days later. The day before his surgery he still had not been given a room and had been sleeping in the emergency room. The housekeeping staff were afraid to enter his room and had been leaving his meals on the floor outside the door. No one had cleaned the room since his arrival. The admitting department stated that they were unable to find room for him. The client believed that he was being discriminated against because he did not have private room insurance coverage and the hospital was unwilling to put him in a room with other patients because of his diagnosis. He was angry and upset, both at his upcoming surgery and at what he perceived as discrimination. This hospital did not have a full time emergency unit social worker and no one was aware of the situation until the patient was overheard telling a

11

friend that he was going to contact the media to complain about his treatment. The patient representative was contacted and was able to successfully mediate on behalf of the patient and the hospital staff in several departments. This example illustrates some of the problems that can occur in health care settings. It also illustrates some concerns about the role of patient representatives in hospitals. Indeed, Miller and Rehr (1983) point out that patient representatives have an ambiguous function within health care settings. Responsible to both the patient and the hospital administration, the patient representative must reconcile the needs of the patient within the capabilities of the hospital.

Social workers have developed a variety of resources to help clients including support or mutual aid groups and outpatient counselling services. As described in this text, social workers are actively involved in hospice services, home health care and community health clinics. In both Canada and the United States, the wide variety of ethno-cultural groups requires an awareness of, and sensitivity to, the health concerns of people with language and cultural barriers (Germain, 1984). Further, patient rights is a growing area of concern for consumer groups in both the physical and mental health fields, and the value base and training of social workers will allow them to play an integral part in protecting the rights of clients.

VII. Historical Aspects

The one area of interest to the new health care social worker about which a general agreement seems to exist is that of the historical development of the field. The forerunner of the contemporary hospital was the almshouse which served the poor, the ill, orphans, the mentally ill and criminals. Originating in England and carried over to the United States, almshouses were essentially regarded as a charitable provider of food and shelter. Medical care was considered supplementary, and, as Rehr (1985) notes, physicians of the day "had no more education than services in an apprenticeship lasting between eight to sixteen weeks" (p. 246).

Rehr (1985) describes several factors which contributed to the transformation of the almshouse to hospital: a growing industrialized economy; increased immigration; advances in scientific knowledge; social reform movements and a growing awareness that there was a relationship between people's health and their environment.

There is widespread agreement that while social workers were engaged in public health care activity during the Settlement House era in the late 19th Century, the legitimization of social work in health settings was only achieved by the introduction of social workers in general hospitals early in the 20th Century by Dr. Richard Cabot, of the Massachusetts General Hospital (Nacman, 1977; Bracht, 1978; Rehr, 1985). The initial function of social work had to do with discharge planning from the hospital and follow-up work in the community (Blumenfield and Rosenberg, 1988). Caputi (1978) has pointed out that social work has followed an accretion process over the decades; that is, the original functions have been maintained while new ones were acquired over time. Miller and Rehr (1983) present the current view that social work has "...the primary function of helping patients negotiate the health care system" (p. 5); thus, the context has changed from a provision of a closely regulated single function to the multiple roles visible today.

A considerable amount of literature exists documenting the historical development of social work in health care settings, in addition to the concern with the frequently ancillary and subordinate status of social workers in health care settings (Stannes, 1967; Nacman, 1977; Watt, 1977; Bracht, 1978; Schlesinger & Wolock, 1982; Wallace et al., 1984; Rehr, 1985; Bywaters, 1986).

VIII. Social Work Education and Health Services

The general competence of new social work entrants to health care settings may be viewed with some suspicion; that is, the degree to which they have been educated and prepared in schools of social work to assume a professional role in a specialized area may certainly be questioned (Borland & Strauss, 1982). There is a continuing tension between social work education, which for some years has stressed the production of generalist practitioners able to operate at a beginning level of professional competence in a wide range of settings, and, for example, social work administrators of organizations charged with delivering health care services. The latter would like to see the development of more specialized forms of social work education, or, failing that, the introduction of post-degree residency programmes (Borland & Strauss, 1982; Wallace, Goldberg & Slaby, 1984).

New social workers may conclude that they are in paradoxical situations whereby they enter the specialized health care field as a graduate of generalist social work education[2] prepared to begin learning specialized practice roles and have the prospect of actually becoming a generalist following four to ten years of experience; i.e., able to function as an expert practitioner, to develop and administer services, to conduct research and to assume a teaching/educational function within the field. In this sense, the gap between education and practice, while real, can also be seen as partially a misunderstanding.

IX. Social Work Roles

Should the new social worker decide to examine the kinds of roles and/or activities available in health care settings, and for which performance might be an expectation, a rather staggering array will emerge. A brief catalogue would include the following:

Administrator	Family therapist
Clinician	Marriage counsellor
Teacher-educator	Team member
Researcher	Collaborator
Advocate	Resource developer
Crisis interventionist	Service planner
Case finder	Enabler
Discharge planner	Facilitator
Membership builder	Mediator
Patient screener	Consultant
Community developer	Assistant
Patient representative	Sustainer
Liaison worker	Negotiator
Organizer	Practitioner-scientist
Innovator	Psychotherapist
Pre-admission worker	Group worker
Supervisor	Assessor

There may well be a number of other available roles not mentioned above (Bartlett, 1961; Lowe and Herranen, 1978; Wokkenstein and Faufenburg, 1981; Lurie, 1982; Schlesinger and Wolock, 1982; Carlton, 1984; Germain, 1984; Ben-Sira, 1987; Rusnack, McNulty, Schaefer & Moxley, 1988). Again, these multiple roles may be seen as a strength or a liability. Such a variety of roles emphasizes the breadth of social work practice in health care settings, yet also points to the difficulty of becoming a skilled practitioner when there are no clearly defined areas of role competence specific to social work practice in health care settings. From one perspective, the notions of social work roles appear in the literature as a great sprawling mass with little coherence or commonality of concepts or terminology. As roles, they are often specific to particular organizations and services. It is obvious that when seen as clusters of activities, a single role, for example, that of family therapist or practitioner, would subsume a good number of the terms appearing in the listing. In addition to the complexity of general role functions, Bracht (1978, pp. 141-154) lists some sixty-one distinct illnesses, from "age-impaired" to "terminal illness" that require specific medical information by the social worker, and about which there is a defined social work literature featuring role functioning.

Perhaps the most generally accepted approach to role functioning follows a phasic or chronological design; i.e., a set of prescriptions for action in which tasks are oriented to what must be done first, then second and so forth. Each phase of practice is specific and is framed in terms of skills. Rosenberg (1983, pp. 140-142) for example, presents a design in which the entry of a patient to a health care organization calls upon the social worker to initially employ entry and assessment skills, then collaborative skills in working with other professionals, followed by contracting skills, intervention skills, outcome evaluation skills and recording skills. Another widely known and popular approach is Haley's (1976) outline of the phases of a single interview; i.e., a social phase, problem definition phase, interaction around the problem, goal setting and the provision of specific tasks for the client(s) to carry out in relation to problem-solving.

The beginning social worker will find that social work roles are sometimes defined in terms of complexes of theories, responsibilities, tasks, skills and knowledge (e.g., consultant, clinician, administrator); sometimes in terms of complexes of activity related to a single general task (e.g., discharge planner); sometimes as the knowledge, skills and tasks related to a specific population (e.g., psychiatric social worker, renal social worker) and sometimes in terms of a single activity (e.g., negotiator, enabler).

One way to understand this is to consider that while the bases of social work theory, knowledge and practice in health care are widely eclectic, there is a high degree of selectivity involved (Monkman & Kagle , 1982). Social workers develop over time and experience what might be termed "packages" of expertise; that is, a particular cognitive organization of an array of knowledge relat-

15

ed to health and illness (which may be constantly reorganized) on a base of relatively constant values common to social work. The beginning social worker may therefore start in a state of personal crisis related to a felt lack of such "packages," but will quickly begin accumulating new theory, knowledge and skills related to health and illness, crisis theory, stress and social support, epidemiology and high risk populations, life-cycle transitions, specific illnesses and the skills of short-term practice. Health settings are learning settings, and in view of rapidly changing knowledge and technologies, everyone is a life-long learner. Again, however, one must stress the necessity of an active stance by the beginner in searching out the opportunities for learning and the development of a number of packages of skillful activities.

The development of social work roles in the health care system has been inconsistent. Historically, social work roles developed largely in response to gaps in health care services. Other professions, notably physicians, have been allowed to define the roles and functions of social work. This has resulted in a lack of autonomy which would allow us to shape and define our unique contribution to health care settings. There is a need for a comparative analysis across areas of social work practice in health care to distil the elements of role commonality.

The health care field is under restraint. As one author noted "Yesterday the magic word was 'audit.' Today it is containment," (Nacman, 1980, p.11). With increasing attention by health care administrators toward quality assurance and accountability, and growing consumer demand for effective, available and accessible health services, it is increasingly important for social worker to clearly define their roles and place within health care settings.

References

Abramson, J., & Mizrahi, T. (1986). Strategies for enhancing collaboration between social workers and physicians. *Social Work in Health Care, 12* (1), 1-21.

Bartlett, H. (1961). *Social Work Practice in the Health Field.* New York: National Association of Social Workers.

Bennett, C. J., & Grob, G. G. (1982). The social worker new to health care: Basic learning tasks. *Social Work in Health Care, 8* (2), 49 - 64.

Ben-Sira, Z. (1987). Social work in health care: Needs challenges and implications for structuring practice. *Social Work in Health Care, 13* (1), 79 - 85.

Berkman, B. G., & Rehr, H. (1973). Early social service case finding for hospitalized patients: An experiment. *Social Service Review, 47* (2), 256-265.

Borland, J.J. & Strauss, M. (1982). Social work education for health care: A blueprint for action. *Health and Social Work, 7* (3), 224-229.

Bracht, N. (1978). *Social Work in Health Care.* New York: The Haworth Press.

Blumenfield, S. & Rosenberg, G. (1988). Towards a network of social health services: Re-defining discharge planning and expanding the social work domain. *Social Work in Health Care, 13* (4), 31 - 49.

Bywaters, P. (1986). Social work and the medical profession–Arguments against unconditional collaboration. *British Journal of Social Work, 16,* 661-677.

Caputi, M. (1978). Social work in health care: Past and future. *Health and Social Work, 3* (1), 9 - 29.

Carlton, T. (1984). *Clinical Social Work in Health Settings: A Guide to Professional Practice with Exemplars.* New York: Springer Publishing Company.

Coulton, C. J. (1979). *Social Work Quality Assurance Programs: A Comparative Analysis.* New York: National Association of Social Workers.

Falck, H. (1982). What is central in social work? *Health in Social Work, 7* (3), 235 - 237.

Germain, C. (1984). *Social Work Practice in Health Care: An Ecological Perspective.* New York: Free Press.

Haley, J. (1976). *Problem Solving Therapy.* San Francisco: Jossey-Bass.

Kerson, T. S. (1982). *Social Work in Health Settings, Practice in Context.* New York: Longman, Inc.

Lowe, J. I., & Herranen, M. (1981). Understanding teamwork: Another look at the concepts. *Social Work in Health Care, 7* (2), 1 - 11.

Lurie, A. (1982). The social work advocacy role in discharge planning. *Social Work in Health Care, 8* (2), 75 - 87.

Miller, R., & Rehr, H. (1983). *Social Work in Health Care.* Englewoods Cliff, New Jersey: Prentice-Hall Inc.

Monkman, M. Q., & Kagle, J. D. (1982). The transactions between people and environment framework: Focusing social work interventions in health care. *Social Work in Health Care, 8* (2), 105 - 116.

Nacman, M. (1977). Social work in health settings: A historical review. *Social Work in Health Care, 2* (4), 407 -418.

Nacman, M. (1980). Reflections of a social work administrator on the opportunities of crisis. *Social Work in Health Care, 6* (1), 11 - 21.

Rehr, H. (1984). Health care and social work services: Present concerns and future directions. *Social Work in Health Care, 10* (1), 71 - 83.

Rehr, H. (1985). Medical care organizations and the social service connection. *Health in Social Work, 10* (4), 245- 257.

Rosenberg, G. (1983). Advancing social work practice in health care. *Social Work in Health Care, 8* (3), 147 - 156.

Rusnack, B., McNulty, S., Schaefer, & Moxley, D. (1988). Safe passage: Social work roles and functions in hospital care. *Social Work in Health Care, 13* (3), 3 - 21.

Schlesinger, E., & Wolock, I. (1982). Hospital social work roles and decision making. *Social Work in Health Care, 8* (1), 59 - 70.

Schlesinger, E. (1985). *Health Care Social Work Practice Concepts and Strategies.* St. Louis, Missouri: Mirror/Mosby College Publishing.

Stannes, C. (1967). Social workers or disposal unit? *Medical Social Work, 19* (8), 267 - 269.

Wallace, S. R., Goldberg, R. J., Slaby, A. E. (1984). *Clinical Social Work in Health Care New Biopsychosocial Approaches.* New York: Praeger.

Watt, M. S. (1977). *The Therapeutic Facilitator: The Role of the Social Worker in Acute Treatment Hospitals in Ontario.* Unpublished Doctoral Dissertation. University of California at Los Angeles.

Weick, A. (1986). The philosophical context of a health model of social work. *Social Casework, 67,* 551 - 559.

Wokkenstein, A. & Faufenberg, H. (1981). Teaching the behaviourial science component in a family practice residency: Social work role. *Social Work in Health Care, 6,* (3), 35 - 49.

Endnotes

[1] The authors wish to acknowledge the insights and support of J. Erickson, MSW, in the preparation of this chapter.

[2] We should note that the difference between the generalist and specialist social work education may consist of only a few courses and a practicum; thus, even "specialist" graduates may find it difficult to either label themselves, or to function immediately, as specialists.

Chapter 2

SOCIAL WORK PRACTICE ROLES IN HEALTH CARE: DARING TO BE DIFFERENT

Michael J. Holosko, PhD

Abstract

The extent to which any professional group can be questioned about what it is doing and why it is doing certain activities is at the core of its professional autonomy. This chapter examines social work practice roles in health care settings from the standpoint of four presuppositions that underpin its practice activities. They are presented as myths that have evolved in health care settings. These are: 1) its legitimacy vs. autonomy; 2) its professional status; 3) its role evolution and 4) its uniqueness.

The main contentions of the chapter are: 1) that social work roles need to be questioned within the context of practice specific and organizational settings and 2) that the sooner social work emerges from the shadow of medicine ineffecting practice, the better. Indeed, social work needs tohighlight its uniqueness and needs to become "daring to be different."

SOCIAL WORK PRACTICE ROLES IN HEALTH CARE: DARING TO BE DIFFERENT

The medical model has had a decidedly mixed blessing effect on the development of social work practice in health care settings. On the one hand, it has inadvertently legitimized social work practice in that, historically, social workers have served patient needs in areas that essentially doctors told them to. Further, they filled gaps in the health care system that were not the domain, concern or interest of other health care professionals; e.g., patient advocacy, community liaising, etc. Indeed, in Mary Richmond's seminal text entitled *Social Diagnosis* (1917), social work and its casework methods became formally hooked on the medical model and its problem-solving approach. In turn, many social workers began assimilating the roles of doctors and nurses in the assessment, diagnosis and treatment of patients.

On the other hand, the medical model has cast a long shadow on the profession of social work in health care settings which has generally hindered its power base, stymied its potential for role development, caused identity anxiety about social work roles and generally compromised its professional autonomy. Ironically, for the most part, social work has not objected to these consequences. Historically, the profession has had "no problem" with plodding along and "figuring things out later" in a completely illogical but comfortable way. Examples of this are numerous in areas such as industrial social work, school social work, rural social work, program evaluation, etc.

However, the health care system as a domain for social work practice is different from all of the above in three main respects:

1) it is more costly;
2) it is more accountable and
3) the likelihood of intervention contributing directly to people either living or dying is implicit in each and every decision made.

As a result, social work practitioners working in health care settings are continually confronted by patients, other professionals and the institutions of care about their activities, roles, functions, worthiness and efficacy, etc. This constant questioning of: what is social work? and, how does it fit into this setting? are daily realities affecting health care practitioners.

Such realities, however, are not generally the concern of social workers practising in the majority of social welfare institutions and agencies; e.g., departments of social service, child and family service agencies, etc.; thus, social workers who practice in health care settings are a unique breed who tend to be very clear about who they are and what they are doing. In short, they cannot afford not to be.

The chapters in this text serve as testimony to the profession stepping out of the shadow of the medical model. They are written largely by practitioners who have not necessarily waited for medicine to inform them about how to evolve, but have "dared to be different" in that social workers have plugged holes in the existing systems by taking initiative to serve patients in need, and have developed, as Erickson and Erickson (1989) indicated, "packages" of operationalized knowledge or skills along the way to serve their own practice needs. Their practice roles, therefore, are clearly separate and unique and complementary to medical ones, and in a number of chapters, readers will note how gargantuan and integral to patient care they have become. In many of these accounts, the "handmaiden to the doctor's" role has become stereotypically reversed [this generalization certainly varies across settings]. Without question, the message is clear: the profession's ability to wean itself from medicine will ultimately contribute to its own professional identity and survival. William James' (1906) classic essay on pragmatism makes the point more succintly as "seeking the difference that makes the difference." Harriet Bartlett (1961) reiterated this by noting that:

> While both medical and psychiatric social work function within medicine, psychiatric social work and psychiatry seem to be largely within the same framework, whereas medical social work and medicine (in spite of overlapping in the social area) seem to be operating in different frameworks. It has not been sufficiently recognized how greatly the problem of integration of service is increased by the degree of such difference; and, at the same time, how much greater is the opportunity to make a significant contribution of something new because of this very difference (p. 131).

Certainly, as race and ethnic relations theory reminds us, our identity about who we are is confronted more frequently when we come in contact with others who are different; thus, at one level, the organizational context of health care practice with its interdisciplinary delivery of service provides the profession with a unique perspective for understanding its focus on a need to be different.

At another level, however, we [social workers] have never seriously questioned a number of practice presuppositions which have kept the profession in medicine's shadow and contributed to its "ideology of conformity," which in turn has limited its potential for professional growth and development. These presuppositions need to be explored as they form the scaffolding for the construction of how practice roles have emerged in health care settings. They can be deintellectualized at this point as simply being myths we have come to believe in these practice settings.

MYTHS ABOUT HEALTH CARE PRACTICE

I. Medical Legitimation vs. Practice Autonomy

As the previous quotation from H. Bartlett (1961) indicated, although some areas of social work practice may overlap in health care settings, outside of helping patients in need, social work and medicine have evolved from very different practice frameworks and, in some instances, may have competing ideologies. Generally, these differences would come to play in the assessment/diagnosis, treatment and follow-up of patients. Specifically, they may become sources of strain in the areas of

1) the organization and socialization process of professional training;
2) perspectives on patient care, illness and role of the health care professional;
3) attitudes toward knowledge and data;
4) attitudes toward and preparation for teamwork;
5) perspectives on the role of the patient and
6) perceptions of social work's function (Mizrahi & Abramson, 1985).

25

Historically, since medicine ascribed "a role" for social work in health care settings; originally it was either

1) "to be the conscience" of the hospital;
2) to provide doctors with social data about patiets or
3) to liaise between the patient, hospital, and/or family — the profession has assured its limited practice autonomy around these roles.

The irony is that such autonomy was dictated by the medical profession's needs and concerns not by social work's needs or concerns; thus, the analogy previously used to being in the shadow of medicine seems apropos.

The companion issue of power-dependency needs to be mentioned at this point. Just as our practice roles have largely been determined by medicine, so has our "power base." Although social work strove to achieve power by taking on the characteristics of the power group (doctors), the profession has neither the resources or credibility (at this time in its history) to become assimilated as such. For instance, many doctors and hospital administrators alike constantly remind social workers and their departments that they are organizationally vulnerable to budget cutbacks, and are often considered a "luxury" to these settings. In short, one can surmise, even in this brief overview, how practice roles have become highly tentative, dependent and non-autonomous, due in large part to accepting the myth that medical legitimization would enhance social work practice autonomy.

II. Social Work is a Profession

The issue of practice autonomy transcends examining social work practice roles in health care settings. Clearly, the struggle for autonomy and professionalism goes on in agencies, health care settings or private practice beyond individual practitioners, to the issue of autonomy as a whole (Caroff, 1988). The optimistic camp suggests it is a profession, and the more reality-based camp suggests it is a semi-profession moving toward becoming a profession.

A careful examination of whether social work is a profession would concur with the latter position (Greenwood, 1957; Toren, 1974; Sainsbury, 1982). Whether one argues the point from its applied knowledge or scientific base, the criteria or attributes of a profession, its theoretical base, the development and utilization of research or its use of practice wisdom — social work is a semi-profession with all of the trappings of a profession (Makris, 1987).

This reality certainly "throws a spanner in the works" when trying to understand how other professions perceive our practice domains and role perceptions; for example, Lister (1980) surveyed the role expectations of 13 different groups of health professions across 36 different tasks, and not one task was seen as identifiable or exclusively the domain of social work. In other words, other health professionals could perform so-called social work tasks as readily as social workers. It is not surprising that often, health care social workers feel like "employees" or "technicians" and not professionals at all. Role confusion? role conflict? role ambiguity? role blurring you say? — indeed.

III. Practice Roles Evolved in Health Care Settings in Deliberate Ways

This is just not the case. One of the greatest strengths of social work has been its malleability, flexibility and adaptation to individual needs and social institutions and social change over time. As needs change, so do practice roles and responsibilities. Over time, practitioners in health care settings evolved roles very different from how doctors or other practioners ever perceived of them. Medical legitimization certainly gave social work a 'foot in the door' of health care institutions. Once in, we evolved in a variety of ways. There are three points to consider in this dispersed role evolution in health care settings: 1) the organizational context; 2) the development of differentiated specialized skills and knowledge and 3) the personal attributes of the practitioners themselves.

Trying to understand how roles and responsibilities of social work are practised in any setting without an examination of the organizational context is remiss. The point worth noting here, is that despite the fact that various units and departments may have the same names; e.g., emergency room social work practice in Hospital A vs. emergency room social work practice in Hospital B, the roles and responsibilities may be very different. Some factors that contribute to such differences include the organizations' perception of social work practice; the resources of the organization; the organizational climate; the competencies of the social work practitioners; administrative support and, interdisciplinary support. Organizational cultures certainly shape the role-taking of all personnel much more than personnel are willing to admit, and social work is no exception.

Although one may convincingly argue that social work is not a specialization (Brengarth, 1981), one must acknowledge that we do have "specialized," "specific" (Bartlett, 1970), or "specialty interests" (Lewis, 1980). Further, we work with specialized patient groups who require specialized care. It seems important, therefore, to identify what such specialized care involves so that social work roles can be better differentiated from other caregiver roles. It is quite appropriate for interdisciplinary roles to overlap, but the questions raised in this context include: a) how are we prepared to practice if they do and, more importantly, b) what is unique about social work practice? In regard to the latter, we need to delineate specific knowledge and skill areas that are unique in more precise ways in order to ascribe the parameters of such specialized practice.

The issue of what personal attributes are needed to effect practice roles in health care settings is more complex than it appears. Its multi-faceted dimensions include examining: 1) the personality characteristics of such practitioners; 2) the personal suitability of such practitioners; 3) the personal attributes that motivate persons to enter schools of social work; 4) their education and training and 5) the personal characteristics deemed to be essential to the professional associations, their standards, and codes of ethics.

One may readily perceive how one social worker's motivation and role expectation could differ drastically from another; thus, the practice roles and responsibilities of social work practitioners are very much attributed to the personal style, personal values and/or personal attributes of the worker. At a very cursory level, and without getting to the generalizable, social work practitioners in health care settings:

1) carry themselves in a professional demeanour (as do the majority of personnel in such settings);
2) are compassionate to patients in need;
3) are not afraid of accountability, as they live with it daily;
4) must be co-operative and team oriented;
5) are able to negotiate systems effectively;
6) have good interpersonal skills,

7) tend to be highly motivated and take initiative and

8) often show creativity in their approaches to helping those in need.

Social work, not unlike other disciplines, has skirted the whole issue of personal suitability for a number of reasons, the most obvious being its legal ramifications; however, as roles and responsibilities of practitioners evolve, and become better articulated, the issue of can this person do this job seemingly will be confronted. We certainly seem to be moving in this direction.

IV. There is Nothing Unique about Social Work Practice

Although there is evidence in the literature to suggest that social work roles cannot be differentiated from other health care practitioners' roles (Lister, 1980), certainly, how we perform our roles is indeed different and unique. The working definition of social work practice articulates the framework and uniqueness of social work (NASW, 1958) as does any introductory text on social work practice. It is no secret that what is unique about social work practice is the *social* part of practice. Practitioners need to reiterate this as "their turf" and promote this to other disciplines or professions. In health care settings, this translates as continuing to move assessments *per se* into psycho-social assessments, continuing to practice within the "person-in-environment" context, continuing to involve family members and social systems in the treatment of patients, continuing to liaise with the community for patient care and continuing the use of holistic and humanistic approaches to understanding people, their problems and needs.

CONCLUDING REMARKS

In order to understand roles and responsibilities of social workers in health care settings (or any setting for that matter), there has to be some questioning of the presuppositions which underpin practice. This chapter attempted to address this issue by examining some of the myths about practice that obfuscate an understanding of the realities of the roles and responsibilities of health care practitioners. Certainly, they are not viewed as exhaustive, but seem to be prevalent with reoccurring presence in many health care settings. The central theme of this overall text is that social work has an important contribution to make in health care systems, one that is usually assumed or consumed by the systems in which it operates. The sooner we [the profession] recognize this reality, the better off we will be. "Daring to be different" from medicine is the message, and the remaining chapters in this text make this case in a very convincing fashion. But I would prefer that you be the judge of that (alas — self-determinism in its classic sense).

References

Bartlett, H. (1961). *Social Work Practice in the Health Field*. New York: National Association of Social Workers.

Bartlett, M. (1970). *The Common Base of Social Work Practice*. New York: National Association of Social Workers.

Brengarth, J. (1981). What is 'special' about specialization? *Health and Social Work, 5*(2), 91-94.

Caroff, P. (1988). Clinical social work: Present role and future challenge. *Social Work in Health Care, 13*(3).

Erickson, R. & Erickson, G. D. (1989). An overview of social work practice in health care settings. In M. Holosko and P. Taylor (Eds.) *Social Work Practice in Health Care Settings*. Toronto: The Canadian Scholars' Press Inc.

Greenwood, E. (1957, July). Attributes of a profession. *Social Work, 2*(3), 45-55.

James, W. (1906). What pragmatism means. In *Pragmatism and Other Essays* (pp. 22-28). New York: Washington Square Press, 1963.

Lewis, M. (1980, June). Discussion of specialization report. Appendix D in *Specialization in the Social Work Profession*. Special Report of the NASW-CSWE Task Force on Specialization.

Lister, L. (1980). Role expectations of social workers and other health professionals. *Health and Social Work, 5*(2), 41-49.

Makris, D. (1987). An assessment of core social work journals from 1980 to 1985 with particular reference to research and practice implications. Unpublished Masters' Thesis, Faculty of Graduate Studies, School of Social Work, University of Windsor.

Mizrahi, T. & Abramson, J. (1985, Spring). Sources of strain between physicians and social workers: Implications for social workers in health care settings. *Social Work in Health Care,* 10(3), 33-51.

National Association of Social Workers. (1958, April). Working definition of social work practice. Report of the Sub-Committee on the Working Definition. *Social Work,* 3(2).

Richmond, M. (1917). *Social Diagnosis.* New York: Russell Sage Foundation.

Sainsbury, E. (1982). Knowledge, skills and values in social work education. In R. Bailey and P. Lee (Eds.), Theory and Practice in Social Work. Oxford, England: Basil Blackwell Publishers Ltd.

Toren, N. (1974). Social Work: The Case of a Semi-Profession. Beverly Hills, California: Sage Publications Inc.

Chapter 3

INSIGHTS ABOUT SOCIAL WORK FIELD PLACEMENTS IN A TEACHING HOSPITAL: PREPARATION FOR GENERALIST PRACTICE

Sonia Busca, RSW

Abstract

This paper highlights various features that characterize social work in a teaching hospital and examines how skills in these areas are transferable to other settings. Students whose placements are in the hospital will have to be proficient in organizational analyses, multi-disciplinary collaboration, interpersonal communication, teaching and community liaison. Skill development in these areas is valuable for the generalist practitioner in all aspects of social work practice.

INSIGHTS ABOUT SOCIAL WORK FIELD PLACEMENTS IN A TEACHING HOSPITAL: PREPARATION FOR GENERALIST PRACTICE

Upon entering a large teaching hospital, the social work student is faced with an array of sights and sounds that would boggle the medically uninitiated. Clusters of lab-frocked individuals, chin in hand, pensively following their leader; names solemnly paged by invisible voices; nurses in pastel-coloured uniforms purposefully bustling from room to room; beeps, buzzes and other unintelligible sounds ringing in all directions. It is understandable that the social work student would question how she will ever find a place in this hi-tech world. In fact the literature has many references regarding how poorly equipped academically students are for hospital practice (Lane, 1982; Berkman, Kremler, Marcus & Silverman, 1985).

Yet year after year, social work students make significant contributions in hospital settings and come away from hospital field placements with greater professional identity, personal strength and wisdom. The purpose of this chapter is to identify some unique features which characterize social work practice in a teaching hospital and to examine how these characteristics prepare the student for such practice. More specifically, this chapter will highlight how the field experience in a teaching hospital may contribute toward skill development that is highly transferable; therefore, in keeping with the solid generalist orientation prevalent in modern practice. As defined by Cossom (1988) the general practitioner in social work is one who has knowledge and skill to intervene in various types and sizes of systems, drawing on a core of generic practice skills and combining a variety of methodological approaches.

Generalist practice was not the concern of the first Canadian Social Service Department opened in 1910 at the Winnipeg General Hospital in Manitoba. A brief retrospective glance will illustrate the evolution of functions and responsibilities of the social worker in this hospital setting. A press release, dated 1910, found in that hospital's archives, summarizes the major tasks of the hospital social worker as one who looks after the material welfare of patients who are about to leave the hospital, ensures that they shall live in proper hygienic surroundingsand have proper clothing and food and arranges suitable occupations (Archives, 1910-1988). Clearly, social work's commitment to the person in relationship to her/his environment remains a concern to the modern professional; however, unlike the early practitioner, who was motivated by the charitable spirit of doing good, current hospital social work practice is informed by the knowledge of social factors and how they underpin individual concerns.

The modern social worker is called upon to intervene in increasingly more complex situations than the social service nurse who was her predecessor, and whose function was to "handle welfare problems" or dispense glasses, elastic stockings or surgical belts (Archives, 1910-1988). Great advances in medicine have increased the life-expectancy of those who live with chronic or life-threatening illness.

As more fragile people are thriving, there is a greater emphasis on their right to dignity and equal participation in society. Concurrently, the use of institutions is falling out of favour on philosophical and financial grounds and more families are expected to look after the ill at home, often with limited resources. As the trend towards smaller, often isolated single-parent or double-income families continues, greater demands will be made on many who lack the social resources to comply. Indeed, along with the many benefits of medical/technological advances, have come considerable social costs. It is into this arena that the hospital social worker has largely evolved, as a counsellor, an advocate, a service broker and an educator, and it is also within this arena that the generalist orientation is most useful for professional survival.

ROLES, RESPONSIBILITIES AND SKILLS NEEDED IN A TEACHING HOSPITAL

The social work student enters a situation rich in learning possibilities. Besides exposure to the core clinical health care issues of the psycho-social effects of illness, disability, injury and loss, there are the broader issues of organizational analyses, multi-disciplinary collaboration, interpersonal communication, teaching and community liaison that shape the character of hospital practice. It is proficiency in this latter cluster of skills that provides the greatest preparation for the generalist practitioner. A discussion of each will follow.

The teaching hospital is a large, highly-complex hierarchical institution, governed by two types of authority: bureaucratic and professional. Its purpose and function are multiple, ranging from the cure and care of the sick, training of medical and other professional disciplines and conducting of research (Robinson, 1973). Carlton (1984) described the institution's complexity as resulting from "the intricate, highly specialized knowledge and skill of each professional and staff member in the organization; and the synthesis of this knowledge, and skill in the provision of services which are often given in collaboration or by health teams" (p. 15). The medical institution is steeped in science as its guiding principle, an orientation often unfamiliar to social work students. The ability to analyse the strengths and shortcomings of the health care system from a social work perspective is a crucial skill for students to learn (Lane, 1982). With the institution being predominantly pathology-oriented, the social worker must regularly check her practice against her own values and professional ethics to ensure that she is true to her own professional orientation. The important awareness that the social worker may develop of the interactional forces at play between hospital and patient, or patients and staff, can be one of her most valuable contributions to the health care team. Students should be encouraged to challenge existing practices and perceptions, while advocating for their clients. Doing this, however, requires mutual sensitivity and open-mindedness toward the client and the institution guarding against alienating the latter and, therefore, rendering efforts on behalf of the former relatively ineffective.

Competence in the analyses of the organization and how it works is invaluable in any social work setting. Understanding how to utilize the power of those who have it, recognizing one's allies and appreciating the impact of the larger social structure on the individual or family are of equal importance within the institution of the hospital, as it is within a grassroots community neighbourhood project. The student in a hospital field practicum has ample opportunity to refine this skill.

The amount of inter-intraorganization collaboration in a hospital is probably unequalled in any other system (Berkman, Kremler,

Marcus & Silverman, 1985). Virtually no social work endeavour is a solo effort, with collaboration occurring informally on a case-by-case basis, on the telephone, over coffee or in stairwells, or more formally in regular *ad hoc* team meetings (Carlton, 1984). For instance, to call and chair a team meeting involving 10 or more people, including doctors, medical trainees, nurses and professionals from allied health disciplines and external agencies, is not an uncommon task for the social worker. Students who are new to a hospital setting have found it useful to interview various professionals with a view to learning about the roles and functions of each discipline, to challenge their own preconceived stereotypes of hospital staff and to begin to build a rapport with the staff with which they will come in contact throughout their field placement. This preliminary groundwork will assist in building the skills necessary for interdisciplinary collaboration: "the capacity to listen, to be respectful, to understand the implications of other professionals' opinions, to be willing to recognize and accept areas in which the expertise of a colleague is unique, and to defer to special knowledge when appropriate" (Mailich & Ashley, 1981, p. 135).

Role/task clarification is a crucial element in reducing conflicts among collaborators (Lowe & Herranen, 1977), and this skill is useful to social work practitioners in many other spheres of practice. To be capable of articulating what one is doing, to be clear about one's strengths and limitations, to negotiate roles with others and to allow one's practice to be on display is of vital importance in any social work endeavour, regardless of setting. Working in an inter-disciplinary system allows the student to compare and contrast her/his role vis-à-vis others and emerge with a stronger professional identity. Interestingly, this very premise is the overriding theme of this entire text.

Interpersonal communication skills are the scaffolding for social work's technical repertoire, and a wide range of skills are necessary in hospital practice to utilize with both staff and clients. Further, situations requiring social work intervention are varied. Events of acute trauma, such as burns or motor vehicle accidents, areas of decision making, as in pregnancy or genetic counselling, or the use of life-support systems, ongoing support through a chronic illness, are examples of the kinds of circumstances that social workers may confront. The most basic commonality here is that their clients are seeking medical services, not social services, and that for the most part the social worker's clients have not referred themselves. This demands that the social workers be proficient in skills of engagement; for example, regardless of whether patients have been referred by other staff who have identified difficulties, or the social worker has defined the need and reached out to the patient, the first contact between patient and social worker is a critical one.

Brill (1973) identified that the results of the engagement process should be:

1) the worker is part of the situation;
2) initial communication channels have been opened;
3) the worker and the client stand together in an approach to a common concern, with some definition of the role of each, based on expression and clarification of the client's expectations and what the worker has to offer and
4) there is agreement on the next step of the process (p. 75).

Once these conditions have been met, the patient has become the social worker's client. In fulfilling these needs, the social worker requires both confidence and flexibilit, for most often the first interview will take place in the patient's room, which is a place fraught with lack of privacy and other professionals competing for time. The student who has worked in a hospital will have had the opportunity to offer services to many patients. As these patients accept or reject her service, she will learn the important elements in beginning a therapeutic relationship. The value of appropriate case beginnings will move with her to other areas of practice.

OTHER GENERALIST CONSIDERATIONS

A teaching hospital is as much a university as it is a hospital and teaching is its vital priority. In this regard, many opportunities exist for social workers to teach through both formal and informal means. Formal rounds, case presentations, speaking to community groups or holding educational groups such as parent training programs are occasions for imparting knowledge and heightening social work's profile. More informally, case discussions with the many medical and nursing students who rotate through the wards can make every contact a teaching contact, to sensitize these students to the psycho-social issues that may affect their patients. Of greatest reward to the hospital practitioner is the teaching of social work students, who are highly accepted in this clinical milieu. Social work students coming from a hospital field placement would hopefully use this exposure to further their teaching and education to workplaces in other settings, be that a life-skills group for prison inmates, or sensitizing politicians to the housing needs of the poor.

Of final consideration in the skills outlined as being useful in generalist practice is that of community liaison/referral. Because clients of hospital social workers bring highly varied, often complex, lives and problems, the social worker needs a vast understanding of the community resources available to assist them. For most, the hospital is a temporary part of one's life, but the reasons one used it often carry very long-term health, social psychological or familial ramifications. The resources of the hospital are eventually finite and then give way to those of community agencies or programs. The social work student should be allowed to thoroughly explore the related agencies to understand their mandates and the breadth of their respective community services. A full knowledge of the social service system is invaluable in all areas of social work practice, as the profession strives to enhance the goodness of fit between people and their social world.

To summarize, the value of a hospital field placement for preparation in generalist practice is obvious. The ability to function competently and critically in a large organization, the comfort in collaborating with others, the skill of engaging people who may not have directly asked for help, recognizing the value of teaching as a vehicle to change and understanding the range of services throughout the community are areas to which the social work student is exposed in a hospital field placement. She may then take these skills and move with ease and competence to other practice settings.

References

Archives. (1910-1988). File held in Department of Social Work, Health Sciences Centre, Winnipeg, Manitoba.

Berkman, B., Kremler, B., Marcus, L. & Silverman, P. (1985). Course content for social work practice in health care. *Journal of Social Work Education, 21*(3), 43-51.

Brill, N. (1973). *Working with People, The Helping Process.* Philadelphia: Lippencott.

Carlton, T. O. (1984). *Clinical Social Work in Health Settings.* New York: Springer.

Cossom, J. (1988). Generalist social work practice, views from BSW graduates. *Canadian Social Work Review, 5*, 297-314.

Lane, H. J. (1982). Toward the preparation of social work specialists in health care. *Health and Social Work, 7*, 230-34.

Lowe, J. I. & Herranen, M. (1978). Conflict in teamwork: understanding roles and relationships. *Social Work in Health Care, 3*, 331-340.

Mailick, M., & Ashley, A. (1981). Politics of interprofessional collaboration: Challenge to advocacy. *Social Casework: The Journal of Contemporary Social Work, 62.*

Robinson, D. (1973). *Patients, Practitioners and Medical Care.* London: Cox & Wyman.

SECTION II
Hospital-Based Practice

Chapter 4

SOCIAL WORK PRACTICE WITH MYOCARDIAL INFARCTION PATIENTS AND FAMILIES IN AN ACUTE CARE HOSPITAL

Joanne Sulman, MSW, CSW
Godelieve Verhaeghe, MSW, CSW

Abstract

This chapter describes the distinct roles and functions that social workers practice with myocardial infarction patients in an acute care hospital. Emphasis is placed on the worker's tasks in assessing patient characteristics, in reducing distressing affect and in promoting compliance with treatment. The family's need for information and support is highlighted, and the development of the social work role on the cardiac service is reviewed.

SOCIAL WORK PRACTICE WITH MYOCARDIAL INFARCTION PATIENTS AND FAMILIES IN AN ACUTE CARE HOSPITAL

"About an hour after dinner my husband complained of a pain in his chest, and he looked real bad. He didn't want me to call an ambulance but I did anyway. They got to the house fast, hooked him up to oxygen and rushed him to hospital. The doctor in the emergency department said he was probably having a heart attack and he would have to be admitted to the coronary care unit. I was terrified."

Myocardial infarction (MI) or heart attack can generate anxiety not only in patients and families but also in social workers new to cardiac care units. In this chapter we will examine the unique features of the client group and outline the nature of social work practice most likely to lead to effective interventions.

THE CLIENTELE

Myocardial infarction patients require acute care that is usually found in a setting where high-technology and an expert coronary care team are available. Our 521 bed teaching hospital, located in a multicultural urban catchment area, is known for its expertise in the medical management of cardiac patients. The core team on the regular cardiac care floor consists of cardiologists, house staff, nurses, occupational and physiotherapists, pharmacists, dietitians and social workers. Patients also have consultants available to them from psychiatry, chaplaincy, psychology and every other specialty in the hospital; nevertheless, the initial impact of life-saving technology in the coronary care unit is the antithesis of compassion. Survival has to take precedence over the immediate feelings of patients and families, and this fact tends to heighten reactions to illness and treatment.

I. Psychological Features

Because a heart attack can drastically alter or eliminate one's future, human beings react with shock, denial, massive anxiety and depression. *Denial* can have a positive or negative effect on physical outcome, depending upon its intensity and time of occurrence (Cassem, 1989). At the onset of symptoms, denial can be lethal; however, in the coronary care unit (CCU) it can promote survival (Hackett & Cassem, 1968, 1979, 1982). When coupled with non-compliance with treatment, denial can again be deadly (Levine & Warrenburg, et al., 1987).

The mobilization of denial provides a defence against the overwhelming realistic *anxiety* that accompanies an encounter with one's mortality. A number of reports implicate excessive anxiety in adverse effects on both the psychological and physical dimensions of recovery (Cay, 1982; Hlatky & Haney, et al., 1986; Taggart & Carruthers, 1981; Levine & Warrenburg, et al., 1987).

Some patients cannot sustain their denial of physical, psychological and social role losses and become *depressed* (Billings, 1980). Depression in the CCU does not appear to correlate with outcome, but in the long-run may signal a poor prognosis (Obier, MacPherson & Haywood, 1977; Hlatky & Haney, et al., 1986).

II. Socio-Demographic Features

Age, sex and social class have an impact on outcome after MI. Older patients cope better with social stress, pain and anxiety than younger ones (Billing, Lindell, Sederholm & Theorell, 1980). In the Framingham study, men were three times more likely to have a heart attack than women, but the prognosis was worse in female patients (Kannel, Sorlie & McNamara, 1979). Other studies suggest that female MI patients are more likely to display anxiety than men (Byrne, 1980-81) and are more likely to come from lower social strata (Kottke, Young & McCall, 1980).

Overall outcome from MI varies directly with socio-economic class. Blue-collar workers are at greater risk for being non-compliant and are likely dropouts from cardiac rehabilitation programs (Oldridge, 1979), and are much less likely to return to work than patients from the highest socio-economic classes (Kottke, Young & McCall, 1980). In the study by Hlatky and his colleagues (1986), low education was the most important independent predictor of work disability. In addition, lower socio-economic class MI patients are exposed to multiple risk factors such as uncertain work opportunities, fragmented social supports, economic hardships and reduced access to information (Ruberman, Weinblatt, Goldberg & Chaudhary, 1984).

III. Behaviourial Problems

In hospital, MI patients present certain clusters of behaviourial problems that indicate a referral to social work is needed. Some patients refuse to acknowledge that they have had a heart attack, want to return to work immediately, or ask for phones and computers to be brought into the CCU. They may try to pull out their IVs and monitors, refuse medication and reject attempts to teach them about their illness and treatment. Often of greatest difficulty for staff are the sexual advances that some patients make in order to reassure themselves that they are not seriously ill.

Another cluster of patients exhibits excessive anxiety. Some are fearful of getting out of bed and are constantly ringing for the nurse. When moved from the CCU to the regular cardiac care floor, they are apprehensive about losing the reassuring presence of intensive care staff and equipment. These patients have trouble absorbing the teaching that staff offer and are therefore experienced as frustrating to care for. Depressed patients are also identified as behaviourial problems as they show little motivation for rehabilitation.

One group may be erroneously defined by members of the multi-disciplinary team as having difficulty: the relatively cheerful patients who comply with treatment. We will highlight this important cluster more intensively in the section on practice roles and responsibilities.

IV. Problems of Families

Families of myocardial infarction patients have a tendency to be anxious rather than composed. Even in their attempts to be reassuring to the patient they can display anxiety. Spouses and children may complain to staff that the patient is not being looked after properly and may refuse to accept information unless it comes directly from the cardiologist. Other families refuse to allow the patient to move out of bed for fear of precipitating another heart attack. Worries about what will happen when the patient comes home are almost universal. These families also experience the common problems that families of other seriously ill patients encounter: the shifts in role, lifestyle alterations, financial burdens and the often profound sense that things will never be the same (Hartman & Laird, 1983; Thompson & Cordle, 1988).

The critical task of social work with MI patients is to assess with accuracy the responses and needs of patients and families, for it is this assessment that will point to subsequent practice roles.

PRACTICE ROLES AND RESPONSIBILITIES

The social worker in cardiac care is a member of a multi-disciplinary team. In conjunction and co-operation with other team members, the worker helps the MI patient comply with medical treatment and rehabilitation measures in order to achieve maximum recovery and a return to a normal lifestyle. For social work assessments and interventions to be useful, ongoing communication with the other team members, particularly nursing and medical staff, is essential. Good communication is achieved by regular attendance at weekly multi-disciplinary rounds where all patients are reviewed. It is further enhanced through consultation with referring staff prior to seeing patients, and by providing prompt verbal feedback and written chart notes documenting social work assessments and interventions.

I. Identification of Referrals

Although anyone in our setting can make a referral to social work through a simple verbal request, most of our referrals come from medical and nursing staff. To identify patients who would benefit most from social work intervention, we developed clinical guidelines and taught them to staff. These guidelines combine four clusters of risk factors with outcome. The key concepts determining outcome are maladaptive versus adaptive responses paired with compliance or non-compliance with medical treatment and rehabilitation measures (Sulman & Verhaeghe, 1985). These can be conceptualized according to four distinct sub-groups with different responses.

Group I consists of people who are at risk for recurrence and cardiac invalidism owing to their incapacitating anxiety or depression. Through their maladaptive attempts to cope with the crisis of their illness they become pathologically dependent and non-compliant with rehabilitation measures.

Group II patients are moderately anxious or depressed but comply with treatment. They are dependent, but not excessively so and have rehabilitation potential; however, their ability to participate in their recovery is tenuous because they have difficulty denying the distressing affect.

Group III patients are characterized by the adaptive use of denial to ward off anxiety and depression (Billings, 1980). They appear optimistic and independent and participate in treatment. They acknowledge their illness without the intrusion of significant emotion. This group displays the greatest rehabilitation potential (Wrzesniewski, 1980; Garrity & Klein, 1975; Byrne, Whyte & Lance, 1979).

Group IV is comprised of patients who react to MI with maladaptive denial. Some refuse to acknowledge that they have had a heart attack and most deny that it will have much impact on their lives. They may speak as if fate alone rather than their own behaviour will determine outcome. Excessively independent, they are notoriously non-compliant with rehabilitation efforts and therefore run a greater risk of complications and recurrence. In Byrne, Whyte and Lance's study (1979) this type of patient numbered half the sample.

II. Social Work Tasks

Not only do these guidelines help to identify patients at risk for a poor outcome, but they also point to distinct roles and tasks. It is important to note that approaches effective with one group of patients may be contra-indicated for another.

With Group I Patients: Patients in Group I need help to manage their anxiety and depression so that they can comply with treatment. The social worker's tasks are to listen empathically to the patient's feelings and concerns, to provide accurate information and to offer encouragement. When indicated, the worker asks the cardiologist to refer the patient for a psychiatric consultation to determine if medication or other treatment is needed. Another recommendation might be relaxation therapy, which could be carried out by social work or by other disciplines such as psychology or occupational therapy. Relaxation therapy reduces anxiety and also acts against depression by promoting a sense of mastery and control (Bohachick, 1984).

The social worker needs to be particularly active during the time that the Group I patient is moved from the CCU to the regular care floor. For staff this change has positive connotations, but for the patient the reduction in medical surveillance may be frightening. Preparation for the transfer in the form of advance notice, information regarding routines on the regular cardiac care floor and plenty of reassurance can go a long way to relieve the anxiety associated with the move.

With Group II Patients: Because Group II patients comply with treatment in spite of their anxiety or depression they are perceived as "good patients." Their compliance may even be credited to the fact that they express their feelings, and staff may be inclined to encourage further exploration of their anxiety and depression. This action, however, is contra-indicated because anxiety and depression have negative physiological consequences. These patients instead need help to reduce distressing effects.

The social worker does this by listening carefully to their concerns and by offering realistic reassurance without encouraging excessive exploration of negative feelings; by providing, in consultation with the team, information regarding what steps the patient can take to regain a sense of control and especially by promoting an optimistic attitude. Because these patients are at risk for becoming Group I patients, they require generous doses of emotional support. If too much anxiety or depression break through, a referral for psychiatric consultation is indicated. Just as relaxation therapy helps Group I patients, it can also be of benefit for Group II patients.

With Group III Patients: Group III patients, who are primarily male, are adaptive deniers whose optimistic attitude and compliance with treatment bode well for a return to a normal lifestyle. The fact that these patients do not dwell on their feelings may become of concern to staff who believe that affective issues are not being addressed. When an adaptive denier is referred, the social worker's tasks are to help staff to see how the patient's denial is working for him, to support his compliance and to encourage his optimism.

With Group IV Patients: Group IV patients are those whose excessive denial prevents them from co-operating with treatment. The members of this group are likely to be men and often are from lower socio-economic strata. In hospital they are eager for discharge and when discharged, they refuse to pace their activity levels. They generally discontinue their medication without consulting their doctors, they continue to smoke, they fail to recognize physical symptoms and they drop out of rehabilitation programs. Their extreme denial puts them at risk for a recurrence.

The goal in working with these patients is to help them regain a sense of control. The social worker encourages care-giving staff to provide them with clear information regarding the rationale for medical protocols. With highly resistant patients, it is useful to enlist the aid of the cardiologist to confront the patient with the consequences of lack of compliance. As much as possible, the social worker should ensure that these patients are involved in decisions about the rehabilitation process. Early involvement in physical rehabilitation is a powerful method for increasing the patient's sense of competence.

Membership in a peer support group can also help to consolidate the rationale for compliance (Boyce, 1981). By reducing feelings of isolation and disability, the peer group encourages patients to participate in rehabilitation and to adopt a more constructive means of re-establishing control.

III. Role With Families

Work with patients can only be effective if families and other social support networks are perceived as crucial to the patient's recovery (Mailick, 1979). The crisis of MI causes a major upset in the family system, and one of the social worker's functions is to help the family regain its sense of stability. Because the patient's survival is indeed at stake, the care-giving team's natural inclination may be to focus solely on the patient and unwittingly to exclude the family. When viewed as passive outsiders, family members are more likely to relate to the patient on the basis of their own anxious assumptions rather than on the basis of accurate information. This creates a barrier between the patient and family and may turn visits into sources of stress rather than comfort.

Family as Part of the Treatment Team: Instead of accepting the family's exclusion, the social worker needs to ensure that provision is made for them to meet with the physician and nurses to ask questions and to receive information about the patient's medical progress. Good communication flow between the family and caregiving staff also allows the family to share its own unique knowledge of the patient and in this way enhances the care that the patient receives.

Information Needs: The family's participation is vital throughout the recovery period. As the patient improves, the family needs specific information about levels of activity, the purpose and effects of medication, recommended changes in diet and smoking habits, methods of reducing stress and resumption of sexual relations. This information can reduce the impact of new anxieties as the family shifts its focus from survival of the patient to long-range adaptation. Part of the social worker's role with the family is to help members obtain and clarify information, and to help them deal with necessary adjustments in their lifestyle (Thompson, & Cordle, 1988).

Affective Responses: Assuming that information needs are being met, the family still must contend with other feelings such as guilt, anger and depression that can impede adaptation. If family members believe that they precipitated the patient's MI, their feelings of *guilt* may prevent them from providing optimal support. Spouses may feel that they should have urged the patient more emphatically to slow down, to change eating habits or to exercise. Since MI's are generally associated with business worries and are not uncommon following arguments, families may feel that they should have done more to protect the patient from life stressors. When these guilt feelings are not dealt with directly, they express themselves as over-protection of the patient and in demanding behaviour toward staff. Social workers help families to examine the realistic basis for their feelings, not only what they have a right to feel guilty about, but also what they have taken unwarranted responsibility for. Family members need to be helped to understand that the patient's vulnerable physical condition was such that the MI could have occurred at any time — if not this stress, then the next. Their realistic guilt feelings can be further reduced by encouraging them to become positive participants in the patient's rehabilitation.

Anger in families can occur as a mask for guilt feelings but also arises in response to the growing awareness of the disruptions that the MI brings to the family's former equilibrium. Family members are understandably reluctant to express their negative feelings toward the cardiac patient for fear of making things worse. Since this concern is a valid one, the social worker can help family members share and understand their feelings and prevent them from going underground or being acted out in a disruptive way toward staff. Families may, however, experience anger about genuine problems with the caregiving system. It is important to identify these problems and to act as an advocate in order to prevent the escalation of these feelings.

Sadness, grief and depression are responses to the loss of what was. Hopes for the future are jeopardized. Along with health and financial stability, the integrity of the family is at issue (Dhooper, 1983). Feelings of anxiety and depression are especially prevalent at the time of discharge, a time when most families expect to be elated. It is as if the grim reality has set in and the change in health of the patient is most evident. To be prepared for this reaction can help family members reduce its impact. They need to know that this response is normal and common during the process of recovery. Reassurance consisting of realistic optimism and ready access to information can help patient and family master this phase.

Community Resources: Financial worries can be an enormous source of stress for patients and their families; therefore it is essential that the social worker address this issue and provide information if required regarding sources of financial assistance. A major support to families of MI victims can be provided through links with community services following discharge. Cardiac rehabilitation programs, cardiac education and support groups, public health nursing and family counselling agencies are underutilized resources that can make an enormous difference to patients and families (Dhooper, 1983). One goal of social work follow-up is to identify and refer families that can benefit from these sources of help. Because high-risk patients are more likely to drop out of rehabilitation programs, continuing support may be required to achieve the connection.

POTENTIAL FOR ROLE DEVELOPMENT

Opportunities for development of the social work role abound in this setting. The social worker's practice arena includes direct work with patients and families as well as interventions in the hospital milieu and the community at large. As an acute care teaching hospital, the setting also encourages roles in education and research.

I. Direct Work With Patients and Families

The social worker initiates regular meetings with the nursing unit administrator and floor staff to identify problem areas in patient care and to discuss possible solutions. The importance of having a close working relationship with the nursing unit administrator cannot be overemphasized. In addition, fostering a good rapport with the cardiologists is helpful, particularly when the worker is co-ordinating the involvement of other disciplines in direct patient care. In order for such referrals to take place and for the consultants' recommendations to be implemented, the support of the staff physician is crucial.

Although families are included more frequently in treatment plans, much work still remains to be done in this area. Social work staff have found that multi-disciplinary meetings with families have been fruitful in clarifying communication, resolving problems and establishing mutual goals.

Similarly, when a particular patient generates feelings of frustration and helplessness among staff, the social worker can be instrumental in initiating a patient care conference to air feelings, to articulate problems and to develop care plans.

II. Team-building

To be an effective team member it is important for the social worker not only to share information about social work roles and functions, but also to be knowledgeable regarding the roles and functions of the other team members. In this way the worker can make informed referrals and can effectively utilize the expertise of other disciplines.

Multi-disciplinary projects enhance patient care and promote identification with the team. On our service, social work participated in the creation of the cardiac rehabilitation manual, contributed the section concerning the management of patients' psychological responses to myocardial infarction and taught this information to other team members.

III. Community Connections

As a natural link between hospital and community, the social worker can play a vital role in reducing fragmentation between the two. For example, the social worker encouraged the participation of the public health nurse in our weekly rounds. As a result of the service's increased visibility, more referrals were made and patient access to this valuable resource was enhanced.

By being active in community programs, the social worker provides a direct service to patients and becomes more knowledgeable about community resources. The social worker in cardiology is a co-leader of a weekly education and support group for discharged myocardial infarction patients and their families. In this eight-week program known as "Heart to Heart", guest specialists in the fields of cardiology, nutrition, psychology and physiotherapy present information regarding heart disease, treatment protocols and rehabilitation.

IV. Education

Social work teaching is part of the multi-disciplinary approach to cardiac education for patients and families. Informal teaching can become more formalized as teams develop rehabilitation protocols. Other disciplines need orientation to the special psychosocial issues of MI patients, and the social worker must initiate and seize opportunities to educate team members.

University-affiliated hospitals may require or strongly encourage the teaching of students in all departments. Our setting is a teaching centre for the faculty of social work, where students learn to work effectively on the cardiac service and, in addition, practice the worker's teaching role with other disciplines.

V. Research

Social work's use of practice theory can add an original perspective to clinical research. The social worker on the cardiac team can recommend avenues for research and, in conjunction with other disciplines, design projects, draft grant proposals, supervise research and report findings.

CONCLUDING REMARKS

Social work practice with MI patients and families has unique features not found in work with other patient groups. The tasks of assessing and identifying the specific needs of each patient are critical ones that lead to distinct social work roles and functions. Beyond the provision of psychosocial support and resources, the social worker can have a positive impact on rehabilitation outcomes with MI patients. This will occur if the worker is able to help patients reduce distressing effects, decrease maladaptive denial and promote compliance with treatment and rehabilitation. For these efforts to be successful, it is essential that families be included in the treatment plan, with special attention paid to their need for information and support in hospital and after discharge.

The social worker on the multi-disciplinary cardiac care team plays a role in linking the patient and family to the community and educates the team about the patient's need for social and community supports. The diverse roles of the social worker with MI patients can best be characterized as generic: direct clinical intervention, advocacy, team-building, staff education, research and development of community resources for rehabilitation. Of these roles, expertise in clinical practice is probably the most useful to the worker and is the basis for effective integration into the team.

CASE EXAMPLE

Mr. H. Smith, a 51-year-old, hard-driving, successful lawyer, was admitted to hospital for treatment of a first MI. He had recently remarried and had three children from his previous union aged 21, 16 and 14 years. In the cardiac care unit Mr. Smith requested telephone access and asked his wife to bring in his files so he could work from his bedside. The moment he was informed that he would be transferred to a regular cardiac care floor he demanded discharge. He declined prescribed medication and refused to follow the schedule for gradually increasing his mobility. His family felt anxious, worried and helpless. Staff were feeling frustrated in their efforts to care for him and were concerned that he was at risk for a recurrence.

The social worker assessed that the patient was employing maladaptive denial to ward off the impact of his illness. The first social work intervention consisted of advocating on behalf of the patient so that he would be allowed to work from his bedside. In this way his sense of control and mastery were enhanced and his demand for an early discharge diminished.

Secondly, the social worker met with the family members on their own to provide them with an opportunity to express their worries and concerns without fear of upsetting the patient. She then arranged a family meeting with the cardiologist that included the patient so that their questions could be answered. At that meeting she recommended a referral for the entire family to the "Heart to Heart" education and support group in the community. She also asked the cardiologist to refer the patient to a highly regarded out-patient cardiac rehabilitation centre. The worker reasoned that the patient would be more likely to comply with rehabilitation in a prestigious milieu that provided peer support.

On follow-up, the patient was continuing his participation in the cardiac rehabilitation program, was taking his medication, had quit smoking, but was less compliant about reducing his work schedule.

References

Billing, E., Lindell, B., Sederholm, M. & Theorell, T. (1980). Denial, anxiety and depression following myocardial infarction. *Psychosomatics, 21*(8), 639-645.

Billings, C.K. (1980). Management of psychologic responses to myocardial infarction. *Southern Medical Journal, 73*(10).

Bohachick, P. (1984). Progressive relaxation training in cardiac rehabilitation: Effect on psychologic variables. *Nursing Research, 33*(5), 283-287.

Boyce, M. (1981). Borgess hospital has outstanding example of cardiac rehabilitation program. *Michigan Medicine,* April; *80*(11) 185-196.

Byrne, D.G. (1980-81). Effects of social context on psychosocial responses to survived myocardial infarction. *International Journal of Psychiatry in Medicine, 10*(1), 23-31.

Byrne, D.G. White, H.M. & Lance, G.N. (1978-79). A typology of responses to illness in survivors of myocardial infarction. *International Journal of Psychiatry in Medicine, 9*(2), 135-144.

Cassem, N.H. (1989). Too much or too little denial plays role in M.I. survival. *The Medical Post, 14*(2) p. 39.

Cay, E.L. (1982). Psychological problems in patients after a myocardial infarction. *Advances in Cardiology, 29,* 108-112.

Dhooper, S.S. (1983). Family coping with the crisis of heart attack. *Social Work in Health Care, 9*(1), 15-31.

Garrity, T.F. & Klein, R.F. (1975). Emotional response and clinical severity as early determinants of six-month mortality after myocardial infarction. *Heart and Lung, 4*(5), 730-737.

Hackett, T.P. & Cassem, N.H. (1979). Psychological aspects of rehabilitation after myocardial infarction. In N. Wenger & H.K. Hellerstein (Eds.), *Rehabilitation of the Patient after Myocardial Infarction.* Chichester: Wiley & Sons.

Hackett, T.P. & Cassem N.H. (1982). Coping with cardiac disease. *Advances in Cardiology 31,* 212-217.

Hackett, T.P., Cassem N.H. & Wishnie, H.A. (1968). The coronary-care unit—an appraisal of its psychological hazards. *New England Journal of Medicine, 279*(25).

Hlatky, M.A., Haney, T., Barefoot, J.C., Califf, R.M., Mark, D.B., Pryor, D.B. & Williams, R.B. (1986). Medical, psychological and social correlates of work disability among men with coronary artery disease. *American Journal of Cardiology, 58*(10), 911-915.

Kannel, W.B., Sorlie, P. & McNamara, P.M. (1979). Prognosis after initial myocardial infarction: The Framingham Study. *American Journal of Cardiology, 44*(1), 53-59.

Kottke, T.E., Young, D.T. & McCall, M.M. (1980). Effect of social class on recovery from myocardial infarction. *Minnesota Medicine,* August; *63*(8), 590-597.

Levine, J., Warrenburg, S., Kerns, R., Schwartz, G., Delaney, R., Fontanta, A., Gradman, A., Smith, S. Allen, S., & Cascione, R. (1987). The role of denial in recovery from coronary heart disease. *Psychosomatic Medicine, 49*(2), 109-117.

Mailick, M. (1979). The impact of severe illness on the individual and family: An overview. *Social Work in Health Care, 5*(2), 117-128.

Obier, K., MacPherson, M. & Haywood, J.R. (1977). Predictive value of psychosocial profiles following acute myocardial infarction. *Journal of National Medical Association, 69,* 59-61.

Oldridge, N.B. (1979). Compliance with exercise programs. In M.L. Pollock and D.H. Schmidt (Eds.), *Heart Disease and Rehabilitation.* Boston: Houghton Mifflin Professional Publishers.

Ruberman, W., Weinblatt, E., Goldberg, J.D. & Chaudhary, B.S. (1984). Psychosocial influences on mortality after myocardial infarction. *The New England Journal of Medicine,* August, *311*(9), 552-559.

Sulman, J. & Verhaeghe, G. (1985). Myocardial infarction patients in the acute care hospital: A conceptual framework for social work intervention. *Social Work in Health Care, 11*(1), 1-20.

Taggart, P. & Carruthers, M. (1981). Behaviour patterns and emotional stress in the etiology of coronary heart disease: Cardiological and biochemical correlates. In D. Wheatley, (Ed.), *Stress and the Heart.* New York: Raven Press.

Thompson, D.R. & Cordle, C.J. (1988). Support of wives of myocardial infarction patients. *Journal of Advanced Nursing, 13*(2), 223-228.

Wrzesniewski, K. (1980). The development of a scale for assessing attitudes towards illness in patients experiencing a myocardial infarction. *Social Science and Medicine, 14A,* 127-132.

Chapter 5

SOCIAL WORK PRACTICE WITH INFERTILITY PATIENTS IN AN IN VITRO FERTILIZATION PROGRAM

Sima K. Needleman, MSW, ACSW

Abstract

The inability to have children stimulates stresses, which can be intensified by infertility treatment such as in vitro fertilization and embryo transfer (IVF), which is being performed in medical centres throughout the world. This chapter examines the psychosocial impact of infertility and demonstrates the role that social workers can play in supporting patients through the course of complicated and anxiety-producing medical treatment in a hospital based IVF program.

SOCIAL WORK PRACTICE WITH INFERTILITY PATIENTS IN AN IN VITRO FERTILIZATION PROGRAM

Infertility has been defined as the "inability to conceive a child after a year or more of unprotected intercourse, or the inability to carry a pregnancy to term" (Garner, 1983). To some degree, infertility affects a large number of people throughout the world. The most recent U.S. government report, which was based on a 1982 survey by the National Center for Health Statistics, estimates that two to three million married American couples experience infertility (*Infertility, Medical and Social Choices*, 1988). Many conditions are known to cause or to contribute to infertility. Forty percent of the time, the problem is the woman's and 40 percent the man's. The remainder of the problems either have no known cause or result from a joint problem (Menning, 1977).

When couples recognize infertility as a problem, they have four choices:

1) to live without offspring;
2) to adopt a child;
3) to make arrangements with a surrogate or
4) to try one or more of the various medical and surgical procedures—the most common of which are: a) drug therapy; b) surgery; c) artificial insemination (either by husband or donor); d) gamete intrafallopian transfer (GIFT) or e) in vitro fertilization and embryo transfer (henceforth to be referred to as IVF).

The last two therapeutic measures (GIFT and IVF), which are often perceived as measures that provide the last hope of having one's own biological child, have much in common but are designed to help people with different diagnoses. GIFT requires open and undamaged fallopian tubes whereas IVF treats women who have blocked or absent oviducts. Both GIFT and IVF are complex therapies consisting of many steps with a chance for failure at each monitored step; thus, patients can oscillate daily between feelings of euphoria when they are responding well and despair when their response is poor. This phenomenon is often referred to as an emotional "roller coaster" (Greenfeld, 1984). The uncertainty and lack of control create an atmosphere of anxiety and a need for crisis intervention and emotional support, roles that social workers are qualified to provide.

THE CLIENTELE

I. Settings

IVF and GIFT can be performed in private, free-standing clinics or in hospital-based settings. Today, many clinics offer both procedures because of their similar protocols. One example of such a program is the Jewish Hospital at Washington University Medical Center in St. Louis, Missouri. This facility is a not-for-profit, non-sectarian, general teaching hospital that is licensed for 628 beds. The program comes under the auspices of the Obstetrics and Gynecology Department and consists of a multi-disciplinary team whose medical director and other physicians are specialists in reproductive endocrinology. Other members of the IVF team are the nurse co-ordinator, whose role is vital to the everyday operation of the program, laboratory scientists and technicians, ultrasound technicians, physician sonographers, a secretary and a social worker.

The program, which is one of many services offered by the Obstetrics-Gynecology Department, does not operate in one centralized area, but rather, utilizes the existing facilities of the parent department.

II. Procedure

Each patient undergoing IVF or GIFT follows a carefully designed protocol (Garner, 1983; DiMattina & Liu, 1987), which includes self-administered daily injections of fertility drugs to stimulate the development of eggs in the ovaries. After a few days of drug therapy, the patient begins daily monitoring by ultrasound to measure the growth of egg-containing follicles and by blood estradiol levels to assess hormone function within the ovaries. When the monitoring indicates that the eggs are mature, the patient undergoes a laparoscopy or an ultrasound-guided procedure to remove the mature eggs from the ovary.

For IVF, the eggs are placed in culture medium in a petri dish. The husband's sperm are introduced six to eight hours later, and the dish is placed in an incubator for approximately 40 hours. During that time, a sperm fertilizes each egg, and cell division occurs. When the fertilized egg has grown to four to eight cells in size, it is transferred into the patient's uterus with the ope that implantation will occur. Eleven to 12 days later, the patient undergoes a pregnancy test.

During GIFT, the eggs are placed in a catheter and the husband's sperm, separated from the eggs by an air bubble, are added to the catheter. Both eggs and sperm are injected into the fallopian tube, which is the normal site of fertilization.

III. Requirements for Acceptance

The Jewish Hospital IVF program requires that the women

1) are legally married for at least 6 months;
2) are younger than 45 and
3) have both an intact uterus and at least one ovary.

Most of the IVF patients have blocked, absent or malfunctioning fallopian tubes; however, other diagnoses are represented as well. Examples are endometriosis, unexplained infertility, ovulation problems and male factor (such as low sperm count). To be eligible for the GIFT program, the woman must meet the above requirements and, in addition, have intact and open fallopian tubes.

It should be noted that since the IVF and GIFT programs are similar in so many ways, comments about IVF patients are true of GIFT patients as well. Also, although infertility is a couple's problem, and the procedure requires sperm from the husband as well as eggs from the wife, it is the woman who takes the medication and goes through the procedures; thus, it is the woman who is considered the patient, and therefore, in the following text, references to the patient will use feminine pronouns.

IV. Demographic Factors

Although infertility knows no socio-economic boundaries, IVF and GIFT are expensive procedures (costing between $4500 and $7500), and they are not covered by all health insurance plans; consequently, in the United States, patients who are served tend to be from middle- or upper-income categories, and the majority of women hold skilled or professional jobs. Typically, the woman is a goal-oriented, hard-working high-achiever. Infertility is incongruent with her life pattern, and she feels helpless, frustrated and out of control; however, husbands are generally supportive and, if necessary, willing to forego having biological children (Batterman,

67

1985). Johnson, et al., (1981) reported that there is an "incredible bond of love and support that binds an infertile marriage together." These authors go on to say that "there is more love and tolerance exhibited in these marriages than in the vast majority of fertile marriages."

Not all infertile couples fit the above profile. Some have a less than optimal marriage, and others are in unskilled or semi-skilled fields. If their insurance company will not cover IVF, they often are willing to save for long periods of time, sacrifice and borrow money for the opportunity to try the procedure.

Although the women in the Jewish Hospital program have ranged in age from 24-44, approximately half have been between 31-35 years of age.

V. Emotional Factors

Regardless of their financial status, infertile people experience similar emotional reactions to their condition. Typically, the couple feels out of control, overwhelmed with emotion and unsure about the future; thus, as stated by Menning (1977), infertility becomes a major crisis and, like other people in crisis, the couple goes through several emotional stages, which are similar to the stages of grief described by Elizabeth Kubler-Ross (1975). Menning explains that first, the couple is surprised. Men and women alike assume that they will be able to reproduce and are unprepared when they learn otherwise. This initial response of surprise is quickly replaced by disbelief and denial. Soon the infertile woman begins to realize that she is different from other people and consequently might isolate herself not only from events that she may find ainful, such as baby showers and family gatherings, but also from insensitive people who make painful remarks (Kane, 1981). Self-confidence and self-esteem suffer (Menning, 1977), and these women often express feelings of being a failure regardless of other significant accomplishments. One infertile woman proclaimed that she was "less than a whole woman."

Another emotional ramification of infertility is anger. Couples have been deprived of a fundamental right and their privacy has been invaded (Menning, 1977). Along with anger, guilt may surface either because of some action or event that occurred earlier in life (such as an unplanned adolescent pregnancy) or because the infertile woman feels that she is depriving her spouse of the opportunity to be a parent (Menning, 1977); thus, infertile individuals become insecure and fear losing their mates. In addition, the strength of the marital relationship is strained by the infertility workup and treatment (Wallis, 1984). Since the timing of intercourse is often prescribed, love-making becomes a scheduled event and consequently not spontaneous and pleasurable (Kane, 1981). Furthermore, the financial burden of fertility testing and therapeutic measures may heighten the pressure on a couple or may be a deterrent to people who either have no health insurance or whose health insurance will not cover the procedures.

Depression is a recurring phenomenon during the long process of the diagnosis and treatment of infertility. Generally, one disappointment has followed another. Often, when told that there is nothing more to try, the couple experience grief in response to a loss that is as great as the death of a loved one. The grief is usually three-fold (Menning, 1977). First, the individuals grieve for the children they will never have. Second, some women grieve because they will never experience pregnancy. Finally, the infertile grieve because they will miss one of life's major roles, that of being a parent. If allowed to work through their grief, Menning (1977) states they will reach the final stage of resolution or acceptance; however, Fleming (1988) suggests that infertility is a chronic illness where the goal is coping and adaptation rather than acceptance. Fleming advocates the use of avoidance and distraction as coping mechanisms and encourages couples to focus on areas where they have pleasure, success and control (Fleming, 1984).

VI. Primary and Secondary Infertility

Infertile women may be divided into two groups: those who have never experienced a pregnancy (i.e., those with primary infertility) and those who have had a child in the past but are presently infertile (i.e., those with secondary infertility). Women in the first category may be married to men who have had children in previous marriages and therefore do not understand their wives' feelings of desperation and failure. Surprisingly, patients with secondary infertility experience the same depth of feeling when their attempts at a subsequent pregnancy are unsuccessful. These women have an additional burden. Those with biological offspring at home feel guilty and greedy in the presence of the women experiencing primary infertility. Others, who became pregnant as unmarried teenagers and either placed their babies for adoption or had abortions, may have difficulty resolving their deep-seated guilt, may feel as if they have given away the only baby they will ever have and are convinced they are being punished.

Because of the vast emotional sequelae of infertility and because "information is one of the best antidotes to anxiety" (Freeman, et al., 1985), te social worker has two goals with infertile patients: 1) to provide both emotional support and grief counselling and 2) to be a source of information about the medical protocol, about alternatives and about support mechanisms.

PRACTICE ROLES AND RESPONSIBILITIES

Social workers, who work with infertile people, are either in private practice or in a medical setting that offers infertility treatment. The primary role, which is to meet the psychological needs of the client, would be the same in either type of practice; however, the opportunity to offer a number of services is greater in a medical setting, such as a hospital-based IVF clinic. According to *Infertility, Medical and Social Changes* (1988), clinics generally provide emotional support in one of four ways:

1) informal counselling by sensitive doctors and nurses;
2) referral to a consultant on a case-by-case basis;
3) inclusion of a professional counsellor who meets each couple on the first visit to prepare the individuals for the anticipated stresses and to discuss community resources and
4) provision of a preventive approach where all participants meet the professional counsellor on the first visit and are followed by that person throughout the experience to focus on ways to reduce stress.

The IVF Program at Jewish Hospital in St. Louis, Missouri, combines the third and fourth approaches mentioned above and demonstrates the kinds of roles and services social workers can provide in a hospital-based setting. The social worker is part of a multi-disciplinary team, works 20-30 hours per week and has a caseload restricted to IVF patients. The worker

1) participates in IVF staff meetings;
2) takes part in patient orientation meetings;
3) performs psychosocial evaluations;
4) provides supportive counselling;

5) is a source of information about resources and alternatives;
6) serves as a facilitator and consultant for a support group, telephone counsellors and IVF newsletter and
7) assists patients with billing and insurance problems.

I. Staff Meetings

In order for an IVF program to run smoothly, staff meetings are held on a regular basis to discuss new developments, changes in protocols and specific cases. The social worker is able to contribute relevant information about specific patients and about the various ancillary services provided to the patients. According to the medical director, the social worker, "more than any other team member, is the 'emotional welfare advocate' of the patient and thereby a 'conscience' in the technology-oriented program."

II. Patient Orientation

Approximately three orientation meetings for patients and their husbands are held each year. At these meetings, the nurse co-ordinator explains the medical protocol, and a laboratory assistant describes various laboratory tasks such as processing semen samples, locating eggs in follicular fluid, putting eggs in culture medium, inseminating and monitoring them and making preparations for embryo transfer. The social worker begins the emotional preparation for the stresses couples should anticipate, mentions the high cost of the procedure with no guarantee of success and discusses the counsellor's function in the program. Next, the worker introduces two couples who have previously participated in the program to share their experiences with the prospective patients. Questions are asked and answered and patients generally develop a clearer understanding of what to expect.

III. Psychosocial Evaluation

"The value of a psychological interview at the outset of the medical infertility investigation has been consistently emphasized in the literature..." (Daniluk, 1988); consequently, at an early stage in the IVF procedure, the social worker interviews each couple to make an assessment of the couple's personal strengths and weaknesses, marital relationship, support networks, unique circumstances, if any, perceptions of infertility, coping mechanisms and how realistic each is about the procedure and its probable outcome. In subsequent contacts, the evaluation becomes more complete. The worker looks for personality traits and relationships that can help or hinder the patient's ability to cope with the stress of the procedure and the possible disappointment of a negative outcome.

IV. Supportive Counselling

Because both the condition of infertility and the IVF procedure are extremely stressful, the second and major undertaking of the social worker is to provide supportive counselling at each stage of the procedure. The worker communicates with the nurse co-ordinator daily in order to receive an update on all patients and, in general, either sees each patient when she comes in for monitoring or calls to show interest and to offer encouragement.

However, people are different and the worker tries to adjust intervention to the particular personality and needs of each patient; for example, some people are open and talk freely about their situation. Others are private and tend to keep things to themselves. For these people, discussing infertility may tend to increase stress. consequently, the worker is always available to the patient but allows the reticent patient to initiate contact.

When couples are receptive to social work involvement, the worker makes an effort to visit after the embryo is transferred. At each of these times, the worker determines how the patient is feeling physically and what her understanding is about the results of the procedure. Some clarification may be indicated. This is generally a time of optimism and encouragement. Even if just one egg is retrieved, the patient is consoled when reminded that it takes just one egg and one sperm to make a baby. On the rare occasion when no eggs are retrieved because of an unforeseen condition such as inaccessible ovaries, the worker attempts to help the patient cope with her grief by allowing her to verbalize feelings, by listening empathically, by encouraging her to take time out to recover before aking any future plans and by reassuring her of continued support and contact. The day of the embryo transfer is a happy day, full of hope and euphoria. This may be the first time that the patient has ever had an embryo inside her body. The main purposes of the social worker's visit are to show concern and to continue to build on the worker-patient relationship so that any needed future intervention will be sought and will be effective. Follow-up phone calls are made at least two or three times during the stressful 12 day waiting period between the embryo transfer and the pregnancy test. If the test is positive, the patient generally returns in two to four weeks for an ultrasound to confirm the pregnancy. If no problems are detected, the case can generally be closed; however, the social worker keeps track of the expected date of delivery and makes occasional follow-up calls until after the baby is born.

When IVF fails, depression usually sets in. At this time, the patient needs a great deal of support to help her accept the failure, to go through the grieving process and to look realistically at the available options. The social worker encourages the patient to ventilate feelings such as anger, disappointment and frustration. An analogy is made between the loss of a pregnancy and the death of a loved one, and the patient is assured that mourning is "normal" and that it will pass. After such an intense episode and the dysphoria following failure, some patients are eager to immediately begin working on an alternative plan while others must distance themselves from thoughts of building a family. For the latter patients, the social worker suggests taking a break and talks about channelling energies into other areas such as redecorating a room or planning a vacation. About a month after the procedure, the patient may be ready to consider alternatives and discussion is initiated by the social worker.

The social worker has to adjust the mode of intervention to the particular response and needs of each patient. In some cases, the patient's reaction to failure is extreme. She may have some deep-seated unresolved problems that may require long term therapy. In these instances, the patient should be referred to appropriate therapists. One example of an extreme reaction was that of Mrs. N., who at the age of 18 was unmarried, became pregnant and placed her child for adoption. During the entire IVF procedure, Mrs. N. was tense and seemed desperate. After the procedure failed, she became despondent, could not sleep very well and found herself dreaming about people she knew becoming pregnant. She often thought about her 13 year old daughter. Mrs. N. initially resisted seeing a therapist but eventually agreed when her symptoms persisted; however, the majority of women in the program seem to have the internal strength and external support to overcome their disappointment and to go on with their lives.

73

V. Presentation of Alternatives

Whenever the procedure fails, the social worker shifts the focus to review realistic alternatives with the couple. Among these alternatives are repeating IVF, which a great many couples opt to do, living childfree, exploring the various kinds of adoption and participating in a surrogate parenting program. The social worker draws upon her acquired knowledge about resources both for surrogacy and for independent and special needs adoption and serves as a resource person for the couple, providing verbal and written information about each appropriate option. At the same time, the patient is referred to the local chapter of Resolve, which is a national support group for infertile couples that provides information, resources, counselling and a "kindred spirit" to couples with infertility problems. In addition, she is informed about publications designed to provide emotional or spiritual support for infertile couples.

VI. Support Groups

Three reasons are given by Goodman and Rothman (1984) for offering support groups for infertile couples:

1) to restore self-esteem;
2) to increase knowledge and thereby gain control in decision making and
3) to reduce isolation.

In the Jewish Hospital IVF program, the social worker and the nurse co-ordinator have always offered a support group specifically for couples who have participated in the hospital's IVF or GIFT program. At these meetings, patients are provided with updated information about the program such as modifications in the protocol, the number of participants, how the program compares with other IVF and GIFT programs and insurance coverage information. In addition, patients are encouraged to share common problems and to ventilate anger or frustration. Some of the subjects that have been discussed at support group meetings are coping with the holidays; the husband's perspective of IVF and ways to help families and friends understand that infertility is a continuous crisis. Often these discussions served as a stimulus to the social worker to prepare some written material for current and future patients.

Attendance at these meetings has been unpredictable. The social worker who held such sessions concluded that those who came either

1) planned to try the procedure again and wanted to be kept up-to-date;
2) had just failed in their IVF attempt and needed to ventilate or
3) had an IVF success and were so grateful to the program that they wanted to continue their ties and "pay back" the program by helping others.

After several meetings with poor attendance, the social worker decided to change the focus from a staff-initiated to a self-help group led by one or two of the enthusiastic, successful IVF patients and serve as a consultant and facilitator for the group. This approach appeared to be better.

Two events in one of the early group meetings later led to a worthwhile therapeutic approach; namely, using patients as a resource for one another. First, two women, who had relinquished parental rights to their only children years before, expressed a desire to meet with each other outside the group. Second, several participants volunteered to provide support on the telephone to any new IVF patient on an individual basis. Matching patients with common obstetrical histories or life experiences and encouraging individuals to provide support to each other can be an effective tool; however, it is essential that the patients involved be carefully screened to ensure that it is not detrimental to the healthy resolution of the other's fertility problem. The fundamental characteristics sought for matching patients are emotional stability, a positive attitude and sensitivity.

In time, this notion of peer support became formalized. Since a number of past participants offered to talk to new IVF patients to help them through their first (and probably most emotionally difficult) IVF attempt, a meeting was held to discuss matters related to peer counselling. Then the social worker prepared two handouts: guidelines for the telephone volunteers and a list of the volunteers' names and telephone numbers for the new patients. This patient-to-patient support effort became so successful and mutually beneficial that it is a permanent part of the support mechanism of the IVF program.

Information and indirect counselling are also provided to IVF patients through patient contacts with one another in the waiting room and through an IVF newsletter. In regard to the newsletter, the social worker was again able to utilize the interest and talents of a successful IVF patient, who is very grateful for her "miracle" baby. This woman expressed interest in helping to produce a newsletter for IVF couples. Soon, she became the organizer, main reporter and editor of a very high-quality IVF newsletter, which is distributed three times each year and is very popular with the patient population. The social worker's role is to write an article for each issue and to serve as a liaison between the editor, the program staff and the hospital printing department.

VII. Insurance Assistance

Questions about insurance coverage, requests for assistance with insurance forms and inquiries from insurance companies are channelled to the social worker, who composes letters or makes telephone calls on behalf of the patient in order to address these matters in an appropriate manner in this area.

POTENTIAL FOR ROLE DEVELOPMENT

The social worker's role could be expanded further to include

1) screening couples prior to admission into the program;
2) leading a therapy group;
3) holding stress management classes;
4) conducting or collaborating in a research project;
5) providing more support for husbands and
6) organizing a professional association of social workers in the field.

I. Screening Couples

Although some IVF programs use psychologists and psychological tests to eliminate prospective patients who are socially or emotionally inappropriate candidates for the stressful infertility treatment, the philosophy of the Jewish Hospital's IVF program has been to accept or reject patients based on medical criteria and to individualize support for emotional needs. Social workers can serve as the professionals who screen couples, as demonstrated by programs, such as Yale-New Haven Hospital (Greenfeld, 1984) and the Hospital of the University of Pennsylvania (Freeman, et al., 1985).

Much is gained from early screening. First, an assessment of the couple's attitudes, expectations and both the present and anticipated levels of stress will help to determine the worker's strategy. Second, serious psychological problems could be identified early and appropriate action could be taken. Third, signs of ambivalence could be detected and might stimulate discussion about delaying or foregoing the stressful IVF procedure until both members of the couple felt comfortable with the decision. Finally, the worker could clarify the financial component and explain that IVF is a big gamble with no assurance of success, pointing out how difficult repaying a huge debt would be with nothing tangible to show for the large outlay of funds.

II. Therapy Groups

In the support group at Jewish Hospital, where new patients are welcome at every meeting, patients do not have the opportunity to resolve problems such as poor self-concept, fear of losing their spouse or acceptance of living without children. If an individual is found to be in need of group therapy, she has been referred to "Resolve", which sponsors small, closed, time-limited support groups led by a professional social worker where the goal is resolution of infertility. A therapy group of this kind could be held in the hospital setting; furthermore, leading a group would be an appropriate role for the hospital social worker.

III. Stress Management

Since stress is a constant companion of infertility, teaching patients ways to cope with stress would be of great value during the anxiety-producing treatments. The Northern Nevada Fertility Clinic in Rent, Nevada, provides prospective couples with a relaxation tape. In addition, the psychologist-consultant associated with the program screens the couple initially and then guides the patient through the relaxation exercises during the embryo transfer phase of the IVF procedure. Not only could social workers be utilized to provide these services, but they could also teach classes or lead workshops in stress management.

s

IV. Research Projects

Due to the unique role of the IVF social worker, he or she is in a position to contribute demographic, social and psychological factors to any medical research being performed at an IVF centre. In addition, the worker could conduct an independent study, evaluating such things as the long term impact of the IVF procedure on the couples' subsequent fertility status (i.e., whether they have acquired children biologically or through adoption; whether they are still pursuing infertility treatment or whether they are resigned to living without children).

V. Support for Husbands

According to Beck (1988), "...part of the problem of many marriages is that there are socially ingrained differences in the thinking and communication styles of men and women. Problems occur because women are taught from the time they are little to discuss intimate problems openly while men have been cautioned repeatedly to remain silent about such matters." Especially in the area of reproduction, "...women tend to be more expressive than men in talking about their pain" (Batterman, 1985). The scarce attendance of husbands at the Jewish Hospital IVF support group illustrates male resistance. Yet, husbands may be as anxious as their wives during fertility treatment. Some husbands have admitted that producing a semen specimen is very stressful for them; consequently, another area that should be addressed is ways to better serve husbands and counsel them through a stressful period in their lives. Given the likelihood that men tend to be resistant to communicating problems, this goal is a real challenge to social work practitioners.

VI. Networking

At professional medical meetings such as the American Fertility Society Conferences, sessions have been held on the psychological component of infertility; thus it is clear that the emotional impact is recognized and that people in the helping professions are active in this field. Yet there is no association of "infertility social workers" as there are "renal social workers" or "oncology social workers." Such an organization could provide an opportunity for sharing of ideas and for professional growth.

CONCLUDING REMARKS

Infertility is a widespread problem with physical, social, emotional and financial ramifications. In spite of many lifetime successes and accomplishments, the typically goal-oriented, high achieving, infertile woman feels as if she is a failure. The amount of stress and self-doubt that accompanies this condition is little understood by the general public. As infertile couples undergo stressful medical procedures to correct their condition, social workers, in many settings, are involved in a number of ways. They provide education about the stressors associated with the medical procedures; make a psychosocial assessment of each couple; offer supportive counselling by encouraging the couples and giving them the opportunity to work through feelings; provide crisis intervention and grief counselling when procedures fail; assist with insurance problems and serve as a source of information about alternatives, support mechanisms and other available resources. Ideally, the role of the social worker could be expanded further to include the screening of couples, leading therapy groups, offering stress management workshops, engaging in research projects, developing new ways to reach out to husbands and establishing an organization for social workers in the field of infertility.

CASE EXAMPLE

Mrs. W. was 39 years old and her husband was 44 when they came to Jewish Hospital for IVF. Despite their ages, their three-year marriage was the first for each of them. Both of their families lived in St. Louis, and they were relatively close to each family. Mrs. W. was an elementary school teacher by profession. Her husband was a businessman who worked for a large St. Louis firm. They had a good marital relationship, communicated well on most subjects and were very supportive of one another; however, their style of coping with problematic life events was different. The husband was a private person who found talking about his problems difficult, while Mrs. W. found comfort in verbalizing her concerns. Since they were married so late in life, the couple decided after six months to begin their family. After one year without success, they sought medical help from a specialist who found that Mrs. W. had endometriosis. She was first treated with medication and then surgery. After that, there was nothing more to be offered except IVF.

Mrs. W. was very anxious when she was first seen by the social worker. All her siblings and friends had children, and she realized that her "biological clock was ticking." She sensed that she might never have children, and consequently, she was feeling desperate. During the IVF procedure, Mrs. W. stated that she felt nervous and that she cried with little provocation. She was told that these symptoms were often side effects of one of the medications she was taking. She was very receptive to contacts with the social worker and seemed to feel better after their discussions. Fortunately, Mrs. W. responded well and went through the entire IVF procedure. What is more, she was among the 25% of women in the Jewish Hospital program rewarded with a positive pregnancy test. Mrs. W. was overcome with joy and wept in the IVF office.

Within two weeks, however, Mrs. W. had a miscarriage, the outcome for half the women with an early pregnancy. Her grief was all-consuming. The worker met with her frequently in order to give her the opportunity to express her feelings and to cry. The worker acknowledged that Mrs.W. felt as if she had been given a gift but that the gift was later taken away. The worker also explained that this was entirely a lonely grief because no one else, other than her husband, could share it with her. An analogy was made between the baby's death and a cut on the finger that hurts so much when it is fresh but that heals in time. Eventually there may be a scar but the pain would subside. Mrs. W. nodded her head, feeling that the social worker understood.

In subsequent meetings, adoption was discussed. This was an option to which she was amenable. Due to her age and her rejection of adopting both a child with special needs and one from a different country, private adoption was the most realistic choice; consequently, suggestions and information were provided. Mrs. W. was asked if she would like to speak with other couples who had acquired children through private adoption. Since she was receptive, two former patients were approached, and both willingly agreed to talk with Mrs. W. Following a friendly exchange with each woman, Mrs. W. contacted an attorney, who was willing to work with her and her husband. Mr. and Mrs. W. came very close to adopting a baby girl, but at the last minute, the biological mother changed her mind.

The adoption experience exacerbated Mrs. W.'s depression; thus, at this point, a suggestion was made that she see a therapist for more extensive, long-term counselling. Mrs. W. took the advice, and, a year later, she called the social worker to say that she finally felt like her "old self again." It had taken one year to fully recover from the miscarriage and from grieving for the children she will never have. She was grateful for her husband and all the other good things in her life, and she was ready to put aside thoughts of parenthood.

References

Batterman, R. (1985). A comprehensive approach to treating infertility. *Health and Social Work, 10,* 46-54.

Beck, A. (1988). *Love is Never Enough.* New York: Harper Row.

Daniluk, J. C. (1988). Infertility: Intrapersonal and interpersonal impact. *Fertility and Sterility, 49,* 982-990.

DiMattina, M. & Liu, J. (1987). Benefits of GIFT for treating infertility. *Contemporary OB/GYN,* October, 145-150.

Fleming, J. & Burry, K. (1988). Coping with infertility. *Journal of Social Work and Human Sexuality, 5,* 37-41.

Freeman, E. W., Boxer, A. S., Rickels, K., Tureck, R. & Mastroianni, L. (1985). Psychological evaluation and support in a program of in vitro fertilization and embryo transfer. *Fertility and Sterility, 43,* 48-53.

Garner, C. (1983). In vitro fertilization and embryo transfer. *Journal of Obstetrics, Gynecology and Neonatal Nursing, 12,* 75-78.

Goodman, K. & Rothman, B. (1984). Group work in infertility treatment. *Social Work with Groups, 7,* 29-92.

Greenfeld, D., Mazure, C., Hazeltine, F. & DeCherney, A. (1984). The role of the social worker in the in-vitro fertilization program. *Social Work in Health Care, 10,* 71-79.

Johnston, I., Lopata, A., Speirs, A., Hoult, I., Kellow, G. & dePlessis, Y. (1981). In vitro fertilization: The challenge of the eighties. *Fertility and Sterility, 136,* 699-706.

Kane, L. R. (1981). Psychological aspects of infertility. *High Hopes: A Forum for Perinatal Social Workers, 1*(4), 12.

Kubler-Ross, E. (1975). *Death: The Final Stage of Growth.* Englewood Cliffs, NJ: Prentice Hall.

Menning, B. E. (1977). *Infertility: A Guide for the Childless Couple.* Englewood Cliffs, NJ: Prentice Hall.

Needleman, S. K. (1987). Infertility and in vitro fertilization; The social worker's role. *Health and Social Work, 12,* 135-143.

U.S. Congress, Office of Technology Assessment (1988). *Infertility, Medical and Social Changes* (OTA-BA-0358). Washington, DC: U.S. Government Printing Office.

Wallis, C. (1984, Sept. 10). The new origins of life. *Time,* 46-53.

Chapter 6

THE ROLE OF THE SOCIAL WORKER IN THE REALM OF HIV DISEASE

Peter Quick, M.S.W., C.S.W.

Abstract

Social work in the realm of HIV disease is often perceived as new. The profession has a tradition of service with disenfranchized, marginalized and have-nots. Social work provides a multifaceted service, encompassing direct clinical work, advocacy, education, and case management. Given the above, social work in the realm of HIV disease is not new. As a profession, social work is well suited to be a key player. From a practice role perspective, there are no standarized methods or absolutes. At the same time, HIV disease is not totally predictable. Psycho-social intervention must be viewed from a developmental framework, permitting the examination of a variety of phases the HIV infected and/or affected person may encounter. The use of case example most clearly delineates the issues, and the role of social work. The need for intervention to be client directed and worker responsive is continually emphasized.

THE ROLE OF THE SOCIAL WORKER IN THE REALM OF HIV DISEASE

In preparing this paper, the focus was to be upon the social worker and his or her service delivery in the realm of HIV disease. The focus was not to be upon a "research" paper, detailing social work theories. My own personal style is reflected here. I like case example as a learning method and as such, the paper uses many of my own reflections and recollections of people with whom I have worked. Needless to say, all names are false and no identifying information is provided. In fact, many case examples are composites of cases. I have seen over 1,000 individuals either infected or affected by HIV disease. They are the ones who have taught me the most, specific to experiential learning. I am truly grateful for their generous "sharing."

THE CLIENTELE

The best description of the HIV Care Programme, found within the flyer for the Programme, states that the HIV Care Programme is a multidisciplinary out-patient treatment facility operated under the auspices of St. Joseph's Health Centre in London (Ontario). The Programme is funded by the provincial Ministry of Health and there is no direct cost/payment for services by the clients. The funding is provided to meet the needs of the HIV infected (those who are diagnosed with the virus) and affected (those who are affected by someone diagnosed with the virus). The Programme is a regional one serving all of Southwestern Ontario (approximately 1.3 million people).

The aim of the HIV Care Programme reflects the mission of St. Joseph's Health Centre — excellence and compassion in patient care. The focus of the Programme is upon the psycho-social and medical aspects of HIV disease, providing psycho-social counselling and support, medical assessments and monitoring, health promotion, and treatment of complications of HIV infection. The care is for the individual with HIV related concerns or problems, as well as for family and friends.

The Programme is based on a medical model. Referrals to the HIV Care Programme are made by a physician. The Programme works on an out-patient basis with scheduled appointments and, in general, is not able or equipped to handle emergencies. It has regular office hours Monday to Friday. However, due to service demands (e.g.: patients who work or educational programs), some evening work is necessitated.

The Programme opened in the Fall of 1989. It moved into its present off-site location in January 1990. The Programme currently has approximately 250 registered patients. The projected number of patient visits for 1990 is 2,150. The Programme serves any persons diagnosed with HIV infection (the classical presentation groups of homosexual, bisexual, hemophiliac, partner of infected person, recipient of blood/blood products, injected drug user, and through perinatal transmission). "There has been no disease in recent memory that has occupied the attention and stimulated the concern of the biomedical community and lay public as has the acquired immunodeficiency syndrome." (Fanci, 1985). By all case reports and projections, HIV disease will continue to increase. The following table gives AIDS reports for Ontario, indicating the progressive, escalating nature of the disease. (Ontario Ministry of Health, 1990)

Year	Number of Case Reports	Accumulative
1982	6	6
1983	13	19
1984	46	65
1985	133	198
1986	175	373
1987	322	695
1988	348	1,043
1989	413	1,456
1990		

PRACTICE ROLES AND RESPONSIBILITIES

In approaching practice roles and responsibilities, two factors need to be considered. The first is standardization. HIV disease is new. All persons involved in the provision of service delivery, from whatever professional bias, maintain that no one holds the absolute answer. There are no standardized methods of treatment. This is positive in that flexibility is inherent and dogma has not been established. On the other hand, many become concerned when no standards exist. The practitioner is often left asking "Is this the right thing to do?... How will I know what will be effective?"

The second factor is predictability. HIV disease is not constant. Some people are diagnosed with this disease and are very well from a psychological perspective. Others receiving the same diagnosis do not adjust well and become quite troubled, even to the point of contemplating suicide or attempting suicide. Differentiality is highly underscored in HIV disease. How is one to respond given a potential life threatening, or actual life threatening, diagnosis? No two people will respond in exactly the same manner although practitioners typically wish for a standardized, predictable response.

Given the above, the preferred method of addressing this area is one which provides a developmental framework. This framework can be utilized to examine the individual, family/friends, groups, community and societal responses. Further, this development framework permits the examination of a variety of phases the HIV infected and/or affected person may encounter. The following phases will be addressed, examining the developmental issues for the individual, the professional social worker's role, and using case examples:

(i)   pre-test

(ii)   test

(iii)   post-test

(iv)   asymptomatic

(v)   symptomatic

(vi)   palliative

(vii)   bereavement

(i) Pre-test

The issue of whether or not to be tested for HIV is highly individualistic. For some, it is a process which one must do. Example: Mary is the wife of John who was diagnosed HIV positive in 1986. John has hemophilia. It is most likely that John contracted the HIV infection through the blood supply (which, in Canada since November 1985, is regularly screened for the virus). Mary and John continue to have sex. Although they use safer sex practices (i.e. condoms and spermical foam with nonoxynol 9), Mary constantly worries that she will become infected. For Mary, the issue of being tested is of paramount importance. She does not want to see her two children, ages ten and eight, become orphans. For Mary, this is a most isolating experience. Some of the family know of John's HIV status and some do not. Those that know are uncomfortable talking about it. For those that do not know, Mary prefers they do not know, for even if they did, she would not choose to talk with them.

The above case example highlights a number of issues for social work intervention: the importance of confidentiality, the need for support, the burden of ongoing/constant concern, and the availability of testing.

For others, the issue of whether to be tested or not is never considered. Example: Joe is 24 years old. He works for a factory. In the spring, the company had a blood donation campaign. Joe, doing as the rest of his co-workers, gave blood. The routine screening of Joe's blood indicated HIV prevalence. Joe was most distressed.

Joe's case illustrates the need for crisis intervention, confidentiality, support, case management/planning, education, and medical follow-up.

Another group is what some refer to as the 'worried-well.' Example: Suzanne is single. For three months last year she was seeing Bob. One month after their relationship ended, Suzanne got an anonymous phone call. The male voice said, "You better get to a doctor.... Bob's got AIDS." Suzanne did consult a doctor and she was tested for HIV. She tested negative. Since this time, Suzanne continues to seek medical attention. She believes she is HIV infected, despite the fact that she has now had five tests, all being negative.

The above case example outlines the need for education, the

need for counselling and support, and the issue of availability of testing.

Finally, one other group should be considered. This is where someone knows that they have been involved in sexual behaviour that can be described as "risky," and the practice of safer sex has not been consistently applied. Example: John is a gay man who is single. Although he is most aware of safer sex practices, he knows that there have been some occasions where he has had unprotected anal sex. Although this has been rare, he is cognizant of the facts. For the past year he has contemplated being tested. He has had some of the symptoms associated with HIV disease. When asked, John has stated, "I won't be surprised to know I am infected." Further he notes, "I now need to know for a fact...I can't live in limbo."

A second example: Harold is married and has two children. He is a salesman and, due to the nature of his work, often travels out of town. During trips away from his home, it has been a regular practice for him to employ prostitutes. Today Harold is scared. He believes that his practices may put him at risk of becoming infected. At the same time, he is lonely and notes that he has no one with whom to talk.

These two case scenarios show the importance of comprehending the patient's recognition of their behaviour, encouraging verbalization, providing support and education, and facilitating medical follow-up.

Social workers have provided their services to the above case situations. It is most probable that social work services will be involved on an ongoing and escalating basis as the issues are far ranging. A well known social work principle is "starting where the client is." For Mary, being tested is so very important, central to her ongoing, day-to-day existence and functioning. For Joe there was no pre-test phase. For Suzanne, she is stuck in the pre-test phase, not able to move forward. For John, the pre-test phase has been a long and difficult ordeal with a certain pre-conceived end or result. For Harold the pre-test phase is filled with anxiety and a sense of isolation.

(ii) Test

The actual test for HIV is simple; blood is drawn and sent to a lab for analysis. The psycho-social issues relating to this phase are found in the methods of HIV test documentation. Although there are various methods, what will be considered here are three: nominal, non-nominal, and anonymous.

Nominal testing, the present method generally used in Ontario when blood is drawn and analyzed, is done by completing a lab slip on which the name, address, date of birth, sex, and "risk group" are noted. The following is the information for the Ontario Ministry of Health by which the patient's risk group is selected: none; referred by blood collection agency; hemophiliac; endemic area immigrant/traveller; homosexual/bisexual male; work place parenteral exposure; sexual partner of AIDS/ARC or anti-HIV positive person; intravenous drug user; blood/blood product recipient; offspring of AIDS/ARC or anti-HIV positive person; and other. The law, as written at present, supports this method.

Non-nominal testing is the same except that no names,only initials, and no addresses are used. Although the law supports nominal testing, non-nominal is the practice adopted and preferred by some.

In anonymous testing, typically, a code is utilized (rather than names or initials). Often the sex, age, and risk group are noted (this is for demographic/epidemiological purposes).

It is noted that the law supports nominal testing, yet non-nominal is used. One centre in Ontario publicly provides anonymous testing. The law, for Ontario, is most likely to change in the near future allowing for flexibility in the methods of test documentation. People need to have options dependent upon the situation at hand. Example: Gordon lives in a community of 1,000 people. Although there is a place for anonymous testing, he would not go there for testing. He knows that his neighbour's daughter works there and would he be recognized. Gordon, given his situation, may choose to have either nominal or non-nominal testing with his family doctor. The issue of confidentiality is imperative for most individuals being tested.

What about the testing of others? While mandatory testing of others is not and should not be possible, there are particular incidents which raise the issue for compulsory or mandatory testing of others. Two examples are a needle-stick injury by a health care worker, or a rape where one has reason to believe there has been a potential exposure to the virus. At the same time, testing others is done and universally supported in such areas as: blood donation, organ donation, or sperm donation. The testing of others is an area of social work involvement outlined in the Section, Responsibilities for Social Workers, below.

A final note on testing should be included. A positive test indicates the presence of antibodies to HIV. This probably means that there is HIV present in the body, the infection is irreversible, and the individual is capable of transmitting HIV to another person.

A negative test means that an individual has not shown, from an analysis of their blood, the presence of antibodies to HIV. This could mean either that the person has not been exposed to HIV or the person has been exposed but has not, as yet, become infected (developed antibodies to HIV). Simply put, a negative test means that an individual is not infected at that time. He or she could become HIV positive (seroconvert) at some future point in time. In some situations, repeat testing is required.

For social workers, testing should be understood within certain confines, given its complex medical/scientific nature. Good medical intervention is important. Social work intervention is equally important and needs to focus largely on the anxiety that is often present during this phase.

(iii) Post-Test

There exists a dichotomy within this phase. One is either seronegative (no detected presence of antibodies to HIV) or seropositive (detected presence of antibodies to HIV).

If one is seronegative, a degree of caution may be required depending on the individual(s) behaviour. Example: Jim and Bill recently met one another. They have been using safer sex practices and are monogamous. The issue is that both want to stop safer sex practices given that they are both equally committed to their relationship. Their first tests done two weeks ago were negative.

The above case indicates a need for support and education, as well as the need for continued safer sex practices. Many would advocate the need for retesting at six months before the cessation of safer sex practices in a monogamous relationship.

Returning to Suzanne, there is clearly a need to provide post-test services from a social work point of view. Ongoing counselling appears to be indicated given her internalized belief that she is HIV infected. Education can be one part of the treatment but, in addition, psychotherapy may be appropriate.

The issues for social work intervention for the seropositive are addressed in the asymptomatic and symptomatic phase.

(iv) Asymptomatic

The asymptomatic phase is one where an individual, although seropositive if tested, is free or relatively free of disease. No one knows how long this phase may last. An individual looks, feels, and medically is well. Individuals may be in this phase for some time, not knowing their HIV status as there has been no testing nor indicators for HIV testing. Example: Cathy is 30 years old. During the past nine years she has had two longstanding relationships. While in the relationships, she did not see other men. Now she is "single" again and dating. She enjoys sex and is somewhat aware of HIV disease. She does prefer that her partners use condoms but, on occasion, has not insisted. While she has engaged in unprotected sex, Cathy does not believe she would ever become infected. Her rationale is that she is engaging in coital sex (no anal sex), she is not "promiscuous," and she will only have sex with men who, to her, seem healthy and fit. Unknown to Cathy, one of her partners was HIV infected and the virus was transmitted. She has been HIV infected for a year. From a medical perspective, she is asymptomatic.

Cathy's case illustrates a commonly held belief that 'it couldn't happen to me.' Social work intervention necessitates the examination of each client's belief systems. This may include religion, cultural, professional, familial, and peer group and/or societal beliefs. The importance of a thorough psycho-social diagnostic workup is apparent.

The asymptomatic phase, from a psycho-social perspective, is often an area of significant involvement. Intensive social work intervention during this phase is common. Example: Donna is a widow and mother of a four year old. She contracted HIV from her husband who used IV drugs before their relationship. He died six months ago. Donna was diagnosed one year before her husband died. Although she has no symptoms, Donna has been receiving counselling once per week for the past year. Her issues range from her diagnosis and potential disease progression, quantity of life, long-term parenting of her child (who is not infected), and grieving of her lost husband.

Another example: Robert is 36 years old. He was diagnosed three years ago. The first two years after diagnosis, he states, "I was fine." About a year ago, he referred himself for counselling.

He perceives that "issues seem to be building...I have night-mares...I don't know what is going to happen." Like Donna, Robert is asymptomatic. He works as a school teacher. His friends and family know of his disease and all are most support-ive. He often says, "I don't get it...I'm better off than so many oth-ers...I feel that I shouldn't complain."

The above case examples are evidence of the need for ongoing counselling. Social workers are in a position to assist Donna and Robert in dealing with a multitude of human realities. As noted earlier, there does not exist a single model or standard. The vari-ety of intervention methods are not disease specific, but rather client directed and worker responsive.

(v) Symptomatic

Within this phase, the individual begins to exhibit symptoms which are directly related to HIV disease. Example: Len was diag-nosed HIV positive in September 1987. After an initial depression, be began to feel more in control. He felt well supported and was able to continue with his life much as it was pre-diagnosis. Len awoke one morning and, during his usual routine of preparing for work, he noticed some purplish marks. He immediately felt panic. He knew that these marks were Karposi's sarcoma (KS).

From an experiential frame of reference, the symptomatic phase is a time where patients' issues are not only within a psy-chological realm. The need for a solid medical knowledge base is of paramount importance. Example: Alex complained for two months that "something was going on." He had been in individu-al counselling for six months. In examining what Alex meant, the social worker discovered that Alex was experiencing decreased ability to do certain tasks. He gave examples of not being able to balance his cheque book, being grocery shopping and not being able to remember what it was that he needed, or finding that he was missing various appointments.

The above case underscores the need to comprehend various aspects of the disease. Is Alex exhibiting symptoms related to HIV dementia? Is Alex exhibiting symptoms related to depression?

For many, symptoms of HIV disease are well known. For some, there may be a sense of "this is the beginning of the end." Example: Barry was diagnosed in 1986. In 1988, his partner died of HIV disease. Last month, Barry had his first bout of pneumocystic carinii pneumonia (PCP). Prior to this Barry had been asymptomatic and had felt fine. Now he has "recovered" from the PCP. However, from a psychological point of view, the onset of the symptomatic phase has shaken the foundation of his existence. Barry often relives the sorrows of his partner's death, being able to visualize his own demise.

Another feature of the symptomatic phase can be hospitalization. The majority of people, for some reason, prefer not to be in hospital. The focus of many HIV clinics is to maintain people outside of hospital. However, despite the best efforts of all, hospitalization may become necessary. For some, this represents a significant milestone. It may also reinforce societal reactions and stigmatization. Example: Margaret was HIV negative and her husband was HIV positive. They knew the risks. Although they both stated that it was not a planned pregnancy, when the 'accident' happened, both did want the baby. Margaret and her husband managed to not focus upon the potential transmission of HIV. Soon after the birth, Margaret began to sense that she was being "watched" and treated differently. Her husband arrived one afternoon and stopped at the nursing station. While waiting, he saw a patient listing on the desk. Margaret's name was in large letters, in red, and contained a notice: "possible AIDS." The reality was that Margaret was being treated differently and that the hospital staff were being extremely cautious in their provision of care. They feared of becoming HIV infected. Margaret was their first patient where HIV infection was a factor.

The above case example highlights that staff reactions do affect the client. Although education for staff can increase their knowledge, experience and skill must also be developed. All of us have attitudes. Some would argue that the above case would not exist in their given place of employment. However education is a process and there are always new staff and new experiences. The need for social workers to be involved on an ongoing basis is clear. Further, many community based agencies are now just beginning to receive referrals for services. Social workers must be involved in educating and advocating for services based upon our clients' needs.

(vi) Palliative

This is a phase of HIV disease that, in many respects, is similar to other work with palliative care patients. The following cases are provided to demonstrate the reality that HIV disease affects all ages. There are no boundaries. The demands for care are great and social work has a vital role to play.

Jane is 18 months old. She was born to a mother who was HIV infected. Jane is in the final stages of HIV disease and is not likely to live much longer. She is in hospital where her care providers are attempting to keep her comfortable and pain free. At the other end of the age continuum Julia is 77. In 1984 she had cardiac bi-pass surgery. The blood she received during the surgery had HIV. She is presently in hospital and is not responding to treatment.

The social worker has been working with Jane's mother. The grief and guilt she feels is overwhelming. The mother oftens states "it's all my fault that Jane's sick.... It is all my fault." Julia's daughter has been seen by the social worker to deal with her sense of injustice. Her daughter states "I can't understand why my mother's sick...its so unfair...this shouldn't be happening."

This phase may present some unique issues for intervention with gay men. Example: Bill was dying. His partner of eight years was asked by the staff physician to get in contact with Bill's family. The partner stated that there was "only Bill and I..Bill hasn't had any contact with his family for the past 12 years. When he told them he was gay, they disowned him." The physician was persistent. His point of view was that Bill was not able to make his own decisions. In addition, he did not perceive that he was able to have the partner as "next-of-kin," and needed to consult with a "blood" relative.

The above case example clearly demonstrates the need for flexibility. Client situations vary greatly. Not all case situations or client's unique needs are going to "fit" neatly into the existing or preconceived service delivery methods.

The palliative phase, in some situations, may be a "double disclosure." For some families, the first time they confront their son's homosexuality is when he is also dying. In such a situation, the role for social work may become conflicting. An example is where the family of origin does not want the son's partner involved in decision-making. Social work intervention needs to be flexible.

A further note on the palliative phase, is that to some extent, palliative care may begin at diagnosis. HIV is irreversible. HIV has no cure. Some patients are acutely aware of their prognosis. Social workers must examine their own issues as countertransference may be present. A false sense of support is not appropriate. Equally inappropriate is too much "reality orientation." A "doom and gloom" outlook can be devastating. It is imperative to achieve an effective and workable balance.

(viii) Bereavement

This phase is one where social work intervention may immediately follow the palliative phase, or may emerge some time later. Social work involvement may be intensive and prolonged. Example: Jerry died one month ago. His partner, while grieving the loss of Jerry, also had to attend to many legal and practical matters. Another issue was testing. Jerry's partner, for a number of reasons, had never been tested for HIV.

The above case outlines the need for social work to provide a multifacted intervention. The issues of support, pacing, education, and practical assistance are inherent.

For others, the bereavement phase is one in which withdrawal is apparent. Some prefer to distance themselves from social work asistance. Some prefer to not use social work intervention, but to use alternate services such as pastoral care. What must be underscored is the fact that social work intervention may not cease with a patient's death. The need to "start where the client is" is continuous.

The bereavement phase need also be examined from a community sense. Many service providers experience grief and loss in an exponential manner. The death of one patient may be felt as a loss of great significance. The reality is, HIV disease is affecting many:

"the worried, the ill, the dying, and the bereaved will occupy social workers' caseloads and continue to touch their personal lives as well. Whole families of intravenous drug users are becoming infected and dying; orphaned children with AIDS languish in inner-city hospitals; gay men die; elderly parents grieve for sons, daughters, grandsons, and granddaughters; and agency staffs are immobilized by the illness of a social work colleague repeatedly hospitalized for one opportunistic infection after another. No setting in any region of the United States will be spared by the pandemic of AIDS that will continue into the next century, according to all the best estimates." (Shernoff, 1990).

SOCIAL WORK SERVICE DELIVERY

Treatment models and service delivery are multifaced. The variety of intervention methods are not disease specific or phase standard, but rather, are client directed and worker responsive. The counselling modalities include: individual; couple; family; group; and community.

Practice experience has suggested three broad categories of service delivery. All begin with a thorough assessment in order to obtain a pycho-social diagnosis.

i) **assessment** - From the assessment, further service may be indicated (see below). Sometimes the assessment indicates that the client currently does not require further social work services. Other times, although social work service is indicated, the client does not want additional service at this point in time.

ii) **short-term services** - These individuals require some type of minimal social work services. Examples could include the following: practical work (such as assistance with finances); brief therapy, such as disclosure of diagnosis to a significant other, contract oriented work (social work services for a prescribed length of time); or crisis intervention with resolution, or possible additional follow-up and/or referral. Some clients do not, at that given time, need (or necessarily want) more. Short-term service may represent an "introduction," to social work as it may be the first time the individual has seen a counsellor.

iii) **Long-term services** - These individuals require and want services of a protracted nature. For some, ongoing supportive counselling is indicated. For others, psychotherapy of a dynamic, insight oriented nature is appropriate.

As has been stated, "starting where the client is" is imperative.

SOCIAL WORK RESPONSIBILITIES

In 1989, the Ontario Association of Professional Social Workers (OAPSW.) published "OAPSW statement on HIV/AIDS: A Social Work Perspective." This statement delineates seven areas for social workers:

(i) **social action and advocacy** - The tradition of the profession includes involvement in social action and advocacy. Social work needs to be active in the prevention and elimination of discriminatory factors related to HIV disease; advocate for resources and services; encourage the development and implementation of educational programmes, both client based and agency/staff based; advocate for policy and legislation changes to improve social conditions; be informed and up-to-date, ensuring the provision of accurate information; and participate in and/or initiate research projects.

(ii) access to and development of services and resources - There is a need for a comprehensive service delivery system. Social work needs to facilitate the process of obtaining access to services and resources; encourage the development of a range of services to meet needs; and promote flexibility in gaining access to service needs.

(iii) HIV antibody testing - Testing for HIV involves numerous bio-psycho-social issues. Social workers need to be "on record" as being against mandatory testing, involved with organ donation, blood donation, or sperm donation; advocate for informed consent prior to testing; advocate for pre-test and post-test counselling; and provide pre-test and post-test counselling.

(iv) confidentiality - Discrimination is a reality. Social workers need to advocate for anonymous and non-nominal testing; and actively maintain confidentiality.

(v) disclosure - Disclosing HIV status and information needs careful consideration.

(vi) reporting - Social workers are ethically responsible to assist in the control of the spread of HIV disease. Having reasonable and probable grounds, to believe that an individual is engaging in activities that put others at risk, social workers are ethically bound to report this information to the proper authorities.

(vii) social worker with HIV infection/AIDS - No social worker should be obliged to disclose their HIV status. Any social worker who is infected should be encouraged to continue to work. All social work employers should be encouraged to support the infected worker and his or her co-workers.

CONCLUSION

What is social work? For me, it has meant working with the "disenfranchised," the "marginalized" and society's "have nots." Social work has a legacy of servicing the "difficult" client, the "multi-problem" client, and the "reluctant" client. Traditionally, social work has provided a multifaceted service: clinical/direct service, education, advocacy, case management, coordination of services, and liaison.

My experience has consistently proven that work with the HIV infected and affected is no different. Social work in the realm of HIV disease, has demanded a variety of services and intervention modalities. Differential use of self has been an absolute necessity. The profession is truly doing work in the uncharted.

In examining the impact of HIV disease, the profession of social work is well suited to be a key player. Our body of knowledge, theoretical constructs, and practice orientation enable us to provide leadership and coordination in the psycho-social treatment of HIV disease. Social workers, in whatever setting they are working, will see increased numbers of individuals, family groups, and communties who are HIV infected and affected. Let us not become isolated or perpetuate denial. Be proactive. Get involved.

References

Fauci, A.S., et al. (1985). The Acquired Immunodeficiency Syndrome: An Update. *Annals of Internal Medicine*, 102, 800-813.

Ontario Association of Professional Social Workers. (1989). *OAPSW Statement on HIV /Aids: A Social Work Perspective.*

Ontario Ministry of Health. (1990) *AIDS Statistics for Ontario and Canada.* Disease Control and Epidemiology Service, Public Health Branch.

Shernoff, M. (1990). Why Every Social Worker Shold Be Challenged by AIDS. *Social Work.* Jan., 5-7.

Shilts, R. (1987) *And the Band Played On: Politics, People, and the AIDS Epidemic.* St. Martin's Press, New York.

Chapter 7

PERINATAL SOCIAL WORK PRACTICE

Catherine J. Cameron, MSW
Randee J. Moir, SSW
Marlene L. Rees-Newton, MSW

Abstract

Perinatal social work is an emerging specialty in the health care field. Within a framework of family-centred care, medical and psychosocial issues dealing with conception, pregnancy, birth and newborn death are the focus of social work practice. Social workers respond to referrals from Antenatal, Delivery Room, Neonatal Intensive Care Unit and Post-Partum Units. Intervention includes individual casework, marital counselling and group work. As integral members of the interdisciplinary team, social workers collaborate in the formulation of a treatment plan. They have a mandate for program development and in-service education within the secondary setting.

PERINATAL SOCIAL WORK PRACTICE

Perinatology has emerged as a specialty in the field of health care over the past two to three decades. Perinatology is a branch of medicine, within Obstetrics and Paediatrics, that deals with the fetus and infant during the perinatal period. The perinatal period is variously described as beginning at the completion of the 20th to 28th week of pregnancy, and ending 7 to 28 days after birth.

At St. Joseph's Health Centre, London, Ontario[1], the area of perinatology is a challenging, progressive field where the expertise of social work has become highly valued. Although social work service had been provided to the various units on a fragmented basis, a major step in program development at this centre took place in 1987, when three full-time equivalent social work positions were allocated to this specialty. It was perceived that a social work team approach would provide improved service and increased continuity of care. Under this new approach, the social worker who completed the assessment during the initial hospitalization would continue her/his involvement with each transfer and/or readmission ensuring service continuity.

Figure 1. Potential Perinatal Admission Sources.

First Admission	Readmission	Delivery Room
Gynaecology —>	Antenatal —>	Mother admitted
Diag: Hyperemesis	Diag: Pregnancy	with premature
	Induced Hypertension	labour
	30 weeks gestation	
Infant admitted to	Mother on	Infant admitted to
NICU	Postpartum —>	Pediatrics
prematurity, —>		6 mos. of age,
		Diag: Failure to
		Thrive

The Perinatal Program encompasses Gynaecology (24 beds); Antenatal (24 beds); Delivery Room (15 beds); NICU (42 beds); Postpartum (62 beds); and Paediatrics (25 beds) (see Figure 1). The focus of this chapter will be on social work practice in the areas of

Antenatal (women with high risk pregnancies, 20-weeks gestation and over), Neonatal Intensive Care Unit (newborns with high risk medical problems), Postpartum (women who have given birth to a premature or full-term infant) and Perinatal Loss (neonatal death or stillbirth).

THE CLIENTELE

St. Joseph's Hospital is the regional teaching centre for high risk pregnancies and births in Southwestern Ontario. There were 4,200 births in 1988, with 800 admissions to the Neonatal Intensive Care Unit (NICU). The clientele served are families in their childbearing years. More specifically, these would include (a) women who are hospital inpatients and their families; (b) parents whose infants are admitted to the NICU or (c) parents whose infants do not survive. Unlike hospitals in large, multi-racial urban cities such as Toronto, Vancouver or New York, the clientele tend to be from white, lower-middle class and middle class socioeconomic groups.

There is a large spectrum of problems and needs presented by this clientele. Social work receives a referral from Antenatal, Postpartum or the NICU if one or more of the following problems are identified:

1. high risk medical situations;
2. evidence of psychosocial concerns or
3. perinatal loss (neonatal death or stillbirth).

I. High Risk Medical Situations

Antenatal. On Antenatal, women may be admitted to the hospital for diagnostic testing or long-term treatment of pregnancy-related complications. Diagnostic testing may result in confirmation of fetal anomalies (e.g., dwarfism), some of which may be incompatible with life (e.g., anencephaly). With pregnancy-related complications (e.g., pregnancy induced hypertension or premature ruptured membranes) comes the threat of premature delivery and admission of the infant to the NICU. Fear, inadequacy, guilt and anger are common responses as parents attempt to deal with uncertain outcomes.

Prolonged hospitalization, combined with medical concerns for both the mother and the unborn child, generally create a disruption to the family system which requires adaptation. The family must draw on resources, both emotional and social, at this time. In a regional centre, individuals are often separated from their families by distance. There are many repercussions of such a separation, including financial pressure, child care issues and marital strain.

NICU. To have an infant admitted to a Neonatal Intensive Care Unit at the time of delivery constitutes a crisis for families. The unique stressors of the NICU environment are often intimidating to parents. They are confronted with a highly technological environment, as well as a diversity of health care professionals. Many parents report their initial visit to the NICU as traumatic. This first glimpse of their baby, who may be attached to life support and monitoring equipment, can trigger a dramatic emotional response.

Identification of high risk medical situations such as the diagnosis of a life-threatening illness, particular syndrome or anomalies create great distress for the family. Parents often describe feelings of confusion when the focus is on the survival of their infant. Grief over the loss of the "perfect child" stimulates feelings of guilt, anger and helplessness. There is additional stress if the infant has been transferred from an outlying community and the mother has remained in the local hospital. The father often feels torn between being with his wife and with his critically ill child. There may also be concern for children at home and related financial pressures. All of the above may create strain on marital relationships and stretch the coping abilities of families beyond their previously tested limits.

Postpartum. Women who enter hospital and give birth to a healthy full-term infant spend an average of three days on the Postpartum Unit; therefore, perinatal social workers responding to referrals in this area must work in an expedient and collaborative fashion with allied health professionals and the client.

There are instances where a baby may be medically sound but the health of the mother is compromised, requiring an extended stay in hospital (e.g., caesarean section or pregnancy-induced hypertension). Conversely, medical complications may be diagnosed with a newborn which are not life-threatening and, therefore, do not require admission to the NICU (e.g., cleft palate, fetal alcohol syndrome, Down's syndrome, etc.). Such diagnoses, however, still create disruption for the family. These parents also feel a sense of disappointment, anger and guilt at the loss of the "perfect" child. They are faced with the task of acceptance and long-term adjustment to the special needs of their child.

II. Psychosocial Factors

Individuals and families have histories and problems that will have an impact on their experiences of pregnancy and birth. Many have the inner resources, in addition to family and community supports, to cope with these events.

There are those, however, who do not have such resources and present particular psychosocial needs that require social work intervention. For example,

1) nnsufficient resources that may include limited support systems; inadequate childcare for siblings; financial constraints that prevent families from visiting or poor financial planning that impedes the parents' ability to provide for the physical needs of the baby upon discharge;
2) parents who have experienced a previous loss: loss of infant, child, spouse or significant other;
3) identification of conflictual relationships with couples or extended family members;
4) patients or families who have difficulty working within the health care system (e.g., relating to hospital personnel, adjusting to long-term   hospitalization, adhering to hospital rules and routines, etc.);
5) patients who are overly anxious, or exhibit bizarre, inappropriate behaviour that may interfere with their ability to problem-solve or
6) single mothers expressing ambivalence regarding whether to keep their baby or place her/him for adoption.

Occasionally, the newborn is the focus of intervention as high-risk social factors have been identified. Birth is a maturational crisis that demands an adaptive response on the part of parents. sPerinatal social workers have a mandate to ensure the safety and well-being of the newborn, and to facilitate and assess the parent-infant bonding process and the parents' capacity to meet the basic needs of their infant at discharge.

The following are examples of such high risk social factors:

1) single teenage mothers and couples who do not have an acceptable plan for meeting the needs of their infant at discharge;
2) arents who may not have the intellectual capacity to parent;

3) Parental history of physical abuse or substance abuse that may place thp infant at risk for neglect or abuse;
4) women who have had children previously apprehended by a child welfare agency due to physical or emotional abuse or neglect;
5) women or parents who have a known psychiatric history that may affect their ability to parent and
6) women experiencing delayed or impaired bonding that may place their infant at risk for future abuse or neglect.

III. Perinatal Loss

In recent years, a perinatal loss has been acknowledged as an event that has long-term effects on the psychosocial functioning of the bereaved family. Whether the infant was stillborn or lived for several weeks, the baby's death is experienced as a tragedy and marks a disruption in the life of the family.

The loss of an infant confronts both parents simultaneously; however, each partner may engage in different styles of grieving that may also be conflicting. Certainly, the socialization process in North American society has conditioned females and males to express feelings differently which further compounds this problem.

While it is recognized that bereaved people experience social isolation by others, parents who have had children die seem to encounter feelings of abandonment more intensely, particularly from other parents who fear that this may also happen to them.

It is recognized that intervention by a perinatal social worker at the time of loss can affect the outcome by reducing the impact of the crisis and influencing positive adaptive responses. This model for intervention is based on the integration of aspects of family systems theory and crisis theory.

PRACTICE ROLES AND RESPONSIBILITIES

The National Association of Perinatal Social Workers (U.S.A.), whose aim is to promote, expand and enhance the interests and role of social work in perinatal health care, was established approximately 15 years ago.[2]

What do these social workers actually do? In a secondary setting they undertake a variety of professional responsibilities.
Specifically, they have a mandate to

1) ensure quality service to families;
2) limit stress associated with hospitalization;
3) ensure the safety and well-being of the newborn;
4) respond to the needs of newly bereaved parents;
5) advocate for the client both within the hospital system and the
   community;
6) positively influence adaptive responses in crisis;
7) act as an inegral member of an interdisciplinary team;
8) pursue continuing education and contribute to the knowledge
   base of perinatal social work and
9) provide education to allied health care professionals.

Specific functions, as with roles, relate both to the family and the
setting.

I. Services to Families

Perinatal social workers provide a full-range of social work services to families including individual casework, brief marital
counselling and group work. Aspects of crisis, systems and
bereavement theories are utilized within a humanistic framework
aimed at facilitating positive adjustment.

Individual casework. Referrals are received from the health care
team or from the patient herself. Initial contact is most often with
the mother while she is an inpatient. If there is a spouse involved,
an effort is made to meet with the couple at least once to assess the
impact of the current situation on their relationship and to gather
relevant history data. If there is no spouse involved, it is desirable
to meet with the patient and her main support person.
Supportive/adjustment counselling is offered to the family
throughout the hospitalization. Where the parent's response is
assessed as requiring psychiatric intervention, a consultation is
requested from the Department of Psychiatry. It is common for the
social worker to facilitate the use of community resources, and to
interpret hospital policies and procedures for the family.

When high risk social factors have been identified that may
place the infant at risk for neglect or abuse, the social worker is
asked to provide an assessment and facilitate a discharge plan.

This includes the capacity to parent, ability to bond with the infant, existing family and community supports and financial resources.

A critical function for social work is in co-ordinating a discharge plan for these high risk families. The social worker is expected to respond in an expedient fashion because the hospitalization is generally brief. Discharge planning involves collaboration and co-operation with hospital staff and community personnel such as the public health nurse, family physician, child welfare and other family service agencies. The social worker usually initiates and organizes case conferences that involve those professionals who will follow the family in the community. This provides a forum for the exchange of information in planning for the infant's discharge.

Perinatal social workers seldom have the luxury of separating assessment from intervention and, therefore, must be skilled in establishing trusting relationships in their initial contacts with families. This is an important step in ensuring co-operation in discharge planning.

Groupwork. The social worker provides a once-weekly group where antenatal inpatients have the opportunity to discuss topics of common interest. These topics vary from session to session and include such concerns as separation from family, management of children at home, early interruption of employment and other psychological or social pressures related to pregnancy or hospitalization.

The Parents' Information Series is a weekly educational support group for families of hospitalized neonates. A multi-disciplinary approach is used and a structured format has been established that also allows for informal discussions. Allied health professionals attend the meetings on a rotating basis and present on a variety of topics. Many families, often intimidated and fearful of emotional support groups, are responsive to the more information-oriented structure. The chronic stress of the "ongoing crisis" of premature birth is addressed in such a format.

Brief marital counselling. The crisis of hospitalization sometimes precipitates marital discord or exacerbates previously existing conflicts. Couples are offered brief marital counselling in an effort to help them through the crisis. Such counselling is goal directed; focusing on the loss of the "perfect" child, providing a safe forum for ventilation of underlying fears, mobilizing their collective strengths, etc. If more severe dysfunction exists, a referral to a community agency is facilitated.

Perinatal loss. When pregnancy ends in either delivery of a still-born infant or a neonatal death, the Perinatal Loss Team, consisting of physicians, nurses, social workers and pastoral care workers, endeavours to respond to the immediate needs of the grieving family. A perinatal loss protocol has been instituted to ensure that certain steps are followed. The protocol is usually initiated by the nursing staff in the delivery room. A referral to both social work and pastoral care is automatic. A social work assessment is completed that incorporates the parents' understanding of events surrounding the loss, individual coping skills, their capacity to mutually support one another and the degree of family and community support presently available.

Social work intervention with the family is aimed at helping the parent(s) accept the reality of the loss, providing adequate information to assist with decision making and ensuring a safe environment for the expression of grief.

In conjunction with nursing staff and a pastoral care worker, parents are encouraged to see and hold their dead baby and to give him or her a name. Newly bereaved parents are offered a booklet on Newborn Death[3], polaroid pictures of their baby, and other remembrances (identification bracelet, name card, lock of hair, clothing). Information is provided regarding funeral arrangements, and financial assistance is requested from social service agencies when needed. Brief follow-up is offered to a limited number of families where indicated, and parents are encouraged to participate in community-based grief recovery groups.

II. Secondary Setting Services

Social workers perform numerous functions related to the hospital setting aside from direct patient and family contact. As members of the multi-disciplinary team, they attend weekly rounds on the various units. At these rounds, cases are screened for possible social work referrals, medical and psychosocial information is exchanged on active cases, and discharge plans are formulated. It is the responsibility of the social worker to keep allied staff appraised of ongoing psychosocial developments both through ongoing consultation and documentation in the medical record.

Social workers also perform an important teaching role in perinatology. In-service education related to family dynamics, bereavement and the role of the social worker is offered to staff at regular intervals. As well, social workers collaborate daily with bedside health professionals to assist with the interpretation and understanding of familial behaviour and coping styles.

Program development and related committee work are also significant social work functions. Social workers are active participants on the Perinatal Loss Committee, the NICU Parents' Information Series Committee and the hospital's Child Abuse Committee.

The health care team in Perinatology is faced with many complex ethical decisions. For instance, questions regarding the continuation of pregnancy when a mother's life is in jeopardy, the uses and termination of life support systems, organ donation from anencephalic infants, treatments of the pre-viable fetus and planning for the care of aborted babies who have lived or infants with AIDS, present ethical dilemmas to all team members, not only the physician who is traditionally seen as the team leader within the medical model. The interpersonal relationships that social workers develop with families allow them to gain insight and understanding into family dynamics, and this knowledge aids in the development of a treatment plan. Social workers, in the role of advocate, convey the needs and wishes of the family to the treatment team; however, at times they face dilemmas regarding disclosure of information; for example, when there is conflict between the needs of the newborn who is potentially at risk for neglect or abuse, and the need of the parents for autonomy and confidentiality.

As hospital employees, social workers must help parents understand hospital policies, procedures and limited resources. The need for parents to have time to deal with the imminent death of a critically ill infant on a life support system must be considered in light of the high cost of such equipment and its clinical effectiveness in the individual case.

As team members, social workers are asked to organize multidisciplinary conferences and meetings to consider these issues, assist team members in their individual bioethical struggles and speak to these issues from a social work perspective at Bioethics Rounds or community conferences.

POTENTIAL FOR ROLE DEVELOPMENT

Aside from the roles and responsibilities previously described in this chapter, there are requests for social work services at St. Joseph's Health Centre that go unanswered due to a lack of funding and insufficient staffing. Because the facility is the high risk centre for maternal care in the region, there are many obstetrical specialists on staff and others who have admitting privileges at St. Joseph's. There are numerous requests to provide social work services to antenatal out-patients where the physician or obstetrician has identified psychosocial problems related to the pregnancy. Parents may need assistance in dealing with diagnostic information concerning fetal anomalies, some of which may be life-threatening. Other patients may be in jeopardy because of chaotic lifestyles, substance abuse, or violent relationships where the expectant mother is physically, and/or mentally abused. At the present time, the Social Work Department does not have a mandate to serve this outpatient population.

For those women who do come into hospital antenatally, there is service provided both on an individual, marital and group basis as described earlier. A need that is not addressed at the present time is group work with long-term antenatal couples. For instance, men may feel isolated and overloaded when their spouse is hospitalized for months at a time, as they are left to cope with juggling the stresses of full-time job, housework and childcare. In some centres, there are evening groups run for couples to help with the pressures brought about by their imposed separation.

Groups could also be offered on the Post Partum units to address the needs and fears of first-time mothers regarding initial adjustment issues. This would include the high number of teenage mothers keeping their babies.

Most parents who have experienced a perinatal death are able to draw upon their own inner strengths and existing support systems to resolve their loss. Others are less fortunate and experience delayed or impaired grief resolution. These parents could benefit from follow-up counselling with their perinatal social worker after discharge from hospital.

Providing service to women who have experienced a perinatal loss under 20 weeks is another area of need. It is now understood that the grief reaction of this population may be as equally trau-

112

matic and intense as experiencing a neonatal death or stillbirth. As stated earlier, there is a protocol established for loss over 20 weeks; however, at present, there are insufficient resources to meet the needs of women experiencing an earlier loss. A committee has prepared a pamphlet for these women that addresses common medical and emotional issues. Unfortunately, there is limited staffing to provide individual casework and many are discharged home to cope with feelings of sadness and emptiness on their own. An effective way of assisting this group of women would be to offer community-based, time-limited support groups.

Some babies are followed through the Developmental Surveillance Clinic which monitors their development for the first five years of life. The role of the perinatal social worker could be expanded in this area. For instance, a successful program is presently in place at Alberta Children's Hospital in Calgary. According to perinatal social workers Loretta Young and Helen Surdhar, the focus of intervention includes: "(a) the loss of 'the perfect child'/periodic grief, (b) existing marital dysfunction which may be exacerbated by the demands of caring for a premature or sick infant, (c) the physical and emotional stress which results from caring for a child in a high risk situation and the subsequent effect on siblings, (d) the mental health status of the primary care giver, (e) the child's immediate and long-term adjustment to repeated medical procedures/invasive therapy. In a number of situations, instrumental tasks in terms of linking these families with appropriate community resources (e.g., relief care), may be all that is necessary." (Young, 1987, p. 8).

Social work at the present time performs an important teaching role by providing regular inservice education to the Units served. The department is presently offering a series of in-services for NICU nurses on "Dealing with Challenging Families." This same program could be modified to meet the needs of staff on other Units since so-called "challenging" families are not unique to the NICU. Additional topics for in-services might include issues surrounding the mandate of child welfare agencies, parent-infant bonding, family dynamics, crisis intervention and normal versus pathological grief. Teaching could focus on helping staff recognize their own interpersonal skills and coping styles that affect their interaction with patients. Another facet of the teaching role could be expanded to include student placements for specialized training of perinatal social workers.

There are unlimited possibilities for research in the field of perinatology. Research initially could be directed into evaluative studies regarding social work effectiveness. Complex areas such as changes in self-concept and self-esteem in long-term antenatal patients, marital adjustment following the birth of a premature infant and ongoing adjustment of families coping with a child with special needs could be examined.

The field of perinatology is rich with opportunity, and one would hope that there will be increased funding for and allocation of social work staff for the expansion of this specialty.

CONCLUDING REMARKS

The field of perinatology is filled with challenges, and places high demands on health care staff including perinatal social workers. In this fast-paced, highly technical society, social workers must respond quickly to demands for service. As integral members of the health care team they must be skilled in dealing with the complexities and politics of the secondary setting.

To work effectively in this area, social workers must have a specialized understanding of the life cycle stages, in particular the child-bearing years; aspects of conception, (high risk) pregnancy and birth; issues surrounding parent-infant attachment and bonding and concepts of bereavement. They need to demonstrate competence in individual, family and group work practice. More specifically, the ability to make an expedient and thorough assessment, while extrapolating possible high risk psycho-social factors, is essential for effective intervention.

At St. Joseph's Health Centre, the unique social work team approach has proven to be a valuable structure. Dealing with the incongruence of birth and death on a daily basis results in accumulated stress. The trusting relationship that has developed among the three workers provides the support necessary to remain energized, enthusiastic and effective.

CASE EXAMPLE

Susan and her husband Frank have been married for 6 years, and have a daughter, Jennifer, age four. The family was relocated to London, Ontario, three months earlier when Frank received a transfer with his banking firm. Due to the transfer, and confirmation of a twin pregnancy, Susan terminated her part-time accounting position. This was their first move away from their families with whom Susan and Frank describe positive relationships. Susan's father however was recovering from a stroke and was still quite dependant on her mother. Frank's parents both enjoyed good health and worked full-time.

The unplanned admission to the Antenatal Unit, suspected problems in the twin pregnancy, worries about childcare, the stress of moving and the unavailability of family contributed to Susan's anxiety. Susan was forthright in describing her stressors to the social worker. She was also concerned about Frank who was adjusting to a new job, complaining of sleeplessness and seemed more irritable.

Susan was tearful and distraught throughout the initial interview. She questioned "why everything was going wrong" and expressed guilt about leaving Jennifer. She was uneasy about the tension in her otherwise stable marriage and felt she was to blame for Frank's distress.

The social worker assured her that her feelings were normal and interventions were aimed at restoring her sense of control. Her concerns for Jennifer were discussed and it was agreed that a joint meeting with Frank would be helpful.

The social worker contacted Frank, explained her role and requested a meeting. Frank acknowledged stress related to childcare, concern about Susan and unanswered medical questions.

During the initial joint interview, the couple cautiously expressed their feelings of disappointment, anger and helplessness. They seemed able to mutually support one another, but the relationship was being pushed beyond previously tested limits. Practical matters were also discussed (childcare, finances) and a second meeting arranged. While the couple continued to wait for results of diagnostic testing, Susan appeared to reorganize and adjust to her hospitalization.

While working with Susan and Frank during this initial phase, the social worker kept members of the treatment team informed of relevant history and the rationale for Susan's behaviour through team meetings and regular charting in the medical record. This facilitated the development of a comprehensive patient care plan by the team.

One week later, testing confirmed that one of the twins had abnormalities that were incompatible with life. The other twin appeared to be in no apparent distress and the medical team opted for conservative treatment: continued hospitalization and careful monitoring.

The social worker found the couple to be in mild to moderate shock following their meeting with the obstetrician, and made arrangements for Frank to stay overnight. Over the next three weeks Susan withdrew, although she developed a meaningful relationship with one nurse. Weekly meetings with the social worker continued, which focussed on their feelings surrounding the impending birth and preparing Jennifer and other family members.

One month after Susan's admission, she went into premature labour and delivered male and female twins. The male twin "Robbie" died at four hours of age. Susan's mother, Frank's parents and Jennifer were present. All saw and held little Robbie. The pastoral care worker prayed with the family. The family accepted polaroid pictures, and other mementos.

Rebecca was admitted to the NICU and required ventilation. The grieving couple were highly anxious about her well-being. Susan appeared mildly withdrawn and there were concerns about her bonding with Rebecca. The social worker met with NICU staff to discuss the uniqueness of the grieving process with the loss of a twin.

The social worker continued to meet with the couple on a weekly basis as Rebecca's progress was slow and unpredictable. The focus of these sessions was on the process of bonding with Rebecca while grieving for Robbie, and on their own relationship beyond their role as grieving parents. Susan and Frank attended the NICU Parents' Information Series sporadically. While neither one was particularly vocal, they appeared to value the information they received.

During Rebecca's two-month stay in the NICU her medical condition improved and the couple seemed to reorganize emotionally. Discharge planning became the focus of social work intervention and the worker consulted with allied health care professionals including the neonatologist, nursing staff, physiotherapist and public health nurse, and a referral was made to the local Infant Stimulation Program. Rebecca was transferred to the Neonatal teaching apartment, where the parents assumed her care for 48 hours prior to discharge.

Three months to the day that Susan was admitted to hospital, Rebecca was discharged home. Rebecca appears to be a healthy baby who may require corrective eye glasses in the future.

References

Anderson, J. (1984). *Counseling Through Group Process.* New York: Springer Publishing Company.

Black, R.B. & Furlong, R. (1984). Impact of prenatal diagnosis in families. *Social Work in Health Care. 9(3).*

Gaffney, K.F. (1986). Maternal-fetal attachment in relation to self-concept and anxiety. *Maternal Nursing Journal, 15(2),* 91-101.

Gardner, S.L. & Merenstein, G.B. (1986). Perinatal grief and loss: An overview. *Neonatal Network,* October, 7-15.

Horner, T.W., Theut, S. & Murdoch, W.G. (1984). Discharge planning for the high risk neonate: A consultation-liaison role for the infant mental health specialist. *American Journal of Orthopsychiatry, 54(4),* October, 637-647.

Kemp, V.H. & Dage C. (1986). The psychosocial impact of a high-risk pregnancy on the family. *Journal of Obstetrics & Gynecological Nursing,* May/June, 232-236.

Kramer, P.D., Coustan, D., Krzeminski, J., Broudy, D. & Martin, C. (1986). Hospitalization on the high risk maternity unit. *General Hospital Psychiatry, 8,* 33-39.

MacNab, A.J., Sheckter, L., Hendry, N.J., Pendray, M.R. & MacNab, G. (1985). Group support for parents of high risk neonates: An interdisciplinary approach. *Social Work In Health Care, 10(4).*

Mahan, C.K., Krueger, J.C., Schreiner, R.L. (1982). The family and neonatal intensive care. *Social Work in Health Care. 7(14).*

Treatment Decisions for Infants and Children. (1986). Canadian Paediatric Society. (June).

Williams, L. (1986). Long-term hospitalization of women with high risk pregnancies — A nurse's viewpoint. *Journal of Obstetrics & Gynecological Nursing,* Jan./Feb., 17-21.

Young, L. & Surdhar, H. (1987). Perinatal follow-up program, Alberta Children's Hospital. *NAPSW FORUM*, 7(4).

Endnotes

1 St. Joseph's Health Centre, located in London, Ontario, 120 miles west of Toronto, is one of three active treatment hospitals in a city of 285,000 people. As a Roman Catholic Centre, owned and operated by the Sisters of St. Joseph's, we celebrated our 100th year anniversary in 1988. The Centre consists of a 500-bed active treatment hospital; 185-bed chronic-care hospital and a 247-bed Home For The Aged. The major program thrusts of the Centre are Perinatology and Gerontology.

2 Standards for Social Work Services in the Newborn Intensive Care Unit and Code of Ethics are available from the National Association of Perinatal Social Workers, 3319 North Youngs Boulevard, Oklahoma City, Oklahoma 73112.

3 Many appropriate booklets on loss are available from Centering Corporation, Box 3367, Omaha, NE 68103-0367.

Chapter 8

SOCIAL WORK PRACTICE WITH CHILDHOOD CANCER

David W. Adams, MSW, CSW

Abstract

Recent treatment advances in childhood cancer have resulted in increasing longevity and more positive cure rates; however, the pathway to survival is often impeded by the impact of the illness and treatment. This chapter examines the impact upon the family members, and social work roles and practice responsibilities. The chapter emphasizes social work's broad spectrum systems approach, its ability to build upon child and family strengths and its focus on health versus illness. In future, social work should use group and community development skills to aid the growing population of survivors.

SOCIAL WORK PRACTICE WITH CHILDHOOD CANCER

It was only about thirty years ago that children and families faced a dismal picture of suffering and death with most types of childhood cancer. In acute lymphocytic leukemia (ALL), one of the most common types of childhood cancer, children usually succumbed to the disease within a few months (Bozeman, Orbach & Sutherland, 1955; Natterson & Knudson, 1960). Today, major advances in medical treatment have resulted in a new era where hope for long term survival and cure predominates in many types of childhood cancer (VanEyes, 1987). For instance, in ALL about three quarters of newly diagnosed children can be expected to receive intensive treatment for two or three years, remain relatively disease free and be long term survivors (Clavell, et al., 1986; Adams & Deveau, 1988); nevertheless, childhood cancer usually develops without warning, threatens lives and strains every aspect of family relationships (Adams & Deveau, 1998). The continuing challenge for caregivers is how to help children and their families endure treatment, maintain their optimism and, hopefully, move on to disease-free longevity (Christ, 1987; Michael & Copeland, 1987).

Throughout the illness, social workers may help the children and families to adapt, problem-solve, build upon their strengths and enhance the overall quality of their lives. This chapter addresses what the clientele must face, discusses the impact of the disease on family members, describes the settings, delineates practice roles and responsibilities, briefly examines the potential for role development and closes with a case example.

THE CLIENTELE

I. Phases of ALL

At diagnosis and in the months following, children may encounter several hospitalizations and suffer from painful medical procedures and side effects of chemotherapy and radiation including: temporary hair loss, weight gain, nausea, vomiting and other sequelae (Adams, 1979). For some children, entry into remission and adaptation to treatment will result in new routines and an opportunity for the family to restore order in their lives. For most, however, the intensity of the treatment provides little respite, and adaptational difficulties continue as children face recurrent infections, hospital stays and extended absences from school and social activities. These events disrupt family life and divert parental attention away from siblings who often feel left out and may react strongly (Spinetta, 1981). Children who remain in remission until their course of chemotherapy ends often continue on to long term survival.

Although long term survival is a relatively new phenomenon, evidence to date suggests that, although one-half of the children bear some emotional or physical difficulties associated with childhood cancer, only about one-fifth have moderate to severe residual problems. In most instances, those who face intense, continuous treatment, radical surgery, intense cranial radiation or were treated in adolescence are included in this category (Koocher & O'Malley, 1981). A small percentage of children may also develop a "second" cancer years later that may be related to the treatment received during childhood (Li, 1977).

For some children, relapse of their disease means that their lives are again threatened. Intense treatment must recommence and problems confronted during the initial treatment period may return. For most, renewed treatment(s) mean many more months of discomfort and disruption to individuals and families. In some instances, the success of further treatment or the implementation of additional measures; e.g., bone marrow transplantation, may renew hope for long term survival and cure. For others, relapse may follow, complete with additional suffering and a need for palliative care. For these children and their families, death often includes months of continuous stress and many disappointments. As one parent stated "...it is so unfair that Cindy had to face so much pain and suffering only to die."

For most families, the anticipation of a child's death may help them to grieve in advance and temper their mourning later on (Comerford, 1974; Rando, 1986); however, emotional suffering often continues indefinitely with varying degrees of resolution. Some survivors, for example, may require emotional support and counselling months or years later; thus, their unresolved grief is triggered by memories of the child emanating from special events such as birthdays, anniversaries or other stimuli (Adams & Deveau, 1984). Diagnosis, remission, long term survival, relapse, dying and bereavement as components of the illness cycle, create benchmarks that have often been helpful in guiding the work of professionals in social work and other disciplines (Adams, 1979). Patterned reactions tend to include a range of feelings, perceptions and behaviours that help to shape the need for specialized intervention; however, prior to examining professional involvement, it is imperative to review the emotional impact upon these children and their families. The next section begins with the parents because they are the gatekeepers for, and protectors of, their children. They are usually the first family members to face the reality of the illness and the role models—and as parents go, so go their children.

II. The Parents

When ALL is diagnosed, children's symptoms may have ranged from a persistent fever, and/or recurrent head colds, to pain or discomfort in their limbs or abdomen. Parents may be totally surprised or have their worst fears confirmed. Most are in shock and absorb very little information during the first week or two after diagnosis. As they begin to understand the realities of the illness and the pattern of treatment, emotional responses often surface and remain prominent throughout the illness (Adams & Deveau, 1984). When this happens, most parents usually worry that their children may suffer and die. Others question if it is worth having them treated at all, especially if they equate their child's illness to experiences with adults having cancer. Most parents also wonder why it is **their** child who is afflicted, and may in turn become extremely angry that the illness is dominating their lives. Most are also saddened by the changes in their children and families, and recognize that life will never be the same again. Some may feel guilty and blame themselves for allowing their children to become ill, and/or for not detecting the disease earlier (Adams & Deveau, 1988).

When active treatment is no longer needed, some parents become anxious. As one mother put it, "The crutch was gone, we were scared and wondered how our child could possibly survive." For most parents, this anxiety subsides if children remain disease free; however, some have indicated that they never forget that the disease may return, although they eventually move the thought to the back of their minds and try to suppress it permanently (Koocher & O'Malley, 1981).

If children relapse, parents often experience renewed anxiety about their child's survival. They may suffer from seeing their children grapple with the illness again; from having to reorganize their lives and from facing strong feelings of sadness and despair because there seems to be no escape from this gripping disease (Christ & Adams, 1984).

When children are dying, parents must address their anxieties about where, how and when their children will die. They often wonder if they are strong enough to face death or if they can manage to provide adequate care for their children at home. The end of a child's life dashes their hopes and dreams and contradicts the natural order of life and death. After death, parents may mourn indefinitely. Deceased children cannot be replaced, and parents have lost a part of themselves, and their differences in experiencing grief may dichotomize marital and family relationships (Rando, 1986; Rosen, 1986). Parents who are also engrossed in their own mourning may fail to recognize the needs of their remaining children who are also grieving.

III. The Child

For children and adolescents, childhood cancer is anxiety provoking to say the least. Children sense changes in everyone and readily recognize that their illness is serious. Young children are especially vulnerable in this regard. From ages one to five, hospitalization may generate severe separation anxiety; for example, their attachment to mother may be threatened if she is unable to remain overnight or stay at the hospital for extended periods. Children in the age range of seven to ten may become extremely distressed with injections and other invasive procedures, and may suffer from mutilation anxiety. For pre-teens, their increased understanding of the implications of the disease and their ability to reason may increase their anxiety about treatment, their self-image and the final outcome. The heightening of their anxiety may mean that even minor symptoms or discomforts become major concerns (Adams & Deveau, 1988).

As children and teens face medical procedures and treatment, they may also become extremely angry. They may resent the restrictions of the illness, become frustrated with treatment programs and release their anger toward the hospital staff, siblings and peers. By the same token, they may be sad. Teens in particular, may be concerned with body changes and require time to withdraw, to contemplate the change and recuperate. They must mourn their losses and find ways to cope with what has transpired. When they do not look the same, are unable to continue to be part of their peer group or cannot continue with regular activities, feelings of loneliness and isolation may add to their sadness. They may miss their friends, feel different and believe that others will easily forget them (Binger, 1969; Adams, 1979; Zeltzer, 1980).

Sometimes when children and teens have experienced intense periods of illness or hospitalization, they may also feel guilty. They may regret that they have been such a burden to their families or have been so irritable and demanding (Adams & Deveau, 1988).

When children and adolescents are dying, their level of understanding frequently parallels their cognitive development. For instance, they are often much more aware of what is happening than adults realize. They need the opportunity to make choices, participate in decision making and remain involved in regular activities as long as their physical condition permits (Karon & Vernick, 1968; Adams & Deveau, 1987).

As children face each stage of illness they may be confronted with many additional problems; for example, low energy levels and poor physical health, together with special difficulties such as learning deficits associated with treatment, may impede their return to school after lengthy absences (Christ, 1987).

At any stage, chemotherapy may make them irritable or tearful. They are continually poked, prodded and injected with substances that usually make them feel acutely ill. At relapse, they are often as disillusioned as their parents and staff as they face the stress of the disease returning. Throughout the illness, children require adult attention, understanding and guidance. If solid emotional support is provided, along with opportunities for children to express their feelings through media such as art or play, they may demonstrate a resilience and courage that far exceeds the capabilities of most adults.

IV. Siblings

When children have cancer, siblings are invariably affected by everything that transpires. Throughout the illness, their anxiety parallels or exceeds that of the sick children. They may worry about the sick child, the changes in the family and whether they or their parents will also contract this dreaded disease (Cairns, et al., 1979; Sourkes, 1980; Adams & Deveau, 1988).

At diagnosis, siblings may be sent to stay with relatives or friends, are often excluded from discussions about the illness and may be left on their own to try and understand what is happening. For young children, this approach may create added stress as they mix fact and fantasy to arrive at their own explanations concerning the child's disease and their role in influencing it (Sourkes, 1980).

Often when siblings are excluded, they become angry due to the loss of parental attention and the changes in their lives. Sometimes they appear to accept what is happening at diagnosis but react strongly during remission, at a time when parents are trying strongly to re-establish family life (Spinetta, 1984). Quite logically, they may expect that when the sick child returns home from hospital, life will be the same as it was before diagnosis. They may be disillusioned when their parents continue to attend to the needs of the sick child, maintain household affair, and/or leave them out. This unintentional neglect frequently leads to behaviour problems or difficulties with discipline (Sourkes, 1980).

When family life changes so radically, siblings may also feel sad. They miss the "fun times" or the family outings, or mourn the loss of attention that their parents have usually paid to their personal achievements and problems. Siblings may also react to the distress of their parents or feel sad that their brother or sister is so sick. Sometimes, siblings have been known to withdraw or isolate themselves from the family or peers or continually daydream. Further, changes in school behaviour often centre around their sadness or anger (Adams & Deveau, 1988).

When children are seriously ill or dying, siblings may be also particularly vulnerable. They may feel quite guilty because they believe that evil thoughts or deeds caused the illness or its return. This cause and effect belief is particularly prominent in children ages five to nine. Siblings who are close in age or of the same sex may also be closely identified with the sick child and their feelings of responsibility may be very prominent (Bank & Kahn, 1982). If a child dies, unresolved issues may add to their grief and create lasting difficulties (Adams & Deveau, 1987; Davies, 1987).

V. The Setting

From diagnosis on, children with cancer are usually treated in a university teaching hospital where care is provided by a multi-disciplinary health care team. The typical team includes a paediatric oncologist, clinic nurse, social worker, child life worker and resident physicians or house staff. Other psychosocial resources such as child psychiatrist, chaplain, child psychologist or occupational therapist, may be available to provide consultation (Adams, 1979).

In this setting, social work has often gained prominence as the principle psychosocial or mental health resource. The profession exemplifies the differences between mental health and health professionals, and is less concerned than health professional colleagues about the details of how the disease is managed, the treatment regimen, compliance with treatment, the provision of medical information and survival (Watt, 1977). The primary social work focus is on helping children and families adapt to illness and treatment; increasing their ability to cope; facilitating their learning and personal growth as part of coping; helping them to communicate with each other and the health care team; assisting them in problem solving and enhancing the quality of life. In many instances, social workers have kept in touch with bereaved families and provided periodic intervention and referral to other resources where appropriate.

The social work role frequently matches Watt's delineation of the social worker as "therapeutic facilitator" (Watt, 1977). The role is not restricted to dealing with either the instrumental or emotional issues, but has a legitimate role in the provision of a holistic approach to the care of the child and family. The strengths lie in the scope of our psychosocial knowledge; the ability to conceptualize the "whole picture" of the impact on children and families; the capacity to "tune in" to their needs without judging them and skill in working with hospital and community systems. Few other disciplines have the range of knowledge and the willingness to work with family systems; patiently assist the family through the long involved process of the illness and treatment; remain nonjudgemental; function as intermediaries and negotiators and become patient and family advocates with systems external to the family.

PRACTICE ROLES AND RESPONSIBILITIES

In performing such functions, social work often plays a key role in the assessment of the psychosocial and environmental components of care. These may include the examination of high risk situations at diagnosis where individual or family problems may impact upon the child's care; the addition of knowledge about social functioning to the team's data base and contributions to, or formulations of, a comprehensive, in-depth psychosocial assessment. In many instances, the involvement of the social worker is facilitated by physician and nurse colleagues who are concerned about child behaviour or family functioning, or the degree of stress which accompanies treatment.

As a follow-up to assessments, practitioners may provide a full range of counselling services that include:

1. helping the child and family explore their feelings, examine difficulties and use their strengths in adapting to illness, treatment and changes during the illness cycle; e.g., relapse, long term survival or terminal care;
2. intervening in crisis situations to help children, teens or families to restore the equilibrium within a short intense time span. This involvement is often associated with medical uncertainties such as completion of active treatment, changes in family situations, social stressors or economic difficulties;
3. in-depth or psychotherapeutic counselling to change the style of coping of children and families and to develop their ability to manage complex, stressful situations. Due to patient volume, some of these problems may require referral to external services; however, in some centres, this approach is used selectively, especially with single parents;
4. helping children and families by providing information or referral to community resources. This may include helping them to understand their feelings about the need for a special resource; for example, it may be difficult for families to accept referrals to social assistance agencies, mental health services or specialized resources that assist with a child's disability;
5. providing supportive counselling or maintaining levels of adaptation. This intervention may help parents cope with the aftermath of decisions about a child's treatment; help multiproblem families to prevent crises and control daily living or enable a teen to return to school or other social systems (Adams, 1979; Tylke, 1980; South Western Ontario Paediatric Oncology Team, 1984; Health and Welfare Canada, 1986; Greenburg, 1988; Adams, 1989, in press).

When one functions as an integral part of a health care team, one frequently provides opinions and influences decision making in areas such as ethical concerns about treatment, team functioning and management of staff stress. In addition, social workers may advocate on the child or family's behalf, improve communication within the team or facilitate the use of other mental health disciplines in assessing or managing a difficult problem.

In the daily work routine, social workers may often heighten the awareness of health professional colleagues and learners about the needs of children and families, impart specialized knowledge and facilitate problem-solving and skill development. Such opportunities may emanate from participation in

a) providing consultation that may assist in re-examining and restructuring plans for care;
b) "on-the-spot" supervision that may increase the sensitivity of learners or help them to intervene more effectively;
c) psychosocial rounds and discussions;
d) formal presentations or seminars within the hospital or the community;
e) discussions about how staff cope with loss, grief or work-related stress and
f) the formulation of psychosocial protocols and preparation of audiovisual teaching materials, articles and manuscripts (Adams, 1989, in press).

As increasing numbers of children and teens have required psychosocial support in the community, social work involvement has frequently moved beyond clinics and in-patient units. More specifically, camps, outings, weekends and other sharing experiences for patients, parents and siblings have been compatible with group work skills and a willingness to help our clientele build on strengths, learn from others and be self-directed. In some instances, social workers have assumed responsibility for committees or task forces directed toward improving the co-ordination of treatment, the quality of care or policies of the government or other organizations. This may encompass liaising with the Cancer Society, Candlelighter parent groups or other community agencies that influence service, education or research in this field.

In a few instances, social workers have also made useful contributions in psychosocial research (Hamovitch, 1964; Kaplan, 1976; Chesler & Barbarin, 1987). Unfortunately, research has not been a major strength of the discipline and much greater emphasis is needed in this area.

POTENTIAL FOR ROLE DEVELOPMENT

In the future, there will continue to be a need for capable social workers in pediatric oncology. As increasing numbers of children become long term survivors who are cured of this disease, even greater attention must be paid to assist them with adaptation to illness and treatment and re-integration into community systems. Social workers may contribute to this process by

a) ensuring that psychosocial support systems are in place at each stage of the illness;
b) helping to strengthen mutual aid and self-help programs;
c) participating in the training of volunteers to compliment roles of professionals stressed by heavy patient workloads;
d) educating teachers, community professionals and the general public about policy changes in survival and cure;
e) influencing policy-makers so that employment, insurance and rehabilitation needs of survivors are me and
f) facilitating the development of parent and lobby groups to advocate on their own behalf (Adams, 1989, in press).

In addition, the profession must place a greater emphasis on program evaluation, clinical study and research. At the very least, social workers in pediatric oncology should have a basic knowledge of critical appraisal techniques. Where feasible, the elements of program evaluation and research methodology should be added to their repertoire. Such increased knowledge should facilitate detailed analyses of caseloads, increase effectiveness of interventions and lead to involvement of more knowledgeable colleagues as principal investigators and collaborators.

CONCLUDING REMARKS

Social work practice with childhood cancer is challenging and demanding for both the patient and those concerned with treatment and rehabilitation. Due to the disease focus, much of the present social work activity takes place in highly specialized hospital settings; however, within these settings, the main focus of practice is not necessarily on the disease itself, but how to cope with it, and its psychosocial, familial and support implications. Different childhood patients present differential needs in this regard and it is important for practitioners to connect with the patient and her/his family early on and support the various complex and multiple needs of these individuals over the course of the disease. As this chapter has shown, the profession has much to offer in treating this growing patient group. As it evolves in its treatment efforts, it appears that the focus may shift from the hospital and its medical needs, to the family and the community and their attendant needs.

CASE EXAMPLE

Fifteen-year-old Jim was extremely ill when he was diagnosed with ALL, thus necessitating an initial one month stay in hospital. At the outset, he was tired, irritable and withdrawn. His parents, Joe aged 36 and Marie aged 35, were in shock. As Marie put it, "Jim seemed so normal up to last week. It's hard to believe he has leukemia." By the second week it was obvious that Jim was extremely upset. Staying in the hospital meant that he was missing his friends, hockey and school. At first, he had dismissed his leukemia as a routine inconvenience. Gradually the awareness that he would be subjected to continuing treatments and would likely lose his hair, became most distressing to him.

From the outset, it became obvious that Marie would be readily available to support her son. She excused her husband's absence telling staff that he was self-employed, it was peak season and he worked long hours as a plumbing contractor. Staff noted that in the first week, Joe visited Jim once and left after a brief period. He was curt with the nurses and the family physician recounted how Joe had berated him for not diagnosing the illness more quickly.

By the end of the third week, Jim seemed more positive and more willing to share his concerns with the me. He discussed the family's problems, his anxiety about his mother's well-being and his regret that he had missed his brother John's birthday. At age 11, John idolized his older brother and Jim felt responsible for him. Jim recounted his remorse about being nasty to John and admitted that, "...he's an O.K. kid, even if he bugs me sometimes." By this time, Marie was beginning to think ahead to Jim's discharge. She worried about his physical condition, his loss of time in school and Jim's tendency to talk less with her than he did prior to hospitalization. She also confided to me concerns about the couple's marriage and the effect of the illness on her husband.

Although the couple had remained together, the marriage had been stormy. Stress increased at times of crisis arising from Joe's frequent job changes and financial distress. Each parent had difficulty managing feelings and communicating with each other. Each had turned to other adults for emotional support. Joe relied on his male friends and Marie turned to her only sister.

By the third week, Joe seemed less angry, but kept his visits to his son short. He declined invitations to a team meeting, leaving attendance to his wife. One week later, immediately prior to discharge, the team firmly requested a session with both parents, resulting in an opportunity for the social worker to begin to work with both partners and to determine goals for further sessions. Joe agreed to return based on the couple's need to work together to help Jim.

It was clear that

a) Jim's illness and hospitalization were amplifying the communication difficulties between his parents;
b) Jim's anxiety focussed on the illness, treatment and the situation at home. One past episode of physical conflict increased his concern;
c) his parent's ability to function had been at an instrumental level and increased emotional stress added to the vulnerability of the marriage;
d) Marie's anxiety about her son was compounded by concern for her marriage and being left on her own to face the illness and treatment;
e) under stress, Joe had always reverted to his boyhood friends, leaving his wife to manage their two sons;
f) Joe had great difficulty expressing his sadness and was plagued with distressing memories about his grandfather's death in hospital from cancer;
g) both parents loved their children, but responsibility for child care and discipline was left to Marie;
h) support from the extended families was limited due to distance and the poor health of grandparents. Marie's sister was the only family member available;
i) the family had moved recently and had few friends on whom they could rely and
j) Jim had maintained contact with old friends, but their ability to visit was limited by distance.

These difficulties were aggravated by

a) Joe's inability to come to the hospital or to take care of John at home;
b) Jim's physical and emotional distress;
c) differences in opinions between the parents at diagnosis about what Jim and John should be told;
d) suggestions from Joe's parents that treatment at another centre would be better and
e) financial stress caused by transportation, meals and other expenses that exceeded the family budget.

The social worker assisted Jim and his family by

a) providing emotional support and being a "sounding board" for Jim;
b) building a relationship with both parents;
c) delineating a baseline psychosocial assessment of family members and the family system;
d) clarifying parental perceptions, needs and interactional problems;
e) ensuring that Jim had opportunity to obtain accurate information and enabling him to do so on his own terms;
f) helping Jim to express his anxiety and cope with intense feelings of fear, anger and sadness;
g) assisting parents to discuss their feelings with each other about what had transpired and their concerns about the future;
h) encouraging Marie and, later, both parents together, to talk with Jim about his illness at Jim's convenience;
i) encouraging the involvement of John in Jim's care both in hospital and clinic, in order to help him understand the illness and treatment;
j) discussing with both partners strengths and weaknesses in the marriage and family;
k) promoting interaction between both parents by modelling, clarifying, challenging, redirecting and empathizing;
l) planning an approach to care that met the needs of the family through the provision of
   1) additional emotional support for Jim and his sibling as required;
   2) individual emotional support for both partners in harmony with nursing staff;
   3) a forum for marital, and later, family, therapy using a systems model with the social worker as facilitator, mediator and negotiator;
   4) opportunities to meet with medical and nursing staff to

address medical and treatment concerns;

5) methods to alleviate instrumental concerns pertaining to finances, transportation, babysitting and homemakers assistance and

6) on-going follow-up as required during Jim's treatment program and subsequent visits.

Over time, the conjoint sessions and individual support to each parent increased their trust in the health care team and maintained order within the household. Jim required additional emotional support at the beginning of the treatment program and struggled with the side effects in the ensuing months. He gradually became more trusting and talkative and seemed more relaxed. He noted that life at home had improved and that his father was present more frequently. Several months after diagnosis, when Jim was more settled, his brother John began to act out. He was involved in fights at school, neglected his schoolwork and was caught stealing from his mother's wallet. In the family sessions that followed, he described his feelings of neglect, anger and jealousy toward Jim. He accused his parents of playing favourites and resented their devotion to Jim.

As time progressed, there were several episodes of high stress that the family managed reasonably well. These included a potential relapse of Jim's disease, which did not materialize; further business difficulties and John's serious bicycle accident. After the intense involvement at the outset and a few family sessions to cope with crises and to monitor progress, contacts became less frequent. Jim finished active treatment and is now two years post-therapy. At twenty, he is attending community college and managing well. His mother continues to worry about his physical status and the couple maintain a reasonable working relationship. John has encountered recent difficulties in school and, in his father's words, "is a difficult boy to control or understand."

References

Adams, D. W. (1979). *Childhood Malignancy: The Psychosocial Care of the Child and his Family.* Springfield, IL: C. C. Thomas.

Adams, D. W. (1989a) (in press). Care of children dying with cancer and their families: Issues, dilemmas, feelings and needs. In J. D. Morgan (Ed.), *Helping Young People Cope With Death.* London, Ont.: King's College.

Adams, D. W. (1989b) (in press). The role of mental health professionals in pediatric oncology. In E. R. Davidson & D. R. Copeland (Eds.), *Psychosocial Education for Health Care Providers in Pediatric Oncology.* Springfield, IL: C. C. Thomas.

Adams, D. W. & Deveau, E. J. (1984). *Coping with Childhood Cancer: Where Do We Go From Here?* Reston, VA: Reston Publishing.

Adams, D. W. & Deveau, E. J. (1987). When a brother or sister is dying of cancer: The vulnerability of the adolescent sibling. *Death Studies, 11,* 279-290.

Adams, D. W. & Deveau, E. J. (1988). *Coping with Childhood Cancer: Where Do We Go From Here?* Hamilton, Ont.: Kinbridge Publications.

Adams, D. W. & Deveau, E. J. (1988). The impact of the dying child on siblings. *Forum, 12*(7), 6-7.

Bank, P. & Kahn, J. (1982). *The Sibling Bond.* New York: Basic Books.

Binger, C. M. (1969). Childhood leukemia—Emotional impact on patient and family. *New England Journal of Medicine, 280,* 414-418.

Bozeman, M. F., Orbach, C. E. & Sutherland, A. M. (1955). Psychological impact of cancer and its treatment, III, The adaptation of mothers to the threatened loss of their children through leukemia: Part 1. *Cancer, 8,* 1-19.

Cairns, N., Clarke, G. M., Smith, S. F. & Lansky, S. B. (1979). Adaptations of siblings to childhood malignancy. *Journal of Pediatrics, 95,* 484-487.

Chesler, M. A. & Barbarin, O. (1987). *Childhood Cancer and the Family: Meeting the Challenge of Stress and Support.* New York: Bruner/Mazel Publishers.

Christ, G. (1987). Social consequences of the cancer experience. *American Journal of Pediatric Haematology/Oncology, 9*(1), 84.

Christ, G. & Adams, M. A. (1984). Therapeutic strategies and psychosocial crisis points in the treatment of childhood cancer.

In A. E. Christ & K. Flomenhaft (Eds.), *Childhood Cancer: Impact on the Family*. New York: Plenum Press.

Clavell, L., Gelber, R. D., Cohen, H. J., Hitchcock-Bryan, S., Cassady, J. R., Tarbell, N. J., Blattner, S. R., Tantravahi, R., Leavitt, P. and Sallan, S. E. (1986). Four agent induction and intensive asparaginase therapy for treatment of childhood acute lymphocytic leukemia. *New England Journal of Medicine, 315,* 657-663.

Comerford, B. (1974). Parental anticipatory grief and guidelines for caregivers. In B. Schoenberg, A. C. Carr, A. H. Kutscher, D. Peretz & I. Goldberg (Eds.), *Anticipatory Grief*. New York: Columbia University Press.

Davies, B. (1987). After a sibling dies. In M. A. Morgan (Ed.), *Bereavement: Helping the Survivors*. London, Ont.: King's College.

Greenberg, C. (1988). *A Study of Childhood Cancer Services in Ontario*. Toronto, Ont.: Pediatric Oncology Group of Ontario.

Hamovitch, M. B. (1964). *The Parent and the Fatally Ill Child*. Duarte, CA: City of Hope Medical Center.

Health and Welfare Canada. (1986). Canadian workload measurement systems: A national hospital productivity improvement program. Ottawa, Ontario.

Kaplan, D. M. (1976). Predicting the impact of severe illness in families. *Health and Social Work, 1*(3), 72-82.

Karon, M. & Vernick, J. (1968). An approach to the emotional support of fatally ill children. *Pediatrics, 7*(5), 274-280.

Koocher, G. P. & O'Malley, J. E. (1981). *The Damocles Syndrome*. New York: McGraw-Hill.

Li, F. P. (1977). Second malignant tumours after cancer in childhood. *Cancer, 40,* 1899-1902.

Michael, B. E. & Copeland, D. R. (1987). Psychosocial issues in childhood cancer. *American Journal of Pediatric Haematology/Oncology, 9*(1), 73-83.

Natterson, J. M. & Knudson, A. G. (1960). Observations concerning fear of death in fatally ill children and their mothers. *Psychosomatic Medicine, 22*(6), 256-265.

Rando, T. (1986). *Loss and Anticipatory Grief*. Lexington, MA: D. C. Heath.

Rosen, H. (1986). *Unspoken Grief: Coping with Sibling Loss*. Lexington, MA: D. C. Heath.

Sourkes, B. M. (1980). Siblings of the pediatric cancer patient. In J. Kellerman (Ed.), *Psychological Aspects of Childhood Cancer*. Springfield, IL: C. C. Thomas.

Spinetta, J. J. (1981). The sibling of the child with cancer. In J. J. Spinetta & P. Deasy-Spinetta (Eds.), *Living with Childhood Cancer*. St. Louis, MO: C. V. Mosby.

Tylke, L. (1980). Family therapy with pediatric cancer patients. In J. L. Schulman and M. J. Kupst (Eds.), *Child with Cancer*. Springfield, IL: C. C. Thomas.

Van Eys, J. (1987). Living beyond cure: Transcending survival. *American Journal of Pediatric Haematology/Oncology, 9*(1), 114-118.

Watt, M. S. (1977). *Therapeutic Facilitator: The Role of the Social Worker in Acute Treatment Hospitals in Ontario*. Doctoral Dissertation (unpublished). University of California at Los Angeles.

Zeltzer, L. K. (1980). The adolescent with cancer. In J. Kellerman (Ed.), *Psychological Aspects of Childhood Cancer*. Springfield, IL: C. C. Thomas.

Chapter 9

SOCIAL WORK PRACTICE WITH PAEDIATRIC BEREAVEMENT PATIENTS

Michael Bull, MSW, CSW

Abstract

This chapter describes a social work bereavement program for pae-diatric patients at the Children's Hospital of Western Ontario. A clientele of children aged 4-18 is treated, and a wide variety of potential presenting behavioural problems is outlined. The practice roles of assessment, counselling, consultation and community organization/education are described within the framework of four tasks of mourning. The need for more accessible bereavement ser-vices for children is discussed and some suggestions are made to help bereaved children at home and at school.

SOCIAL WORK PRACTICE WITH PAEDIATRIC BEREAVEMENT PATIENTS

THE CLIENTELE

The Children's Hospital of Western Ontario (CHWO), a paediatric treatment centre for Southwestern Ontario, provides tertiary health care for children with critical, chronic and life-threatening illnesses. CHWO is recognized for its specialized treatment in a wide range of areas including emergency medicine, critical care, oncology, genetics, endocrinology, cardiology, transplantation, cystic fibrosis, neurology and orthopaedics.

Social work services are provided to this 100-bed facility by a staff of three MSW social workers. At CHWO, bereavement follow-up and counselling have always been recognized as an important component of social work services. The death of a child is acknowledged as a risk factor in families (Krupnick, 1984; Rando, 1986; Schiff, 1977; Worden, 1982), and grief counselling may prevent many of the negative effects of such a loss. Unfortunately, as in many acute care settings, crises and inpatient situations take priority and may leave little opportunity for effective bereavement follow-up; furthermore, there is a realization that many bereaved children, particularly those who had a parent or sibling die, are receiving little or no bereavement counselling.

As a result, in 1987 two social workers initiated a program for bereaved children. The goal was to provide assessment and counselling in situations both related to CHWO (e.g., the death of a sibling) and previously unrelated and referred cases from the community (e.g., the sudden death of a parent). This service was introduced in a low-profile manner, as it was perceived that the potential demand could exceed the limited number of service hours available. In fact, over two years, a steady flow of referrals has been received and the service has been recognized for its specialized focus and importance.

The children seen ranged in age from 4 to 18, with an even mix of boys and girls. Some young adults had been seen as an adjunct to the service, as the intent was to keep the referral criteria as flexible as possible given the limited alternative services in the community. Referrals have been received from family physicians, school boards, public health nurses, the police, family consultants, children's treatment centres, Bereaved Families of Ontario and through word-of-mouth.

It is interesting to note that few referrals have come from within the hospital; i.e., regarding children bereaved by a death occurring at the hospital. This and other experiences suggests that there is value in separating bereavement services and acute-care medical services. Specifically, some bereaved persons seem to need or appreciate distancing from the setting where their loved ones received active care, especially after a long illness; for example, some bereaved initially find it difficult to return to the building associated with the acute care. As well, clinically, it may be helpful for bereavement counselling to be provided by someone unassociated with the pre-death treatment. Grief work, then, is part of a new beginning in a sense.

The children referred are seen primarily on an individual basis, as group counselling has not been offered, largely due to the orientation of the two social workers. Further, children have been seen in sibling groups or conjointly with a parent. The length of treatment has ranged from one assessment session to regular sessions occurring for over a year.

Normal office space has been moderately adapted for the bereavement program. A play corner was created by the addition of a child-size table and chairs, along with a variety of art supplies and toys. These items include crayons, coloured pencils, markers, large sheets of paper, board games, a play hospital, a doll house and a punching clown. Carpeting allows for more comfortable play on the floor if necessary. For adolescents and young adults, a traditional office set-up is used with art supplies available, as needed.

The losses experienced by children can vary considerably in both content and intensity. Referrals to the program have included

1) sudden death of parent through accident or illness;
2) parental death after prolonged illness ;
3) death of family members through murder-suicide;
4) perinatal death of a sibling;
5) sudden, accidental death of a sibling and
6) death of grandparents through illness or accidents.

Other potential losses for a child include a stillbirth or miscarriage, the death of a teacher or classmate, a pet's death or even the death of well-known public figure, such as Terry Fox, John F. Kennedy or the crew of the Challenger.

Referrals are made to the program usually because of a parent's concern about how a child is coping with a death, or because a child's behaviour has brought her/his grief to the attention of a caregiver; e.g., a teacher. Parents frequently express a desire to prevent any long-term negative effects for the child, but are uncertain about what to expect or how to respond. Older children and teenagers may recognize their own need for counselling, perhaps precipitated by a developmental crisis, such as missing the adult identity model in adolescence if a parent has died.

Children are more likely to show their grief behaviourally, and behaviourial changes or problems are themselves often the presenting problem. These behaviours may include

1) sleep disturbances	- dreams/nightmares - fear of going to sleep - wanting to sleep with parents
2) school difficulties	- deterioration in grades - increased absenteeism - difficulty in concentrating - emotional upset at school
3) regressive behaviour	- bed wetting - thumb sucking - reliance on old toys, blankets - increased dependency
4) somatic complaints	- stomach aches - headaches - symptoms similar to the deceased
5) emotional liability	- moodiness - increased crying, tearfulness - fearfulness - angry outbursts
6) death theme activity	- play focussed on killing, death - increased talking about death or the deceased - attachment to dead person's possessions, clothing, etc.

7) "other" behaviours   - running from home
                             - defiant or delinquent behaviour
                             - suicidal thoughts or actions

Behaviour changes often occur in the period shortly after a loved one's death; however, some behaviours may be evident much later. Some children do not want to impose their grief on their "already-upset" parents, so they wait until it is "safer," i.e., after their parents' acute grief has subsided. Somatic complaints in bereaved siblings often have presented about one year after the death of a brother or sister. As well, behaviourial changes may occur later as a child moves into another developmental stage and re-examines the loss from a different perspective and with different coping skills.

For the family and the bereaved child, these behaviours may be very troubling and upsetting. Parents and other caregivers often need reassurance that the child's behaviour does make sense within the context of grieving. Further, they need information about children's grief and support in how they are responding to the child. Grieving children need an opportunity to focus on their loss in a non-threatening and accepting environment. This "special" opportunity allows the child to more fully express her/his grief and to develop skills for regaining some control of what often seems "uncontrollable"; i.e., the permanent loss of a loved one.

PRACTICE ROLES AND RESPONSIBILITIES

A social worker's roles and responsiblities are determined by the needs and goals of the client. Several authors discuss stages or phases involved in grieving, but the model presented by Worden (1982) seems readily understandable and applicable in grief counselling. Worden (1982) identified four tasks faced by the bereaved:

1) to accept the reality of the loss;
2) to experience the emotional pain;
3) to adjust to the environment without the deceased and
4) to withdraw and re-invest emotional energy.

While this model is described primarily for adults, it does generally apply, with some adaptations, to children as well.

These adaptations are determined by three differences in children's grieving processes (Krupnick, 1984). First, children grieve over a longer time frame than adults. As they proceed through different developmental stages, children will, in a sense, "regrieve," i.e., experience the loss in different ways in relation to new cognitive and coping skills. Similarly, due to limited ego strengths in relation to the intensity of grief, children will grieve in "spurts," thereby extending the overall time frame. Second, grieving children will tend to split their emotions from the content. For example, a child may talk nonchalantly about her mother's recent death with little evidence of grief, yet s/he may become disproportionately tearful when asked to straighten up her/his room. The experience and the feelings are separated, again as the child's defence against the intensity of grief. Finally, children need a normal routine and neutral environment to provide the security which allows them to risk facing their grief. The potential stress and disorganization which can occur after the death of a family member may impede a child's grieving, or postpone it until the family system is more stable.

Social work roles and responsibilities with the grieving child will be discussed under the categories of assessment, counselling, consultation and community education and development.

I. Assessment

Assessing the nature and progress of a child's grieving is an important role for a social worker. Grief, generally, is not well understood and this is even more so with children's grief. For many children and their families, this will be the first experience with the death of a significant loved one. They have little with which to compare this experience, to know whether they are coping "normally." A common question for the bereaved, trying to deal with this new and intense situation, is "Am I (or my child) going crazy?" The social worker plays an important role in assessing the family's situation in relation to the known information and guidelines about grieving.

In the program at CHWO, the assessment process begins in the initial session, which usually involves the parent(s) and the child. The parent is often seen first by the two social workers in the program so that a history of the death and the child's reactions can be obtained. (With regard to very young children, the parent may be the only one seen.) An intake sheet has been developed and is completed with the parent in this first interview (see Exhibit A, p.139). This sheet documents information about the family system, data related to the loved one's death and specific behaviours that are causing concern. This data sheet is retained in the social work chart and serves as part of a data base for research.

After the parent is interviewed, the child joins the social workers and parent for a brief discussion regarding the death and the purpose for the initial interview. The child is then seen individually by one of the social workers, while the parent is interviewed further by the second worker. This team approach has proven useful in attending to the separate needs of the child and the parent, and in obtaining assessment information from two perspectives. It also recognizes that, while the primary focus is the child, the parent also has experienced a loss and will have her/his own grief issues which will affect the child.

In the assessment interview with the child, the social worker seeks to determine the child's understanding of the death and her/his ability to cope with this loss. The child is encouraged to "tell the story" about the death, including events leading up to the death, the actual death, and events post-death; e.g., the funeral, family changes, etc. These expressions may be facilitated through the child's use of art and pictures and by having the child complete a "family tree" genogram. The family tree is helpful in identifying other family deaths, and also reinforces for the child a sense of family apart from the current loss.

The assessment aims generally to determine the child's progress with the four tasks of grieving. Areas to be explored more specifically include

- the extent of the child's support system;
- the child's involvement prior to and at the time of death;
- previous losses or deaths;
- behavioural changes or symptoms;
- physical symptoms;
- any "unfinished business" (issues left unresolved due to the loved one's death);
- concurrent stressors;
- the child's emotional expressiveness and
- the child's general age-related functioning.

The questions child will ask or strggle with when a loved one dies are:

1. did I cause this to happen? [guilt feelings]

2. will it happen to me? [one's own mortality]
3. who will take care of me now? [security, changed relationships]

While bereaved adults face similar issues, children's egocentricity no doubt intensifies the importance of these concerns. The social worker should try to assess how problematic each of these areas might be for the child.

This assessment process may take from one to three sessions. In some cases, it may be determined that there are no significant difficulties in the child's grieving, at this time, and the parents can be reassured about their handling of the situation. These families are advised of the ongoing availability of the service should issues arise as the child grows. In other cases, specific difficulties may be identified and a counselling contract established. Worden (1982) differentiates between grief counselling and grief therapy. The former is defined as counselling which assists with uncomplicated or "normal" grieving, while the latter refers to psychotherapy directed at complicated or "abnormal" grief. The assessment should attempt to identify which type of grieving process is occurring and therefore what treatment is indicated.

One point of note here—it is sometimes easy for both parents and professionals to label a death as the cause of all presenting problems in a child. It is important for the social worker to be aware of this and try to distinguish between grief responses and behaviours that are related to other individual or family problems. The assessment plan should reflect these distinctions so that the appropriate treatment is provided. A disservice is done to the child and the family if the misperception about a death's significance and impact is reinforced in the assessment process.

II. Counselling

The goal of grief counselling is to assist the child in working through difficulties with the tasks of grieving. Because of the longer time frame for children's grieving, the social worker will likely not be involved through the entire process or with all tasks; however, the counselling role will be discussed in relation to each task.

Accepting the reality of the loss: A useful way for the child to work on this task is through the telling and re-telling of the story about the death. The social worker can direct the story through enquiries about the pre-death period, the death itself, the funeral visitation and ceremony, and the wake. By listening to how the child describes the death and the deceased, the social worker may determine how the child perceives of the loss in terms of finality and permanency. Does the child say the words "died" or "dead," or use euphemistic terms like "gone" or "away"? Does the child speak as if the person is still alive and will return? The social worker, allowing for age-related perceptions of death, may correct misperceptions about the reality of the loss. Having the child draw pictures of the death, the funeral or the dead person can assist in making the death more real, more concrete, and also further clarify how the child sees the death.

If the social worker is involved with a child and family prior to or at the time of a death, s/he can play an important role in encouraging and advocating for the child's involvement in the death-related activities. As a general rule, children should be asked whether they wish to be part of visitation, funeral and/or other activities. Their response, whether positive or negative, should be respected. Children often will want to participate, but will also set their own limits. The child's involvement in these activities assists greatly in her/his understanding and acceptance of the loss' reality, and may facilitate long-term grieving.

Experiencing the emotional pain: At certain ages (e.g., 9-10 years), emotional expressiveness is less likely to occur. The social worker, then, needs to facilitate the feeling component of grief while being respectful of the child's limits.

The social worker, however, can assist the child in gaining some control in how feelings are experienced. With each telling of the story of the death, the child gains a clearer perspective and the sadness can be diffused/diminished. Asking a child to bring in photographs and mementoes of the deceased facilitates remembering and focusses feelings. A memory book can be developed with the child or given to the child to complete. Some children respond to an offer to visit the gravesite with the social worker. Older children can be assigned the "homework" of keeping a journal about their feelings, or writing prose or poetry about their grief.

One tool that helps children focus on their feelings in a structured way is the "grief train." Grieving is described to the child as a kind of journey, with several stops or stations along the way, each representing a different feeling. The child draws the train, the track and the various stations, labelling them with the appropriate feelings. The child, in concretizing the feelings, can gain some control while being given the image of progress toward less painful feelings as the "grief train" moves along.

It may well be that much of a child's emotional expression will occur outside of the counselling sessions. The social worker may work with the family to establish an open environment at home, one in which the child's feelings will be accepted and understood. Bedtime, for example, is often a time when a child will discuss the loss or show some feelings. Parents can be assisted in attending to and talking with the child at such times. Books with themes of loss can be recommended by the social worker for use by parents at home. Lists of appropriate books can be found in various sources (e.g., Grollman, 1976; Lombardo & Lombardo, 1986; Schneider, 1985).

Adjusting to the environment: The social worker's role in this area may not be as significant with children as with adults, who seem to face more role changes after a loved one's death. However, any changes in family routines will affect the child, and the social worker can work with the family to re-establish routines. For instance, a young widower and his children may benefit from the social worker's efforts to obtain child care assistance for the family, while a young widow may need some support in learning to drive or to be more effective as a disciplinarian. The children, too, may require support in understanding and accepting new roles and responsibilities that allow the family to cope better.

As family roles are adjusted, the social worker may assess whether children are not assigned roles beyond their capabilities. For instance, in families with older children and adolescents, there may be a tendency to parentify the child through inappropriate expectations and responsibilities. The social worker may assist the parent(s) in establishing a suitable balance without overburdening the child and increasing family stress due to the child's resentment.

As the family's functioning changes, the child may need reassurance from the social worker that the survivors will be able to adjust and cope effectively; however, perhaps more difficult for children than role changes are changed relationships. What they gave and received with the deceased is now missing; what they received from the survivors is now changed and, in a sense, is also lost. The social worker can assist the child in grieving these secondary losses and, as discussed below, in seeing new ways of having relationship needs met.

Withdrawing and reinvesting emotional energy: This task refers to the child's ability to "let go" of the relationship with the deceased, while still remembering, and establishing new relationships. The social worker explores with the child any "unfinished business" and helps the child resolve these issues. Such business might include not being able to say "goodbye" or "I love you"; negative feelings resulting from a fight; a child's fantasy that s/he did something to cause the death. By re-examining such issues with the social worker, the child can have misperceptions clarified and begin to balance the positives and negatives in the relationship with the deceased. Specific tasks, such as selecting a favourite keepsake, drawing a "good bye" picture or writing to the deceased can help in the letting go process.

With regard to reinvesting in new relationships, the social worker plays an important role as a transitional significant other for the child. Within this relationship, the child can experiment with being close and trusting after the hurt of the loss. Children will readily seek a substitute for the deceased as a way of filling their emptiness and having their needs met. The social worker can help the child to keep such efforts in balance with the importance of the relationship to the deceased. The child can be helped to move toward constructive relationships with teachers, step-parents, other family members, Big Brothers or Big Sisters, friends, etc.

III. Consultation

In reality, the majority of bereaved children will not be seen in a clinical counselling setting, such as described above. The social worker, then, can play an important role for many other bereaved children as a consultant to those who work with or have access to such children. To a large degree, the CHWO program developed as a response to the many consultation requests that were being received. Schools, bereaved family organizations, children's aid societies and camp programs are among the resources with which consultation has occurred.

Consultation with schools and agencies has often taken place in case conferences. Like the parents, those who teach or work with bereaved children often have had little experience with grief, and appreciate the reassurance and suggestions which the social worker can give. The social worker can help them explore their own anxieties, questions and perhaps fears about dealing with death. These professionals often have an established helping relationship with the child, and it is appropriate for them to be the primary resource for the bereaved child. To assist them, the social worker can provide periodic consultation and resource material.

As well, the social worker can act as a consultant to families who do not feel the need for counselling. Several parents who have called the program, have requested information about grief, or have asked about available resources. In addition to telephone consultations, the program has provided families with reading materials from its library.

IV. Community Organization and Education

There is a significant educator role to be played by the social worker in this area. In the experience of the CHWO program, there is a real interest in the general public and among helping professionals to learn more about children's grief. Because education about grief and bereavement counselling is virtually non-existent in most professional education or training, many of those on the "front line," when faced with a bereaved child, find themselves without adequate information, direction and/or support.

Education requests have been received from teachers, physicians, parent groups, hospice workers, child welfare professionals, clergy members and social work students. Teaching activities have included small group in-services, workshops at professional conferences and involvement in the planning and presentation of major educational events, such as the internationally recognized death and bereavement conference held annually at King's College in London, Ontario. In these activities, the social worker can present the psychosocial/ systems orientation characteristic of social work and advocate for the inclusion of such frameworks in teaching activities.

In addition, considerable opportunity exists for social workers in the areas of publication and research about childhood bereavement. Social work literature in this field is not extensive; single-case studies and program descriptions, in addition to more extensive evaluative research, can be valuable contributions to the profession. One of the social workers in the CHWO program published the results of a research study on children's anniversary grief responses (Plotkin, 1983), and this article has gone as a reference in other subsequent publications (Krupnick, 1984). Another CHWO research project on bereaved families hired a social worker as the research co-ordinator, a key player in the effective collection and organization of data.

In the area of community organization and development, social workers may be active on committees, advisory boards and/or planning groups. Organizations such as Bereaved Families of Ontario and Compassionate Friends often welcome social workers as professional advisors and support resources. In the London community, the involvement of one social worker with Bereaved Families of Ontario (an organization for families whose child has died) has resulted in the initiation of a group for bereaved siblings. Several social workers also have been integral in the development of a proposal for a bereavement service in London. This service, based on the St. Mary's Grief Support Center in Duluth, Minnesota, would provide bereavement programs across the community and region, including services for children. This project illustrates the major impact that community-oriented social work efforts may have in this field.

POTENTIAL FOR ROLE DEVELOPMENT

Interest in the areas of death and bereavement is clearly growing, and with it, the potential for social work practice with bereaved children. Helping the bereaved is preventive intervention, and perhaps the greatest challenge is to increase the accessability of services to bereaved children. The model utilized at CHWO is limited in its ability to reach the many children who experience a loss by death. Efforts to improve and increase services to bereaved children may be maximized by foremost targeting the child's natural environments: home and school.

In the home, parents need more help in understanding and responding to their bereaved children. Parents describe behaviours and reactions in their children that are strange and confusing. Yet, in a recent review of literature about children's grief, the author found that the current resources for parents are very limited. Only a few resources were found that clearly described the wide variety of possible reactions in children (e.g., Fleming, 1985; Krupnick, 1984), and these came from the professional rather than the popular literature. There is clearly a need for concise, parent-oriented information in this area. Such a resource could range from a one-page handout to a more detailed booklet, tape or video on the subject. Information could be directed at parents through more popular media such as newspapers, magazines or television. Social workers may organize seminars or courses for parent groups, or develop "grief hotlines" which parents could call for information and assistance. Social workers may work with other professionals who have ready access to bereaved families, such as funeral directors and the clergy, to facilitate the provision of parent information early in the grief process.

Social work is also expanding its involvement into health care areas that directly impact families in which a death has occurred. Palliative care services, hospices, home care programs and nursing homes are increasingly employing social workers, who have the possibility of working with bereaved children and their families. Even within the more traditional settings, such as hospitals, cancer clinics and family medical centres, there remains untapped opportunities to help bereaved children. The challenges for social work are to maintain a family system orientation and to recognize that, with the death of any individual, there are probably children who are now bereaved.

Schools are an ideal setting for assisting bereaved children, and some exciting developments are currently taking place in this regard. Increasingly, schools are offerring support groups for children who have experienced a loss. One such program, Rainbows for All God's Children and Spectrums,[1] is an Illinois-based curriculum that is spreading throughout Canada and the United States. Rainbows (for younger children) and Spectrums (for adolescents) train facilitators to work with small groups of children within their own schools. Facilitators include teachers, social workers, psychologists and others. Similar programs are developing in many school systems and individual schools.

Many school boards are also developing crisis response teams to go into schools when a death occurs. In the event of the traumatic death of a student, parent, teacher or other staff member, the response team may be asked into the school to assist the students and staff with their immediate grief reactions and also with the initial planning for a school-based response. School social workers are active members on many of these teams, together with acting as case consultants in relation to individual bereaved children.

In man cases, the school setting is ideally suited to identifying and responding to the needs of bereaved children due to (a) the amount of time spent daily in contact with the child and (b) the prolonged nature of this contact over time. Indeed, a child's school performance is very often a significant indicator of emotional difficulty (Krupnick, 1984). Health care and school social workers can examine ways for monitoring the progress of a bereaved child through subsequent school years, for, as was discussed earlier, the child's grieving is an ongoing process. Review mechanisms could be annual case conferences that may include parental input, in-service training with a child's new teachers and case documentation that allows consistent transfer of information about the child's loss. Such monitoring can also improve services to the child by reducing the likelihood of subsequent crises.

There is also a need to develop, refine and evaluate specific approaches and techniques in conducting grief counselling with children. Little seems to be written about the relative benefits of group work with bereaved children as compared to individual counselling. For instance, how can a family group be worked with in a way that meets the needs of the bereaved child and the other family members (e.g., Warmbrod, 1986; Worden, 1982)? Children's facility and comfort with non-verbal techniques suggests that these techniques may be refined and applied to grief counselling (Segal, 1984). Further, how can drawing tasks (such as the "grief train") and story telling, for example, be best utilized? What techniques work best in helping children resolve unfinished business? These are some of the practice and research questions that social workers can be actively involved in addressing.

CONCLUDING REMARKS

Bereavement counselling is focussed largely on the prevention of individual and social problems, and nowhere is this more crucial than with children, who are in the midst of their development. Yet, in many ways, bereaved children are a "hidden" population. Not only does society prefer to avoid the pain of the bereaved, but it often ignores or misunderstands the grief of children. The challenge for social work, then, is to identify the many opportunities for working with bereaved children in health care and other settings, and to risk touching the pain associated with grief, recognizing that the bereaved, with guidance and support, will recover.

CASE EXAMPLE

Paul, eight years old, was referred for bereavement counselling by a children's mental health centre. Paul's brother, Greg, had died unexpectedly at age two when Paul was three years old. While Paul and Greg were playing at home, Greg collapsed and died soon thereafter from an undiagnosed neurological disorder. Paul, after the death, showed signs of seizuring and Paul's mother, a single parent, became highly anxious about Paul's health. The stress of Greg's death and stress about Paul resulted in a brief psychiatric admission for their mother. Behavioural and social difficulties exhibited by Paul were often seen by his mother as his reaction to Greg's death and, in fact, Paul would verbalize this when under stress.

At time of referral, five years after the death of his brother, Paul was exhibiting marked behaviourial changes at school, difficulties in going to sleep and of most concern, suicidal ideation. For example, both at school and home, Paul had twisted pieces of clothing around his neck, stating that he wanted to die and be with Greg. Paul had verbalized this wish in the past but had not acted on it.

In an interview with Paul, he stated that he was increasingly missing his brother and found himself thinking about Greg during the afternoon at school. He indicated that he thought about where Greg was, what he was like and what they might do together if Greg was alive. Paul's ability to relate to his brother was complicated by the fact that the family had no pictures of Greg, and Paul had been very young when Greg died. Interestingly, Paul came to the first interview holding a teddy bear that had been Greg's.

Paul responded well to drawing assignments and, over a period of 2-3 sessions, was asked to draw pictures of his family, himself, Greg and the scene at the time of Greg's death. These pictures tended to be generally pleasant in nature but included themes of lost relationships (e.g., Greg was not included in the family drawings) and guilt about Greg's death. One piece of unfinished business for Paul was that he had never visited the gravesite due to his mother's emotional difficulty in making such a visit. Paul drew a picture that he could take to the cemetery when he did visit, an activity the social worker had offerred to do with Paul.

The school, which had been instrumental in identifying some of Paul's current difficulties, convened a case conference at the initiation of the school social worker. It was agreed that Paul would be included in a social skills group at the school and would receive some remedial attention. These activities were seen as ways of improving Paul's self-image and of refocussing his thoughts through the long afternoons. Paul's teacher also had some books with death themes that she planned to read to the class to stimulate some general discussion and create an environment that might facilitate Paul's expression about his loss.

Paul's renewed difficulty around Greg's death seemed to have been precipitated by his changed awareness, as he moved into a different developmental stage, about the meaning of the loss. The loss of a brother, playmate and best friend became more acute as Paul grew older and experienced social difficulties in other relationships. He seemed to be struggling, too, with what his brother looked like and was like, as Paul's memories and reminders of Greg were limited. Paul's drawings seemed to act as a concrete link with Greg, and Paul seemed to value these memories he created. The cemetery visit performed a similar function and relieved some of his mother's anxiety as she was not ready to meet Paul's need due to her own grief. Paul's suicidal thoughts may, in fact, have been prompted by a coincident crisis within the family, but this area continues to be monitored by the mother, the school and the bereavement social worker.

It is anticipated that, due to Paul's complex family situation, he will need counselling for some time. One challenge has been, and will be, to not label Paul's difficulties as simply a result of Greg's death. Similarly, many of Paul's responses seem to reflect his mother's anxiety and unresolved grief. The school social worker is working with his mother to support her in efforts to parent Paul and to help the mother with her own grief. This attention and assistance tothe mother is no doubt vital in stabilizing and strengthening the family system, rather than trying to "fix up" Paul.

Exhibit A

BEREAVEMENT INTAKE QUESTIONNAIRE

Name:_____

Date:_____

Referring
Person:_____

Presenting Problem: (as stated)_____

_____

Parents:_____

Marital Status:_____

Address:_____

Phone:_____

Children:	Name:	Age: (birth date)	Grade:
1.			
2.			
3.			

Name of Person who
Died:_____

Relationship: (to children)_____

Cause of Death:_____

Date of Death:_____

Concerns about Children:

Sleep Disturbance_____   Behaviour Problems _____

Eating Problems _____   Withdrawn Behaviour_____

School Problems _____   Excessive Saddness_____

Crying _____   Other _____

No specific concerns_____

References

Bull, M. A. (1988). Death in the family: Structure and stresses, crises and coping. In M. A. Morgan & J. D. Morgan (Eds.), *Thanatology: A Liberal Arts Approach*. London, Ontario: King's College.

Fleming, S. J. (1985). Children's grief: Individual and family dynamics. In C. A. Corr & D. M. Corr (Eds.), *Hospice Approaches to Pediatric Care*. New York: Springer.

Grollman, E. A. (1976). *Talking About Death: A Dialogue Between Parent and Child*. Boston: Beacon Press.

Krupnick, J. L. (1984). Bereavement during childhood and adolescence. In M. Osterweis, F. Solomon & M. Green (Eds.), *Bereavement: Reactions, Consequences and Care*. Washington: National Academy Press.

Lombardo, V. S. & Lombardo, E. F. (1986). *Kids Grieve Too!* Springfield, IL: Charles C. Thomas.

Plotkin, D. (1983). Children's anniversary reactions following the death of a family member. *Canada's Mental Health, June*, 13-15.

Rando, T. A. (1986). *Parental Loss of a Child*. Champaign, IL: Research Press.

Schiff, H. S. (1977). *The Bereaved Parent*. New York: Crown Publishers.

Schneider, P. L. (1985). The topic of death in children's literature. In S. V. Gullo, R.Patterson, J. E. Schowalter, M. Tallmer, A. H. Kutscher & P. Buschman (Eds), *Death and Children: A Guide for Educators, Parents and Caregivers*. Dobbs Ferry, NY: Tappan Press.

Segal, R. M. (1984). Helping children express grief through symbolic communication. *Social Casework, 65*, 590-599.

Warmbrod, M. E. T. (1986). Counselling bereaved children: Stages in the process. *Social Casework, 67*, 351-358.

Worden, J. W. (1982). *Grief Counselling and Grief Therapy: A Handbook for the Mental Health Practitioner*. New York: Springer.

Endnotes

1 Rainbows for All God's Children, Inc., 1111 Tower Road, Schaumburg, Illinois 60173.

Chapter 10

SOCIAL WORK PRACTICE IN FAMILY CENTRED AIRWAY MANAGEMENT

Jean M. Lawrence, MSSA, ACSW

Abstract

The role of the social worker has expanded readily in response to changes in the provision of health care services. This chapter will illustrate the roles and responsibilities of the hospital-based social worker who provides services for families of infants and children with airway management problems. This pediatric population requires an apnea monitor, oxygen therapy, a tracheostomy or mechanical ventilation to monitor, assist or sustain respiratory effort. Social workers provide crisis intervention, supportive counselling and community resources for these families, and serve as educators and advocates in the hospital and the community to emphasize the diverse and complex needs of these young patients and their families.

SOCIAL WORK PRACTICE IN FAMILY CENTRED AIRWAY MANAGEMENT

The role of the social worker in the health care setting has expanded readily in response to changes in the health care industry. Two of these changes are the increased availability and use of high-technology treatment modalities, and the shift from hospital-based to home-based family care for many chronically ill patients. This chapter will focus on the multiple roles of the hospital based social worker who provides services to families of infants and children with airway management problems.

THE CLIENTELE

Children with airway management problems make up a large percentage of those children who are identified as technology dependent. In the Technical Memorandum, *Technology Dependent Children: Hospital v. Home Care,* the technology dependent child is defined as, "one who needs both a medical device to compensate for the loss of vital body function, and substantial and ongoing nursing care to avert death or further disability" (1987, p. 3). Within the context of this chapter, the phrase "airway management" will be used to identify the treatment needs of those infants and children who require an apnea monitor, oxygen therapy, a tracheostomy or mechanical ventilation to monitor, assist, or sustain their respiratory effort.

The data on the actual number of children who require ongoing airway management are difficult to obtain on a local, state or federal level. Funding for their care is provided by different sources, including the Division of Services for Children with Special Health Care Needs, Medicaid and private health and automobile insurance companies. In addition, airway management problems re secondary, treatment related and are associated with a wide variety of primary medical problems. The Office of Technology Assessment estimates the prevalence of the following pediatric populations in the United States for 1987:

1. children who require ventilator assistance .680 to 2,000
2. children who require other device-based respiratory or nutritional assistance (tracheostomy tube care, suctioning, oxygen support and tube feedings) 1,000 to 6,000 and
3. children who require apnea monitors 6,000 to 45,000

According to Donar (1988) the etiology of chronic respiratory failure requiring mechanical ventilation, a tracheostomy or oxygen therapy can be divided into three categories: Respiratory Distress Syndrome (RDS)/ Bronchopulmonary Dysplasia (BPD); congenital anomalies such as tracheal bronchial malacia, diaphragmatic hernia and esophageal atresia and neurological and neuromuscular diseases such as encephalopathy and myelomeningocele. In a study of a ventilator dependent population at Children's Hospital of Philadelphia, Schreiner, Donar and Keltrick (1987) found that infants under one year of age with chronic respiratory failure, most often associated with BPD secondary to prematurity, made up most of the ventilator dependent population. Those children over one year of age experienced respiratory failure or insufficiency as a result of neuromuscular disease spinal cord injur, and restrictive pulmonary disease.

The number of children requiring long term respiratory management is increasing due to several factors. These factors include the increased rate of survival of very low birth weight infants who are at risk for long term respiratory and central nervous system sequelae (McCormick, 1985); the aggressive treatment and rehabilitation of children who sustain traumatic injuries and the potential for long term survival of children with progressive neuromuscular diseases and congenital anomalies. In the past, children who survived with these illnesses and disabilities spent extended periods of time in acute care hospitals or in nursing homes where their respiratory problems and other medical needs could be managed by health care professionals. Recently, the site of post-acute care for these medically fragile children has begun to shift from the high-tech environment of tertiary-care hospitals and extended-care facilities to the home environment.

Factors that have influenced this shift include economic and demographic variables, and public and professional acceptance of home care (Haddad, 1987). Changes in public policy, including *Public Law* 96-272 (*Social Security Act*, 1935), and 94-142 (*Education of the Handicapped*, 1970), which have focussed on the "least restrictive environment" for the care of children with special medical and developmental needs, have also emphasized the need for home care for high tech children (Hockstadt and Yost, 1989).

The decision to discharge an infant or child who requires continued airway management is one that health care professionals need to make co-operatively with the family, legal guardian, or foster parents who will be the primary caregivers. A child cannot be discharged until the medical condition is stable. For the ventilator-dependent patient, this would include a stable airway, consistent oxygen requirements, safe levels of oxygen and carbon dioxide in the blood and adequate nutritional intake (Schreiner et al., 1987). The decision making, discharge planning and teaching should be carried out with input from a multi-disciplinary team of professionals who have provided care for the patient and family during the hospitalization. The primary caregivers are key members of the decision-making team since they will ultimately be responsible for implementing and co-ordinating the plan in the home after discharge.

Taking home an infant or child who requires airway management is stressful for the caregivers, and requires adjustment and adaptation. The degree of stress and the amount of adaptation is based on the coping skills and support system of the family, not just on the type of technical assistance required by the child. Discharging an infant on an apnea monitor or with home oxygen therapy is becoming more common, particularly for premature infants being discharged from Neonatal Intensive Care Units. Stressors associated with the use of apnea monitoring may include the family's perceived need for constant watchfulness, feelings of confinement, social isolation and guilt (Dean; 1986, Desmarez, Blum, Montauk, & Kahn, 1987). Families with infants on home oxygen therapy are often concerned about their infant's health and weight gain, and about their ability to transport their infant with the necessary equipment, and their ability to handle emergency situations (Young, Creighton and Sauve, 1988).

Caring for a child who has a tracheostomy or who requires mechanical ventilation often necessitates major lifestyle changes. As emphasized by Fanconi and Bolthauser (1986) in their letter to the *Journal of Pediatrics*, many parents and guardians are capable of learning the technical skills needed to provide home ventilation, but they must be able to cope with the many challenges which accompany their technology- assisted child into their home. These challenges may include a loss of privacy, limitations on their social life, loss of a wage earner if that parent is needed to care for the child at home, disruption in sleep patterns, limitation on their time spent with other children in the home and the decision not to have additional children. These families must learn to cope with the presence of professionals in their homes, including skilled and private duty nurses from one or more nursing agencies. Frequent visits by durable medical equipment providers may also be necessary to service and restock the child's medical equipment. Families must be able to elicit support from extended family and friends to provide respite when nursing care is not available because of scheduling problems, lack of adequate insurance coverage and the universal shortage of nursing care. Additional stress may result from the redefinition of roles of the family members and health care providers. Hochstadt and Yost (1989) state that:

> Often this struggle is not recognized as a role or boundary problem but is played out as a control struggle. The family perceives that they know what is best for the child and can modify or change the health care regimen as they see fit; the home health care providers perceive that they are the health care professionals and know what is best for the child (p. 7-8).

The hospital-based social worker may serve these patients and their families in different ways throughout the course of the hospitalization and after discharge. Ideally, the social worker should meet the family early in the admission, particularly when long term airway management is required. This may be at the times of the delivery of a premature or handicapped infant, the admission of the child for a traumatic injury or acute infection or the diagnosis of a neuromuscular disease. The social worker can meet with the family throughout the course of hospitalization and serve as a key member of the multi-disciplinary health care team, particularly during times of crisis. After discharge, the hospital social worker may serve as a link between the hospital-based medical care providers and the community in which the patient and family live. The role of the social worker may vary throughout the family's different phases of adaptation to the illness or disability, with the social worker assisting the patient and family to cope emotionally, socially and financially with the infant's or child's medical condition

PRACTICE ROLES AND RESPONSIBILITIES

In order to provide optimal services for families of children with airway management problems, the social worker must function as a member of the team of health care professionals, including physicians, nurses, physical therapists, occupational therapists, respiratory therapists and discharge planners who provide care for these young patients during their hospitalization and after discharge. The social worker in the health care setting has many different roles and responsibilities, with the ultimate goal being to facilitate the family's ability to cope with the infant's or child's medical condition and make the necessary decisions regarding the child's care, both in the hospital and after discharge. Shelton, Jeppson and Johnson (1987) assert that "because the ultimate responsibility for managing a child's health, developmental, social and emotional needs lies with the family, health care systems must enable families to function as primary decision makers, caregivers, teachers, and advocates for their children" (p. 4).

Families of children with airway management problems may present a wide variety of problems and concerns, including adjustment to illness or disability, changes in family dynamics and marital relationships, changes in financial status, need for community resources and respite care for their child. The social worker must help the family to obtain the necessary resources for the child and reinforce the competence of the parents in carrying out these tasks (Healy and Beck, 1987).

One of the roles of the social worker is to evaluate the support system and coping skills of families in order to give the health care team insight into the family and its coping methods in times of stress and crisis. Families may be coping with problems that developed within the family system prior to the onset of disease or disability, and that may be exacerbated by the child's illness. Such problems may include alcohol or drug abuse, emotional illness or instability, marital problems and abusive or neglectful family environments. These problems may compound the family's ability to cope effectively with the illness or disability, particularly if the etiology of the child's condition is related to one of these problems. Examples include the premature delivery of an infant precipitated by the effects of cocaine use, or an injury sustained by a child in a motor vehicle accident caused by a parent's driving under the

167

influence of alcohol or drugs. Couples with marital problems may plan a pregnancy in order to save their marriage, only to find that they are unable to cope with the additional stress of having a premature or handicapped newborn. Such issues need to be evaluated early in the hospitalization to ensure that the family is able to cope with the patient's illness or disability, to make the necessary decisions in the best interest of the child or infant and to provide adequate care after discharge.

The social worker, in collaboration with other members of the health care team, should work with families to assist them in addressing these problems. Assessments must be made in a nonjudgmental manner to prevent alienation of the family who are often ill at ease in the high-tech medical environment. The supportive therapeutic relationship that the social worker develops with the family may be used to encourage the family to seek additional counselling or treatment related to their specific problem or concern. Interventions may include alcohol and drug treatment, psychiatric evaluation, marital counselling and parenting skills training. In addition, the hospital staff needs to be aware of any cognitive deficits, lack of reading skills and communication barriers such as hearing, vision or language problems so that information is conveyed in a manner that is understood by the family. This may necessitate the use of foreign language interpreters and materials printed in the language understood by the family. It may also include the use of sign language and the provision of equipment with visual alarms that can be recognized by a hearing impaired parent.

In some cases, it may become necessary to make a referral to Child Protective Services. Such action is appropriate if it becomes evident that the family is unable or unwilling to address specific problems that may either endanger the safety of the patient or siblings, or prevent the development of an adequate discharge plan. If a referral is made, the social worker should continue to assist the family in developing a plan that would be least disruptive to the parent/child relationship and that would assure that the child would receive the necessary care in a safe and supportive environment. If, after a complete assessment is made by the health care team in collaboration with Child Protective Services, it becomes evident that the child with airway management problems cannot be provided with adequate care by the family because of psychological, social or environmental factors, foster care placement may be considered. In rare circumstances, adoptive placements may be necessary if parental rights are terminated.

If foster care placement is necessary, the social worker's role should expand to accommodate the needs of the foster family. The social worker will need to provide support and information for members of the foster family to help them determine whether they will be able to provide ongoing care for an infant or child with airway management problems. The social worker assists the foster family during the adjustment process and emphasizes the child's developmental and health care needs. Finally, the social worker will educate the foster family about the community resources that are available, and will serve as the hospital liaison with the foster care agency. At the same time, the social worker should continue to provide support and advocacy for the natural family during this process since, in most cases, the long-term goal is to return the child to its family when problems can be resolved.

Throughout the child's hospitalization, the social worker provides ongoing support for the family, which includes the patient, together with the patient's parents, siblings, grandparents and other members of the extended family. In her article on the emotional effects of the NICU hospitalization on the family, Sumrall (1987) notes that siblings frequently fear both for their own health and for that of their parents. She also calls attention to the fact that siblings may feel isolated from their parents, who may spend a great deal of time at the hospital and who continue to focus attention on the chronically ill child after discharge. Gallo (1988) emphasizes the need for open communication between the patient and the healthy siblings, and adds that the siblings may need to be encouraged to discuss their feelings, particularly if they perceive that the parents are already overburdened. The social worker may provide assistance by educating the parents on how to deal with the verbal and behaviourial manifestations of guilt, fear, anger and that which may be displayed by the healthy siblings. The social worker can assist parents in responding to the questions and concerns expressed by extended family members, and should be available to meet with these family members if the need occurs.

The social worker should take into account that each family is different and that emotional response to illness and disability varies from family to family. It is important to recognize that each family brings to the situation its own strengths, weaknesses and diversity, and that it will use a wide variety of coping mechanisms in adapting to the situation (*Surgeon General's Report*, 1987). Finally, the social worker must realize that families may respond differently to social work intervention. Some families may accept services related to concrete needs, such as information about community resources, but may not be receptive to counselling or emotional support. The needs of the family may change throughout the course of the hospitalization, and the family will need to know that the services provided by the social worker will remain available even if they are declined earlier in the hospitalization. Families require time to identify their needs before they begin to address them. Therefore, it becomes important to adapt the style of intervention to the needs of the individual family. In her article, "The Parent/Professional Relationship: Complex Connections, Intricate Bonds," Iris (1988) notes the risk associated with the parent/professional relationship:

> No matter how successful I believe my children to be, or how normal they appear, the services and treatment provided by professionals serve as a visible manifestation of my children's special needs. The very presence of the professional emphasizes our vulnerability (p. 9).

An important part of providing support for families of medically fragile children is to put them in touch with another family with a child with a similar medical condition. This may be done on an informal basis, or through organized parent support organizations. These organizations may be sponsored by individual hospitals, or they may be organized by parents in the community. Such organizations can provide emotional support, reduce the family's sense of isolation, provide families with additional information about educational programs available for their child and help families cope with the day to day questions regarding living with a child with specialized health care needs. Such organizations also encourage increased communication between parents and professionals, enhance public awareness of children with special health care needs and support legislative action that promotes improved standards and payment for health care and related support services for these children and their families.

In addition to addressing the psycho-social needs of these families, the social worker must also provide concrete resources and referrals for community resources. This role may differ from hospital to hospital based on the job description and role responsibility of the social worker. In some hospitals, the role of the medical social worker does not include a discharge planning component. A different social worker or registered nurse co-ordinates home care needs, evaluates insurance coverage and arranges for durable medical equipment and skilled nursing care. They may also make referrals for early intervention programs, respite care and community support services. If this role is separate from that of the medical social worker, the social worker must work in collaboration with the discharge planner to ensure that the family's psychosocial and emotional needs are addressed in the development of a home care plan. Input from other professionals who have worked with the patient and family during hospitalization is also important. After discharge, the hospital social worker may serve as a resource for the home care agency if concerns arise about the adjustment to the home care plan, family dynamics and coping skills. Sumrall (1987) emphasizes that parents may be surprised after discharge by their ongoing emotional reaction to the NICU experience, and she states that "just as medical follow-up is important for the high risk infant, supportive follow-up for the family serves the purpose of reinforcing the parents' adjustment" (p. 73).

The social worker may also serve as an educator in the health care setting. The social worker may provide orientation for new nursing staff and residents, in addition to providing ongoing in-service training for hospital staff on the social, emotional and developmental needs of infants and children with airway management problems. The social worker may emphasize the need to focus on the family as the centre of care, and illustrate how the illness of the child impacts on the entire family. Social workers should participate in educational programs sponsored by other members of the health care team to increase their understanding of the medical treatment and nursing care provided for these young patients. The emphasis should be on a free exchange of information between disciplines in order to identify and address the many needs of these patients and their families.

POTENTIAL FOR ROLE DEVELOPMENT

The delivery of health care services for the pediatric population continues to become more focussed on the patient as an integral part of a family with diverse psycho-social and developmental needs. Consequently, there is increasing importance placed upon the social worker's skills of psycho-social assessment and therapeutic intervention, along with the social worker's recognition of the roles of illness and disability as stressors on the family system. The role of the social worker has continued to expand to meet the needs of children and families in the complex health care system. The most commonly recognized roles of the hospital-based social worker involve the provision of crisis intervention, supportive counselling and referrals for community services. Social workers interface with a wide variety of agencies and service providers in the community to organize a continuum of services for patients and familes, during the hospitalization period and after discharge.

The roles of educator and advocate may not be as well recognized. The social worker may serve as an educator within the health care system, providing in-service training for other health care professionals on the psycho-social implications of chronic illness and disability. The social worker may also offer this training for professionals who provide home care health services. The social worker is in the position to facilitate collaboration between parents and health care professionals so that parents can educate professionals about their diverse social, emotional, developmental and health care needs. The University of Iowa has published guidelines for the education of physicians, therapists, social workers and families, entitled *Improving Health Care for Children with Chronic Conditions* (Healy & Lewis-Beck, 1987). Healy and Lewis-Beck's (1987) guidelines provide a comprehensive overview of the needs of patients and families, and are intended to "promote active family involvement, better communication and collaboration between family and professional care givers, access to health care information for families, and the development of individualized service plans" (p. iii).

The social worker may serve as an advocate within the health care setting to facilitate communication between health care professionals and families, and to assist families in locating and obtaining necessary resources. Because the social worker is in direct contact with this technology-assisted pediatric population, the social worker is in the position to use professional knowledge and experience to influence the development and implementation of programs and services, both in the hospital and in the community (Shelton, Jeppson, & Johnson, 1987). The social worker may also become engaged in policy development and legislative action through involvement with local and state organizations that advocate for the health care needs. The role as a direct service provider enables the social worker to identify the diverse strengths, coping skills and unmet needs of the medically complex population of infants and children with airway management problems and their families.

CONCLUDING REMARKS

The impact of recent changes within the health care system has necessitated the expansion of the social worker's role to meet the complex needs of children and families. This chapter has discussed some of the roles and responsibilities of hospital-based social workers who work with the families of children with airway management problems. These children comprise a large percentage of the technology-dependent pediatric population, and are often graduates of neonatal and pediatric intensive care units. The social worker functions as a member of a multi-disciplinary team of health care professionals to identify the psychological, social, developmental and financial needs of these families. Further, social workers use their skills to establish ways to address these needs within the context of comprehensive health care plans for patients and their families.

CASE EXAMPLE

Baby Girl R. was born to a sixteen-year-old single female at approximately thirty weeks gestation. The infant remained in a neonatal intensive care unit in a large community hospital for three months. At that time, she was transferred to a neonatal intensive care unit in a pediatric hospital approximately seventy miles from her home for repeated failure to wean from the ventilator. A diagnosis of subglottic stenosis with complete upper airway obstruction was made. She remained in the pediatric hospital for two weeks and then was transferred back to the referring hospital. During the infant's initial stay at the pediatric hospital, her mother called or visited on a daily basis. Her mother was trying to complete her education while her daughter was in the hospital, since she had been in the eleventh grade at the time that Baby Girl R. was born.

Five weeks later, the infant was transferred back to the pediatric hospital, and surgery was done for the placement of a tracheostomy. Baby Girl R. remained in the pediatric hospital for two and one half months, during which time her mother learned to do tracheostomy care, CPR, and operate the apnea monitor and suctioning equipment. Several days after surgery, her mother had been told that a second caregiver would need to be trained for back-up, and that they would need to have a home phone for emergency use before the infant could be discharged. Ms. R. had indicated that her mother would be the second caregiver, but it soon became apparent that the maternal grandmother had not scheduled discharge training, that she had made no attempts to have a phone installed in her home and that her home was being renovated because it did not meet housing codes. Based on these concerns, a referral was made to Child Protective Services when Baby Girl R. was four and one-half months old because she required specialized home care and medical follow-up, and L.R., her mother, was receiving no support from her family. The father of the baby had not been involved since early in the pregnancy.

Up to this point, the social work roles had been family assessment and support for the teenage mother with a medically fragile child, collaboration with the health care team to communicate psycho-social concerns and obtain information about the health care needs of the infant, communication with the public health and skilled nurse care agencies that had done the initial home assessment and collaboration with the home care nurse to develop a plan for home care that could be submitted to the state for a Medicaid Waiver.

After Child Protective Services became involved, a friend of the family stated that she would allow the mother and her infant to stay in her home, and that she would learn to assist with the baby's care. Although there were some problems with compliance during discharge training, the infant was discharged three weeks later after both her mother and her second caregiver had successfully completed the discharge training and their home had been evaluated by a nurse from the skilled nursing agency.

Approximately four months after discharge, after failing to keep several appointments for medical follow-up, the infant was readmitted for re-evaluation of her airway. At the time of readmission, the Protective Service worker informed the hospital social worker that the infant could no longer live in the home to which she had been discharged because of family conflicts. There had also been reports by the skilled nursing agency that on several home visits, the apnea monitor had not been connected to the infant, and on one visit the equipment had been found in the closet. A petition was filed n Juvenile Court, and the judge ordered the maternal grandmother and two of Ms. R's sisters to learn to care for the infant, which had since been removed. Ten days later,

174

a second petition was filed making the infant, then nine months old, a temporary court ward, and authorizing foster care placement for the infant because the maternal grandmother and the two aunts repeatedly failed to participate in the discharge training that had been scheduled at their convenience. Ms. R. was not able to develop any other plans for the infant's care.

During eight months of social work contact with this family, first on the neonatal intensive care unit and later on the surgical floor, it became increasingly apparent that intense family conflicts made it impossible to develop the support system that would have been necessary to keep Baby Girl R. at home. Ms. R.'s sister and mother stated that they wanted her to have the pregnancy terminated, but that she had refused. Ms. R. blamed the baby's medical problems on her emotional stress caused by her family during her pregnancy. The family only began to recognize and verbalize these feelings after the infant was made a temporary court ward. Although there was never any question that this family had the intellectual ability to learn the technical aspects of the infant's care, the hospital staff concluded that all of the infant's medical needs, including the use of an apnea monitor and daily tracheostomy care, together with consistent medical follow-up, would not be met given the multiple conflicts in this family system. Further, the staff concluded that failure to provide adequate care could be life threatening for this infant. The hospital social worker stressed the need for Ms. R. to have regular contact with her daughter in foster care, and for her to have parenting skills training, continue her education and for the family to participate in counselling.

References

Dean, P. G. (1986). Monitoring an apneic infant: Impact on the infant's mother. *Maternal Child Nursing Journal, 15*(2), 65-76.

Desmarez, C., Blum, D., Montauk, L. & Kahn, A. (1987). Impact of home monitoring for sudden infant death syndrome on family life. *European Journal of Pediatrics, 146:* 159-161.

Donar, M. E. (1988). Community care: Pediatric home mechanical ventilation. *Holistic Nursing Practice, 2*(2), 68-70.

Education of the Handicapped Act of 1970, 20 U.S.C. S 1400 (1975).

Fanconi, S. & Bolthauser, E. (1986). Outcomes of home mechanical ventilation [Letter]. *Journal of Pediatrics, 108* (5 pt. 1) 791.

Gallo, A. M. (1988). The special sibling relationship in chronic illness and disability: Parental communication with well siblings. *Holistic Nursing Practice, 2*(2), 28-37.

Haddad, A. M. (1987). *High Tech Home Care: A Practical Guide.* Maryland: Aspen Publisher, Inc.

Healy, A., & Lewis-Beck, J. A. (1987 a). *Guidelines for families: Improving health care for children with chronic conditions.* Iowa City, Iowa: The University of Iowa.

Healy, A. & Lewis-Beck, J. A. (1987 b). *Guidelines for Physicians: Improving Health Care for Children with Chronic Conditions.* Iowa City, Iowa: The University of Iowa.

Healy, A. & Lewis-Beck, J. A. (1987 c). *Guidelines for Social Work: Improving Health Care for Children with Chronic Conditions.* Iowa City, Iowa: The University of Iowa.

Healy, A. & Lewis-Beck, J.A. (1987 d). *Guidelines for Therapists: Improving Health Care for Children with Chronic Conditions.* Iowa City, Iowa: The University of Iowa.

Hochstadt, N. & Yost, D. (1989). The health care-child welfare partnership: Transitioning medically complex children to the community. *Children's Health Care, 18*(1), 4-11.

Iris, M. A. (1988). The parent/professional relationship: Complex connections, intricate bonds. *Family Resource Coalition Report, 2*(17).

McCormick, M. C. (1985). The contribution of low birth weight to infant mortality and childhood morbidity. *The New England Journal of Medicine, 312*(2), 82-90.

Schreiner, M. S., Donar, M. E., & Kettrick, R. G. (1987). Pediatric home mechanical ventilation. *Pediatric Clinics of North America, 34*(1), 47-60.

Shelton, T. L., Jeppson, E. S. & Johnson, B. H.(1987). *Family-Centred Care for Children with Special Health Care Needs* (2nd ed.).

Washington, D.C.: Association for the Care of Children's Health.

Social Security Act of 1935, 602 U.S.C. S 402 Title IV (1980).

Sumrall, B. C. (1987). The emotional effects of the NICU on the family. *Schumpert Medical Quarterly, 20*(4), 67-75.

U. S. Congress, Office of Technology Assessment (1987). *Technology-Dependent Children: Hospital v. Home Care — A Technical Memorandum* (OTA-TM-H-38). Washington, D.C.: U.S. Government Printing Office.

U. S. Department of Health and Human Services (1987). *Surgeon General's Report: Children with Special Health Care Needs.* (DHHS Publication No. HRSD/MC 87-2). Washington, D.C.: Division of Maternal and Child Health.

Young, Y. L., Creighton, D. E. & Suave, R. S. (1988). The needs of families of infants discharged home with continuous oxygen therapy. *Journal of Obstetric, Gynecologic and Neonatal Nursing, 17,* 187-193.

Chapter 11

SOCIAL WORK PRACTICE WITH VENTILATOR-ASSISTED PATIENTS

Linda B. Fischer, MSW

Abstract

Increasing numbers of patients require on-going ventilatory support. New technology, increased government spending and a growing perception that the chronically ill are able to live in the community has made it possible for ventilator-assisted persons to reside in their homes. The social worker is a vital member of the multidisciplinary team, responsible for the comprehensive psychosocial assessment, co-ordination of hospital and community health care professionals and on-going therapeutic interventions with patients, families and staff.

SOCIAL WORK PRACTICE WITH VENTILATOR-ASSISTED PATIENTS

"Ventilator-assisted individuals require mechanical ventilation either continuously or for a predetermined period of time during each day and/or night" (Leasa, Personal Communication). In planning for a ventilator-assisted patient's care and potential for a discharge home, important considerations include the medical, emotional and psychological stability; the home, financial and community resources and the degree of patient motivation. Emotional disturbances and interpersonal conflicts can be aggravated by the presence of the ventilator patient in the home. The intimidating respiratory equipment and the inevitable intrusion of strangers in the home complicate this difficult lifestyle adaptation.

THE CLIENTELE

Hospital Intensive Care Units (ICUs) are a significant practice area for social workers. Nowhere is a family in more obvious crisis than when faced with the life-threatening illness of a loved one who may be unresponsive and dependent on highly technical equipment. Using the crisis model for intervention, a social worker can significantly lessen the trauma experienced by such a family.

Social Work can provide needed intervention at the time of the crisis in ICU. The assessment of and help with the family's perception of the circumstances, the coping mechanisms used by this particular family and the supports available to them are integral components of the health care team's efforts in caring for and treating the patient. The social worker can decrease the intense emotional experience inherent in a patient's ICU hospitalization and significantly improve the family's adaptation and management of the crisis.

Ventilator patients are identified to social work through regular contact with nursing and medical staff, and attendance at interdisciplinary rounds in the I.C.U. To date, the five ventilator-assisted patients who have been discharged to their homes came to the attention of Social Work in this way. Diagnoses included

Duchenne's Muscular Dystrophy, COPD/Chronic Bronchopleural Cutaneous Fistula, Amyotrophic Lateral Sclerosis, Brain Stem Disease secondary to infection and Incomplete Quadriparetic. "Assisted ventilation is required to maintain or improve quality of life which has been compromised by an underlying disease process or injury such as severe lung disease, neuromuscular disease, lack of ventilatory drive, skeletal disorders or past trauma" (Ontario Medical Review, 1986).

> "Often respiratory failure develops slowly, allowing time to consider the pros and cons of long-term mechanical ventilation. In other cases a medical crisis may force a decision at a point when the patient is confused, impaired or otherwise unable to communicate. If so, the choice must be made by a close relative or designated representative. Ideally, a decision for long-term ventilator care should be made only after the patient's acute respiratory failure has been corrected and the patient can participate intelligently in the decision-making process" (American College of Chest Physicians, 1984).

The complex issues involved must be thoroughly examined by the attending physician, with the assistance and input of the social worker, in order to ensure an informed and knowledgeable decision by the patient and family.

I. Home Ventilation

The emotional stability of the patient is vital to the success of home ventilation. "The psychologically stable patient who is motivated to improve the quality of life and who enjoys the support of others at home, should strive to be as independent as possible" (American College of Chest Physicians, 1984). Consequently, an understanding of the patient's emotional and social functioning prior to hospitalization is important in the assessment of a treatment and discharge plan for the patient.

Patients and families frequently exhibit anxiety with regard to the patient's hospitalization and discharge plans. These fears need to be identified and alleviated through therapeutic intervention, education and instruction in the use of equipment and care of the patient. Supportive family members who are actively involved in the care of the patient seem to reduce the patient's anxiety, in addition to their own (Daley-White & Walsh-Perez, 1986).

When planning for a discharge to home it is necessary to include the patient and the family in the process. Family members, although certain that they want their loved one to return home, often experience ambivalent emotions and thoughts about their ability to manage the patient's needs, or the respiratory equipment. Families must be allowed the opportunity to discuss these concernst and to have their anxieties reduced through education and on-going supportive/therapeutic interventions by social work and other health care disciplines.

An important task of the social worker in this initial stage is to assess the dynamics, relationships, supports, motivations and wishes of the ventilator patient and the family.

An on-going function of the social worker throughout the home care selection process is to communicate this assessment and other concerns to the members of the interdisciplinary team. The social worker becomes the voice of the patient and family when they find it difficult to share their own feelings and thoughts.

PRACTICE ROLES AND RESPONSIBILITIES

A critical part of the selection process for discharging to a home is the assessment and evaluation of the patient's current and projected needs and the patient's and family's ability to manage these needs. A primary concern is the patient's right to make decisions with respect to her/his well-being. There must be an underlying consideration for the quality of life to which the patient is entitled. This is linked to the goal of attaining a comfort level for all persons involved in the home care plan, including the patient and family. Therefore, the decision to be placed on long-term mechanical ventilation requires frequent discussions between patient and families with the attending physician and social worker.

I. Ethical Considerations

Complex ethical considerations usually arise from the introduction of a life support system (Ontario Medical Review, 1986). Members of the health care team, individually and as a group, struggle with the quality of life issues both as a concept and as they pertain to the idividual patient. Team members have a responsibility to identify and deal with their feelings in order to be of greater assistance to the patient and family.

Mechanical ventilation can be perceived as a life of doom, restricting the social, emotional and physical existance of the individual and his/her family. An informed decision is based on the realistic and comprehensive outline of what the patient might expect upon discharge. Patients and families may require repeated explanations and will need a sympathetic and supportive approach. An essential function of social work is to obtain a comprehensive psycho-social assessment. It is necessary to understand the family's history, patterns of interaction, goals, supports and beliefs in order to fully appreciate and assist in their decision-making. Patients and families are seen together and individually to allow for therapist-patient relationship building, and confidential discussions.

An integral function of the social worker in the role of "team builder" includes the co-ordination of hospital and community professionals in addressing the patient/family needs and the facilitation of these on-going supports. The social worker ensures that the patient and family are represented in discharge planning meetings.

The advocacy role of social work guarantees that members of the team are aware of the patient/family's current level of adjustment and of their position in the planning process. This advocacy role was highlighted at the Health Centre in the case of a 51-year-old woman who had presented with COPD/Chronic Bronchopleural Cutaneous Fistula. The patient's spouse expressed the strong desire to have his wife return home. It was interesting to note the reactions from members of the team based on their own beliefs and values. Initially team members refused to acknowledge that the husband would be intellectually or physically capable of understanding and managing her care in the home. Through careful exploration and education the team was able to plan realistic goals for this couple and to effect her successful discharge home.

Once it has been decided that a patient will be discharged home, case conferences are held at least every second week. These meetings, which are held in the patient's room with family and selected health care members participating in the process, are designed to delegate tasks and to ensure consistency in treatment planning. The conferences allow all participants to evaluate the plan in process, and to be aware of the feelings that the patient, family and team members are experiencing.

The social worker is active in the assessment of the patient's and the family's financial status, including income, pension plans and insurance packages through employer or private establishments. The majority of families are unable to care for their family member without comprehensive financial assistance.

The Assistive Devices Program of the Ontario Ministry of Health expanded its financial coverage in 1986 to include home mechanical ventilators under the category of respiratory equipment. This means that 75% of all equipment costs are covered through this government program. The social worker still must be active in obtaining the remaining 25%, which usually consists of contacting employers, insurance companies, social service organizations and service clubs.

Support to staff remains an on-going social work function. It is imperative that staff be sensitive to the different types of families and their coping mechanisms. Members of the health care team bring their own feelings and beliefs to their work, and they should be given the opportunity to discuss and differentiate their feelings from those of their patients. Social work must recognize the difficulty and strain in caring for these patients and be attuned to staff needs.

Prior to discharge the social worker is responsible for the notification of emergency and critical service providers including the police, fire, hydro, ambulance and telephone companies. This ensures that, in the event of a major power black-out, the home ventilator patient will be taken to the emergency department of a local hospital immediately.

Following the discharge home, the social worker normally meets with the patient and family every two weeks in their home to assist with the re-integration into the home and community. Both the patient and family are encouraged to be as independent as possible. Over time social work contact decreases; however, the network remains in place should on-going or periodic service be necessary. In London, Ontario a social worker is currently employed with the Home Care program. The Intensive Care social worker often facilitates the transfer of on-going casework to this community-based social worker.

POTENTIAL FOR ROLE DEVELOPMENT

There exists a need for co-ordinated, long-term ventilatory programs. Such programs would ensure that candidates for home mechanical ventilation would have access to multidisciplinary health care teams committed to the goal of assisting individuals attain their potential. Resources within such programs would include detailed assessments, specialized training, community liaison, financial assistance and clinical/medical follow-up.

Programs must address the changing and ambivalent feelings of patients and families as they struggle with the adaptation of mechanical ventilation and changes in lifestyle. Patient and family concerns often decrease with exposure to structured educational programs and training.

Ventilator-assisted patients represent a complex population that deserves comprehensive and frequent intervention from social work as they prepare for their new life. It is hoped that St. Joseph's Health Centre will eventually obtain space and funding for a 5-6 bed unit in which psychosocial assessments, counselling and discharge planning could occur. This unit would consist of several disciplines geared to specializing in the care and planning for such patients and their families. Such a unit could offer ongoing training and experience for staff and students committed to working with ventilator-assisted patients. This familiarity and expertise would undoubtedly ease anxiety for the patient, family and health care team.

This unit could also serve as a relief unit for families caring for a ventilator-assisted patient at home. Frequently families do not permit themselves to take time away from their responsibilities, nor do they have access to alternative facilities for their ventilator-assisted family members. Should a patient require management of more acute medical problems than can be provided for at home, this facility would be designed for short term readmissions.

Due to the increasing number of ventilated patients, it seems likely that a Ventilator Outreach Team, which would work from this proposed specialized unit, would be necessary to assess patients in regional hospitals. This team, comprised of the attending physician, respiratory therapist and social worker, would meet with patient, family and members of the regional hospital patient care team. If appropriate, this patient could be transferred to the

Health Centre where the plans would be initiated for home placement.

A positive staff attitude can influence the emotional well-being of the ventilator-assisted patient and family. Programs must focus on the enhancement of the individual's potential while allowing for set-backs and realistic limitations. Care required by ventilator-assisted patients may overwhelm staff, and result in serious problems for the patient. Social work would be responsible for the regular scheduling of staff in-service sessions to look at the emotional needs of ventilated patients and their families in addition to their own reactions and feelings.

Society's awareness of the special needs of ventilator-assisted patients is continuing to increase. Indeed, the present mood suggests that this population will become a special-interest group that will eventually develop into a provincial or national association. In support of this trend, social workers may be called on to act as advocates, to educate community groups, to do research and to assist with publications. Policy makers within the health care system will need to be approached for increased program funding. Research, particularly directed at the social/emotional needs of this group, will be a serious responsibility for social workers practising in the field to undertake.

CONCLUDING REMARKS

"We want an individual to lead a relatively independent or productive life, even if he or she requires chronic ventilatory support. We believe that the home environment will enhance an individual's potential, improve their physiologic and emotional well being, and overall enhance their quality of life" (Leasa, Personal Communication).

The hospital multidisciplinary team, with the patient and family, determines suitability and feasibility of home ventilation for individuals. When this has been established the process of psychological reconditioning and reintegration into the community begins. Within the realistic limitations of the patient's physical condition, the social worker aims to enhance the emotional and social well-being of the patient and the family.

A well co-ordinated interactive team approach is essential to deal with the medical, technical, psychosocial, organizational and financial issues that affect the discharge of a ventilator-assisted patient. The social worker is an active member of this team, providing therapeutic and practical intervention to patients and families, and acting as resource and support to staff.

Social work will continue to have an important role in the development of new programs for the ventilator-assisted patient. These courageous patients and their families may serve as a role models for other severely disabled individuals who may wish to reside at home.

CASE EXAMPLE

Mr. A., a 34-year old man with Muscular Dystrophy, was admitted to the St. Joseph's Health Centre Intensive Care Unit in early 1985 for intubation and ventilation. He had a diagnosis of respiratory failure secondary to pneumonia.

Mr. A. had been living independently in a downtown apartment before his admission. He had been a computer analyst with a large corporation prior to going on a long term disability pension as a result of his chronic disease progression. Although confined to a wheelchair, Mr. A. had continued to be actively involved in his career, hobbies and travelling.

As Mr. A.'s condition stabilized in the ICU he began to express concerns for his future lifestyle on a ventilator. The attending physicians felt that due to his progressive disease state, he would now require lifetime institutionalization. London did not offer long term care for ventilator-dependent patients and the closest appropriate facility was 200 km away, with a 5-year waiting list.

Mr. A. strongly objected to any plans for institutional placement. Instead he began to challenge the medical system by presenting a plan to return home with commuiysupports. He recognized that he required continual care, but felt that this could be accomplished in his own home.

By March 1985 Mr. A. only required the ventilator at night. He began to request leaves of absence from ICU and, while a nurse initially accompanied him on these outings, within weeks Mr. A. was able to go on his own.

The physicians and patient care team began to seriously consider the feasibility of a return home given Mr. A.'s motivation. A planning committee comprised of the ICU nursing manager, the attending physician, the Intensive Care social worker and two respiratory therapists was developed.

Initial obstacles were examined by this group. If home ventilation was to be the objective, it was felt that Mr. A. might be transferred to a general medical floor while a discharge nursing plan was developed. This posed a challenge for the team as a ventilator-dependent patient had not been cared for outside of ICU.

The expense of home ventilation was another crucial consideration. Social work and respiratory therapy worked together to list all necessary equipment needs and to obtain funding sources. Community resources such as Home Care, the Muscular Dystrophy Association and Respiratory Services were all contacted to elicit their co-operation and support for our venture.

Throughout this process it was vital that Mr. A. be given every opportunity to be part of the planning and to discuss his feelings. The social worker met regularly with Mr. A. as he struggled with his anxiety, depression and ambivalence. Family members were also contacted; however, in this case practical support from this source was limited.

Mr. A. was medically stable at the time of his transfer to a general medical floor. This interim environment was viewed as a way to assist him in preparation for discharge, by gently weaning him from the constant care of the ICU. As Mr. A. was the first ventilated patient cared for outside of the critical care environment in the history of the Health Centre, nursing staff from the floor were predictably anxious. The social worker was able to assist with communication between the medical floor and ICU by encouraging regular meetings and ensuring adequate training and support.

Mr. A. experienced periods of anger, depression, withdrawal and overt frustration. Although he remained firm in his desire to return home, he questioned the intrusion of community and hospital services into his home and the subsequent loss of his privacy. His fear of institutional life, if the plan was not successful, was frequently expressed. The social worker and Mr. A. had established a positive therapeutic relationship, and daily contact was provided to allow him the opportunity to express his fears and concerns.

The Committee was expanded to include community resources such as the Home Care Co-ordinator and a representative from a nursing agency. Mr. A. was also a member of this committee. Weekly meetings were held to facilitate consistent planning and goal-setting. Tasks were assigned to the disciplines involved. Social Work continued to be Mr. A.'s primary emotional support, in addition to co-ordinating the funding sources for the home care plan. Nurses in the community were trained to use the respiratory care equipment by nurses and respiratory therapists in the Health Centre. A home assessment was completed by the occupational therapist to ensure access, mobility and power availability.

Professionals involved in Mr. A.'s care at home included 24-hour nursing care, funded through Mr. A.'s health insurance package; respiratory therapists through the Home Oxygen Program at the Health Centre; the Intensive Care social worker, as Home Care community social work service was unavailable at that time; a Home Care Co-ordinator and a representative from the Muscular Dystrophy Association with whom Mr. A. was well acquainted.

Mr. A. was sent home on a 48-hour trial leave of absence and as this was successful he was discharged home on June 20, 1985.

Mr. A. experienced predictable stages of adjustment following his discharge. He developed and utilized a variety of coping mechanisms to manage these feelings, and it was not unusual for him to withdraw from or criticize his caregivers unexpectedly. Mr. A.'s anxiety and depression appeared to be directly related to the dramatic change in his lifestyle. The monthly tracheostomy changes done in the hospital were also a major source of anxiety for him, as he feared that coming to the Health Centre might lead to a permanent stay.

Mr. A.'s anger focussed on

(1) his long stay in the hospital;
(2) being ventilator dependent;
(3) the physicians who had suggested institutionalization;
(4) delays of discharge caused by a system unfamiliar with home ventilation and
(5) the hospital for "abandoning" him upon discharge.

While Mr. A. wished to be at home and establish independence, he also felt a need to be protected and taken care of within the hospital setting. Once he understood his confusion and the complexities of his ambivalence, he was able to constructively manage his anger. Of utmost importance to him was his strong need to maintain control over his decision making. The loss of privacy was difficult for Mr. A. but he learned that it was acceptable to make demands, and the nurses in his home became increasingly sensitive and accepting of his need for time alone, or with visitors.

Mr. A.'s ventilator dependency rendered him restricted in

selecting activities for his enjoyment. All interests to be pursued outside his home entailed careful planning, and initially it seemed easier for Mr. A. to isolate himself at home. Over time he was able to try outside activities, which was helpful in his reintegration into the community and to his sense of self-worth.

What has proven beneficial to Mr. A. in his recovery seems to be distance and time away from his hospitalization, continued support from friends and community professionals in his care and the opportunity to freely discuss his feelings. Mr. A. has now been at home three and a half years, and appears to have an independent lifestyle with the continuing aid of nurses and respiratory therapists. Social work and other support services continue to be available to him as he or the Home Care nurse identify a need. Mr. A. has taken long distance vacations (with a private duty nurse), has resumed evening classes at the local college and is an active member of his housing co-operative.

References

Daley-White, K. & Walsh-Perez, P. (1986). Your ventilator patient CAN go home again. *Nursing, 16,* 54-56.

Fuchs-Carroll, P. (1986). Caring for ventilator patients. *Nursing, 16,* 34-40.

Gilmartin, M. & Make, B. (1983). Home care of the ventilator-dependent person. *Respiratory Care, 28* (11), 1490-1497.

Home ventilation: Status in Ontario. (1986) *Ontario Medical Review,* 14-17.

Kopacz, M. A. & Moriarty-Wright, R. (1984). Multidisciplinary approach for the patient on a home ventilator. *Heart Lung, 13,* 255-262.

Leasa, D. *Long-Term Ventilatory Care Program.* (Personal Communication).

The American College of Chest Physicians. (1984) *Mechanical Ventilation in the Home.* 4-15.

Pierson, D. J. & George, R. B. (1986). Mechanical ventilation in the home: Possibilities and prerequisites. *Respiratory Care, 31:4,* 266-270.

Sivak, E. D., Cordasco, E. M. & Gipson, W. T. (1983). Pulmonary mechanical ventilation at home: A reasonable and less expensive alternative. *Respiratory Care, 28,* 42-49.

Winters, C. (1988). Monitoring ventilator patients for complications. *Nursing, 18,* 38-41.

Chapter 12

SOCIAL WORK PRACTICE IN A WOMEN'S HEALTH CARE CENTRE

Deborah MacLean-Brine, RN, BSW

Abstract

This chapter describes a specific obstetrics and gynecology outpatient clinic and the role of the social worker who provides service to this unit. As this type of complete women's health care clinic is relatively unique, the author describes the functioning of the specific unit, rather than making broader generalizations about other medical facilities. The reader will find that an extensive range of issues including teenage pregnancy, adoption, abortion, sterilization and sexually transmitted diseases are addressed by the social worker in this area. A case study provides an example of a young, single woman moving through the process of making a decision about her unplanned pregnancy and the case examines the issue of voluntary pregnancy termination.

SOCIAL WORK PRACTICE IN A WOMEN'S HEALTH CARE CENTRE

The Women's Health Care Centre (WHCC) operates out of Victoria Hospital, an 840-bed general teaching hospital that is a member of the London Health Sciences Centre in London, Ontario, Canada. The WHCC is an outpatient clinic designed to meet the obstetrical and gynecological needs of women from adolescence to post menopause. The clinic provides service for approximately 6,500 visits per year.

The WHCC team consists of five primary and five secondary obstetricians and gynecologists, one full-time social worker, a head nurse, five registered nurses trained in obstetrics and gynecology and one unit clerk. Both in-hospital and community health care professionals are utilized for consultation where appropriate.

The WHCC is a self-contained unit attached to the hospital in-patient service areas. The clinic is comprised of a reception office/nursing station, patient/family waiting room, two consultation offices, four examination/treatment rooms, head nurse's office, staff lounge and, beyond a second set of privacy doors, an inner suite of rooms where patients receive and recover from therapeutic abortions.

The social work office is located just outside the WHCC, halfway between the clinic and the general day surgery services. This location allows the patient to be removed from the immediate clinic setting where the pace is often hectic and where the environment is by nature very medically oriented. The office has been decorated in warm colours with soft lighting and provides enough space to sit four people in large, comfortable chairs placed in a living room-like setting for convenient conversation. It is anticipated that this environment provides the patient, if only for 30 - 60 minutes, the opportunity to be in a comfortable, quiet, totally private milieu conducive to counselling.

THE CLIENTELE

The WHCC serves individuals from the ages of 12 to 75, but the patient population primarily falls between the ages of 15 and 35. Women present themselves in the clinic, via self-referral or referral from a community health professional, with any type of obstetrical or gynecological need. The women's issues addressed in the clinic recognize no intellectual, racial, marital or socio-economic boundaries, for the issues related to human sexuality and the functioning of the female reproductive system cut across all social barriers and impact upon each woman in a unique manner.

I. Services

A woman may arrive at the clinic with no concrete idea of what is happening to her, only that there has been a change in her body's normal functioning. She may present with an ambiguous complaint or concern such as pelvic pain, nausea, weight change or amenorrhea (no menses). She may be anxious and fear the worst about her condition. In response, the WHCC team utilizes a broad range of tests, assessments, diagnoses, procedures and treatments to identify and if possible arrest these problems.

The following are the primary services provided by the WHCC team to address their female patients' needs:

- general gynecological assessments including pap smears and pelvic examinations for vaginal infections, bleeding or irregular menses;
- colposcopy examinations: the diagnosis of abnormal pap smear findings (pre-cancerous cells) and appropriate treatment plans;
- diagnosis and treatment of sexually transmitted diseases;
- teaching of reproductive functioning and contraception including mutual choice of most appropriate method and application of such;
- confirmation of pregnancy;
- Rh Negative blood screening and appropriate treatment of antenatal patients;
- antenatal care during pregnancy;
- amniocentesis where indicated;
- post-partum follow-up care of mother for six weeks after delivery;
- assistance with arrangements necessary to place an infant for adoption.;

- termination of first trimester pregnancies (12 weeks gestational age or less);
- consultation, examination and bookings for sterilization or sterilization reversal;
- urodynamics; bladder function studies and subsequent recommendations for treatment and
- referrals for genetic counselling, dietary counselling, ultra sound and pre-natal education classes.

A patient may receive any combination of these services depending upon her presenting problem and assessment of the OB/GYN consultant. Further, a patient receiving these services may be referred by the WHCC staff for social work consultation and/or intervention.

Both the normal, healthy, reproductive functions of a woman's body and the malfunctioning or diseased parts of her reproductive system are closely entwined with and often inseparable from a complicated network of deep emotional responses and previous belief systems. It is at this crossing of mind and body that the role of the social worker is most clearly defined. In the clinic, the patient receives competent medical attention from the doctors and nurses caring for her. Questions can be asked and concise medical information is provided when possible. However, the facts and information may be shocking, disappointing and/or frightening. Further, the situation may require that a major decision regarding a procedure or surgery must be made by the patient. A number of personal issues must be addressed in order that she feels competent to make the best decision for herself, with subsequent results that she feels she is prepared to accept.

The range of problems presented to the social worker covers a broad expanse of issues. The social worker provides both emotionally supportive counselling as well as concise, factual information for her client. The following points will highlight the primary issues of concern for patients experiencing an unplanned pregnancy as these cases comprise the majority of the social worker's caseload.

II. Primary Issues of the Pregnancy in General

- patient's emotional adjustment to the pregnancy confirmation and gestational age;
- emotional and social issues relating to the circumstances of her conception; i.e., age, marital status, extramarital relationship,

sexual assault, failed sterilization, first sexual experience, incest, etc.;
- informing important others of pregnancy or in some cases ensuring that specific others do not know of the pregnancy,;i.e., father of pregnancy, parents, etc.;
- ambivalence over decision about a plan for the pregnancy;
- her OB/GYN history; i.e., previous pregnancies, live births, miscarriages, stillbirths, abortions, years of infertility, etc.;
- failure to utilize contraception or failure of method utilized;
- her relationship with the father of pregnancy and partner if not the same person, parents, siblings, friends, associations, etc.;
- previous beliefs about premarital sex, contraception, unplanned pregnancy, single parenting, adoption, abortion and the source of origin for these opinions; i.e., parent, religious background, education system, etc.;
- financial situation;
- emotional bonding to pregnancy to date and personal desire to parent now or in the future and
- the very special needs of the underage patient (15 years or younger), and the older patient (over 40 years).

III. Primary Issues of Carrying the Pregnancy with Intent to Parent

- relationship with the father of the pregnancy, family and important others; i.e., ostracism or rejection by partner or parent;
- emotional preparation for responsibility of parenting;
- early marriage or single parenting or late life parenting;
- financial concerns such as maternity benefits, unemployment insurance, general welfare, mother's allowance, parental financial support, paternal financial support, previous debts, etc.;
- housing concerns such as a teen leaving home, acquiring and furnishing an apartment, locating facilities for unwed mothers, subsidized housing, etc.;
- the psychological preparation and adjustment to the stages of pregnancy, amniocentesis, the labour and possible avenues of delivery, breast feeding versus bottle feeding, the normal progression of the post-partum period, etc.;
- continuation of education or employment during pregnancy and after the birth;
- paternal visitation rights and

   – prenatal education and layette needs.

IV. Primary Issues of Carrying the Pregnancy with Intent to Place Infant for Adoption

– previous experience with adoption; i.e., patient herself was adopted or knows of another's experience in placing an infant for adoption;
– emotional preparation for carrying pregnancy, delivery and separation from infant and long-term post-adoption adjustment;
– legal issues and choice of adoptive parents;
– social issues in regard to her ability to cope with the opinions of others;
– involvement of the father and the maternal and/or paternal grandparents in the patient's decision and contact with infant once born and
– her future relationship with the father of her infant.

V. Primary Issues of Termination of the Pregnancy

– previous experience with abortion; i.e., her own pregnancy(ies) or that of others;
– inner conflicts arising from personal moral, ethical or religious beliefs about abortion.;
– clear understanding of the therapeutic abortion procedure; i.e., fears, misconceptions, physical response and recuperation;
– emotional adjustment to having terminated a pregnancy and coping with the ramifications of decision;
– possible risks and complications of procedure and potential for affecting her childbearing ability in the future;
– pregnancy denial and requests for midtrimester therapeutic abortions;
– future relationship with father of pregnancy and future partners in regard to the abortion experience and
– request for pregnancy termination following successful conception after reversal of sterilization.

VI. Other Issues Presented for Counselling Include Sterilization (Tubal Ligation/Occlusion):

- patient's age, marital status, obstetrical and gynecological history and extenuating circumstances;
- comprehension of purpose of procedure, means by which sterilization is performed, clarity of intent for permanence and clarification of common misinformation in regard to reversal;
- acceptance of consequences of decision in light of various possible future life scenarios;
- physical and emotional response to sterilization and
- if appropriate, partner's attitude toward patient's decision.

Sterilization reversal (Tubal reanastomosis):

- patient's purpose in undergoing the reversal; i.e., for psychological reasons or for desire to become pregnant;
- patient's change in opinion, social situation or life circumstances that have brought about desire to resume fertility;
- expectations of success of procedure, understanding the complexity of procedure and ability to cope with emotional response to failure of procedure and
- if appropriate, partner's attitude toward patient's decision.

Contraception:

- previous attitude, religious beliefs, lack of knowledge, misinformation, understanding of reproductive functioning, fear, etc.;
- responsible sexuality;
- underage patient requesting contraception without parental consent and
- non-compliance to method of choice.

Sexually transmitted disease:

- emotional response to diagnosis, adjustment to treatment and/or living with disease and social ramifications;
- responsible sexuality, preventative measures, etc.
- consequences to partner(s).

Amenorrhea:

- non-physical reasons for cessation of menses;
- psychosocial issues requiring assessment to assist in diagnosis and
- eating disorders such as anorexia nervosa, bulimia nervosa, and chronic dieting in the obese patient.

Further issues addressed in counselling:

- sexual assault, incest, sexual dysfunction, menopausal depression, premenstrual syndrome (PMS) and pelvic inflammatory disease (PID).

PRACTICE ROLES AND RESPONSIBILITIES

The role of the social worker is to identify the psychosocial issues inhibiting a woman's ability to adjust to and cope with the various issues related to her obstetrical and gynecological health care. The social worker uses her clinical skills to engage the patient in addressing identified areas of concern, with a view toward enhancing the psychosocial functioning of the patient, thus promoting a healthier adjustment to changes inherent in the obstetrical or gynecological issue/illness and/or procedure/treatment process. She provides her patient with the emotional support required to assist her in undergoing an obstetrical or gynecological assessment, receiving and accepting diagnosis, and following through with necessary treatment or surgery. Further, the social worker provides supportive follow-up counselling to assist the patient with post-operative or treatment adjustment.

Unlike most other hospital settings, the patients referred to the WHCC are not always ill. In fact, many patients are very healthy but present with concerns about their ability to cope with their particular condition. Each individual approaches a solution to her problem based upon her own personal needs and circumstances. For example, a woman may be seen for pregnancy confirmation. She may be very happy that she is pregnant and anxiously looks forward to having a child and being a mother. However, there may be complicating, extenuating circumstances that make a smooth emotional progression through the pregnancy very difficult. Her socio-economic situation plays a large factor in her antic-ipated comfort with and ability to fulfil her role as mother. Another woman may be devastated in learning that the results of her pregnancy test are positive. Although carrying a healthy fetus, she may, for a number of reasons, feel that she cannot carry this pregnancy to term. Thus, two women, in the same physical condi-tion (healthy first trimester pregnancies) are functioning from very different sets of circumstances, beliefs, priorities and goals. Although their decisions may be at opposite ends of the continu-um, in that one plans to keep her pregnancy and the other plans to terminate hers, the basic emotional needs of the two women are very similar.

When dealing with unplanned pregnancy, the social worker must examine each of the patient's options with her, encourage her to examine those options she has overlooked and assist her to appreciate the inappropriateness of certain options to her situa-tion. Each of these steps must be included for the patient to per-ceive her decision as being objective and responsible. In addition, the social worker provides all the necessary information crucial for the patient to make a competent decision, ensures that she has access to resources that are available to her in the health care facili-ty and her community and creates a therapeutic environment in which a trusting relationship will develop. It is important that the social worker supports the patient in making her decision and, once made, provides her with whatever emotional assistance she needs to see the objective through to the finish. Further, the social worker supports the patient in addressing and coming to terms with the emotional ramifications of her choice. For instance, fol-low-up support is equally offered for the post-partum patient keeping her infant, the patient who has placed her infant for adop-tion and the patient who has terminated her pregnancy.

When dealing with an unplanned pregnancy, the social worker must appreciate that the woman is in the difficult position of choosing one of the three preceding options, none of which she wants to face. The fourth option, the one she desperately wants, that is not to have conceived, is not available to her. It is the author's opinion that when making their choices, many women who choose termination do not do so automatically or casually. Only when they have assessed that there is no personally feasible way for them to keep or place an infant do they turn to the third option of abortion. They generally do not welcome it or feel com-fortable with it, but see it as a means to an end. Although her intel-lectual reasonings may point to abortion as a specific woman's best option, the social worker must be alert to the emotional pain the patient may experience at giving up what might have, at another time in her life, been a joyous experience. It may be difficult for the abortion patient to understand that her grief reaction, and her sense of loss and emptiness, can mirror that of a miscarriage reaction, even though she has voluntarily given up the pregnancy. The fact that intellectual reasoning does not remove emotional pain must be addressed in counselling. The social worker assists the patient in understanding that no decision is made in an emotional void and that she will experience some inner emotional response to her decision no matter how sure the patient is of its "rightness" for her. It is certainly clear that all women do not suffer grief reactions in anticipation of, or in response to, abortion, but each woman should be given the opportunity to personally investigate her feelings, accept them, learn how she may integrate them and make peace with them in a supportive, non-judgmental, therapeutic relationship.

The means by which the social worker carries out her role in this particular OB/GYN outpatient clinic are unique and in some ways not unlike the Emergency Department in that there is a high percentage of crisis intervention work that takes place. One of the qualities crucial to the social worker performing competently in this area is her ability to be flexible, to swing with minimal confusion and stress with whatever issues arise in a given clinic day. An often heavy schedule of bookings for physicians, usually 20 – 30 patients per half day, is made by the unit ward clerk as referrals come in from the community and other physicians' offices. Priority for medical consultation is given to patients with issues requiring immediate attention. It is the objective of the WHCC that a patient receive consultation within one week of referral, and often it is sooner.

The patient or referring source is required to at least minimally describe the primary concern of the patient at the time of referral in order that the OB/GYN physician has some idea of what direction to take the questioning in determining whether a patient may be a contraception consult, a therapeutic abortion request, an annual checkup, a new obstetrics patient or a woman who is feeling very ambivalent about her unplanned pregnancy. As the physicians move through the schedule of patients and address their various needs, they also assess the patients' emotional responses to their individual situations. The physician may refer any patient s/he believes would benefit from social work intervention in relation to their presenting problem or adjustment to required treatment or care. However, due to the limited social work resources and the high demand for service, the physicians are required to priorize their referrals. For example, although it would be ideal for all women undergoing pregnancy termination to receive supportive counselling prior to their abortion, numbers of patients and resources do not allow it. Thus, in order to provide high quality service to those most in need, criteria for referrals for therapeutic abortion counselling were developed by the social worker. In brief, but not in order of importance, the priority requests include patients 17 years of age or less, patients having had one or more previous abortion(s), sexual assault patients with resultant pregnancies, patients who learn that their pregnancies are too advanced to undergo an abortion at the facility, patients who are ambivalent or in a crisis about their decision, patients with very unusual circumstances at the consultants' discretion and of course all patients who personally request counselling.

The WHCC social worker functions independently with a great deal of autonomy, yet is a vital member of the OB/GYN health care team. Thus, it is the social worker's responsibility to take her own referrals and make her own bookings for assessments, consultations and counselling appointments. She receives referrals both from the WHCC staff and directly from physicians in the community who will be referring a patient for medical care in the WHCC. As many of the women served are under a great deal of stress and are often attempting to keep their situation completely confidential, the worker's schedule is constantly being changed and altered to meet patients' individual needs.

The social worker may find that it is most beneficial to sit within touching distance from the patient, keeping notetaking to an absolute minimum, as the patient must perceive the social worker's total involvement in what is often her painful tale. Due to the highly emotional nature of the issues this client group is attempting to deal with, the social worker must be prepared to cope with and address a substantial degree of crying while her patients express their sadness, fear, anger, disappointment and often, relief at having found help. The tears may be for their unborn fetus, their own shattered plans for the future, their shame in having behaved irresponsibly, breaking religious beliefs, the loss of their relationship with the father or the anticipated disappointment of their parents.

The initial stage of the counsellor-patient rapport will be developed within the first five minutes of the interview simply in the way in which the social worker invites the patient into her office, begins to introduce herself and her role and inquires about the patient's perception of the purpose of the session. This rapport in the beginning phase is crucial to the success of the interview as contact is often crisis oriented. In cases with only one session in which to address a wide range of issues, the social worker does not get a second chance to establish a connected relationship.

Although there is variance in process depending upon the nature of the referral, it is generally the social worker's function to provide the referral source with a psychosocial assessment from the first interview by assessing the patient's major strengths, significant issues, available financial and material resources, and her emotional support system.

The social worker identifies the issues appropriate for medical social work intervention in the OB/GYN setting and also provides the necessary information and referrals for issues to be dealt with by other social services in the community when appropriate. The social worker formulates and implements an appropriate method of intervention based upon the psychosocial assessment and the woman's presenting problem, utilizing such modalities as individual and relationship counselling (dyads such as girlfriend/boyfriend, wife/husband, daughter/parent), and such therapeutic approaches as problem solving, crisis intervention, stress reduction and relaxation therapy.

The social worker supports and encourages her patients and their partners or parents where appropriate to articulate their needs and explore their emotional responses and also assists them in problem solving through the development of a therapeutic relationship. The social worker's ability to move from one patient's belief and priority system to another's, and back again, is crucial to successful counselling in this area. Further, as the very nature of sexual issues occur in a wide range of social contexts and circumstances, the social worker must be able to deal with complex details regarding the patients' relationships in a non-judgmental manner. For instance, in the case of unplanned pregnancy, the patient is not seeking advice from the social worker, but rather the necessary tools by which she can make the decision she will best be able to live with under her specific set of circumstances at this particular point in time.

In extended care cases, where contact is longer than five days, the social worker provides ongoing assessment and recommendation to the OB/GYN health care team as to the patient's adjustment to the focus of the intervention and identification of the patient's changing needs.

The social worker advocates where appropriate on behalf of her patient based upon knowledge that has been acquired during the assessment and ongoing counselling. Further, the WHCC social worker develops with her patient a follow-up plan where appropriate, prepares her for counselling termination and sets a discharge plan in co-ordination with the OB/GYN health care team.

POTENTIAL FOR ROLE DEVELOPMENT

There is great potential for further development of the social work role in this type of medical setting. The WHCC has proven to be one of the most advanced OB/GYN outpatient units in Ontario. However, even in this setting, the clients receiving social work service are but the neediest and dysfunctional in terms of coping with the issue of concern. These women are but the tip of a much larger client population who just by the highly emotional nature of their problems should be given the opportunity to address the psychosocial effects of their issues in addition to receiving excellent physical care from a medical facility.

The obvious starting point for extension of social work service is increased funding, but even prior to that, the hospital administration and referring physicians must develop a deeper appreciation and recognition of the dual focus of many of these obstetrical and gynecological issues. It is not enough to relieve a 17-year-old of an unwanted pregnancy, provide a 15-year-old with birth control pills, sterilize a single woman or place an 18-year-old's baby for adoption. To say that we provide the best physical medical/surgical care for these female patients is not enough. If the goal of assisting the patient to the healthiest adjustment possible is to be met, then all women receiving obstetrical or gynecological care should be given the opportunity to address the issues surrounding their particular circumstances with a competent social worker, well versed in the specific medical situation in addition to her therapeutic counselling skills.

To date, all issues concerning patient psychosocial adjustment to specific medical conditions have been addressed by the social worker in individual, couple or family sessions. The patient has been viewed as responding to a given situation in a very unique way based upon her specific set of circumstances at the point at which the problem had impact upon her life. However, the author is of the opinion that a follow-up support group format could be effective in adjustment to specific issues such as therapeutic abortion, miscarriage, adoption and premenstrual syndrome. These groups would not take the place of individual counselling but could be a supplement to highly personal information addressed in counselling. In each of these instances, there is strength to be mutually acquired by learning through the group that one is not alone with one's emotional response or one's physical reaction to an experience or condition the members share in common. The social worker cannot fulfil this need for her patient but she can facilitate the opportunity for her patients to voluntarily meet together. Thus, the utilization of support groups is high on the priority list for the development of the WHCC social work role in the early 1990s.

Further expansion of the social work role in the 1990s will hopefully include a formal recognition of the needs of the male partner and thus more extensive counselling services for the father of an unplanned pregnancy. At this time, any man requesting social work service in regard to his partner's pregnancy is provided with emotional support and counselling around the issues resultant from his partner's decision about the pregnancy. Consent from the female patient is obtained and clear lines of confidentiality are determined. However, very few men request this service, perhaps fearing that they will be criticized for the woman's condition or that they are not entitled to recognition of their emotional response to the pregnancy and/or termination. It is the author's opinion that there are many men who receive no support during this difficult time and that many quietly experience the emotional impact of their pregnancy and the decision that they were powerless to make long into their futures. It is anticipated that this expansion of service on a more formal level would include male contraceptive teaching, sexually transmitted disease and responsible sexuality.

The WHCC social worker has always placed a high level of importance upon the preventative/educational component in each counselling session. In situations where improved knowledge, understanding or judgment could have made a difference in the patient's issue of concern, the social worker not only assists the patient with psychosocial adjustment but perceives her responsibility further to include the provision of factually correct information and the development of psychological tools that the patient may choose to utilize in the future to prevent a recurrence of a similar problem.

The WHCC team has, over the past two years, begun to carry the "prevention through education" theme through to community outreach programs, recognizing that there are high-risk groups who are repeatedly seen in the WHCC and who upon assessment have not had sufficient and/or appropriate information necessary to make the decisions essential to responsible sexual behaviour. In response to this need, the social worker and head nurse of the WHCC have begun to provide community education programs to groups who have primary involvement with specific high-risk populations. These information sessions have been provided in such settings as the local Contact Crisis Centre, the Detention Centre and University Health Services Centre.

However, over the past year it became apparent that although these group presentations and discussions were beneficial to those small numbers addressed, it was not serving the purpose of having the maximum impact upon those most in the position to absorb and implement new sexual behaviours and attitudes. Most of the individuals in the early community education groups were women with well established behaviourial and attitudinal patterns.

Thus, the most recent attempt at community education is a project which has been entitled "The Adolescent Outreach Program" and is a collaborative effort between Victoria Hospital, the London Board of Education and the Middlesex-London District Health Unit. The Chief of Obstetrics and Gynecology at Victoria Hospital, the head nurse of the delivery room and WHCC and the social worker of the WHCC were involved from the earliest stages in planning this program for senior secondary school students in the city of London. The concept of an educational package presented by the joint effort of these three publicly funded groups (medical facility/health care provider, education facility and public health educator) was very positively supported by the community. The theme of "responsible sexuality" is carried throughout the educational kit. The classroom teacher and public health nurse jointly present the information to the students over six sessions. The class then participates in a tour and discussion of the specific areas of the hospital (WHCC, labour and delivery, post-partum, newborn nursery and pediatric critical care unit) presented in the teaching sessions, which include human sexuality, fetal growth and development, the process of child birth, teen pregnancy and parenting, the concept and application of contraception and sexually transmitted diseases. Again, the social worker is involved in the planning and facilitating of this preventive, community-based approach to health care that recognizes the very valuable educational tool found in "hands on experience."

Future plans for the WHCC encompass a concept of a facility that would provide an even greater range of services for women. Such issues of concern as eating disorders, breast health care, sexual dysfunctioning, premenstrual syndrome and infertility have been discussed and examined as possible areas in which the clinic could expand to provide even more complete women's health care.

There is no doubt that the role of the social worker in women's health care will continue to develop in new and exciting ways in the 1990s in each of the planning, facilitating, service provision and evaluation stages.

CONCLUDING REMARKS

The opportunity for a female social worker to practise in a women's health care centre is most fulfilling both professionally and personally. The issues addressed are those that reach women at the deepest part of their being and require them to examine themselves, their feelings and their beliefs in ways they may never have previously imagined. The social worker plays a critical role in emotionally assisting her female patients through what often appears to be a complicated progression of frightening, dehumanizing, painful and confusing experiences, even though each may have been presented as being a specific and necessary component in her care. It is most often the social worker who assists the patient to understand and integrate her experience.

The social work position in outpatient OB/GYN health care is relatively new in that it was created through a Social Work Department initiative only six years ago in 1982, when the administration and physicians agreed that women required more than excellent physical care in response to these sensitive issues. Today, the relationship between physician, nurse and social worker is finely tuned. The psychosocial assessment and supportive counselling provided by the social worker are often seen as crucial to the success of a patient's experience and adjustment.

It is anticipated that community education toward responsible sexuality will continue to be a primary focus in the 1990s and the social worker in women's health care will undoubtedly play a vital role. Further, the social work role will require forefront involvement in the strong push toward preventative health care both within the facility, through the WHCC and within the community through public education and outreach programs.

CASE EXAMPLE

Ann was a 20-year-old single college student who made a self-referral to the WHCC requesting a pregnancy test because her usually regular menstrual period was two weeks late. After examination by the doctor, Ann was determined to be 6-7 weeks pregnant and when asked if she had made any decisions about her situation, she broke down and wept in despair. Ann was offered the opportunity to meet immediately with the WHCC social worker to discuss her circumstances and the various options and resources available to her both through the WHCC and the community. Ann gratefully accepted the offer, stating that she was extremely confused, and she proceeded through the interview process to give the following social history.

Ann graduated from grade 12 at the age of 18 and was now in her second and final year at a college in the city. She lived near the college in an apartment that she shared with two other female students. Ann had grown up and lived in a close relationship with her natural parents and younger brother in a small town about 60 miles away. She had met 22-year-old Peter, the father of her pregnancy, through a friend during her first month living away from home and had dated him seriously for the following year and a half. Peter had graduated from grade 12 four years previously and had since been contentedly working full-time in his father's business. Ann had remained a virgin throughout high school and had her first sexual experience with Peter after they had been dating about six months. Although they had always used condoms during intercourse, she had thought about going to get birth control pills, but with the demands of school and the apparent success of what they were using for contraception, she had procrastinated. Ann had told both Peter and her parents of her fear that she was pregnant because she felt that they also needed time to prepare themselves. Their responses had contributed to her sense of confusion and dismay. Although Peter had told her that he would support her no matter what her decision, he had gone on to say that he had never believed in abortion and that he felt that it would be best if they were to get married and have the baby. On the other hand, Ann's parents were very distressed about the possibility of their only daughter's pregnancy. They told Ann that they felt that abortion was the only option for her and that having the baby at this time and in this way would only ruin her life and that of the child.

Prior to learning of her pregnancy, Ann's plans for the future had been to finish college and begin the full-time job she had already acquired through her co-op program experience. Although her family had attempted to assist her financially, their own income was limited and she had, therefore, acquired a substantial amount of debt through student loans and fully realized her responsibility in repaying this debt. Ann had imagined herself as working for several years, doing some travelling and then perhaps marrying and starting a family in her mid to late twenties. She had been thrilled with her relationship with Peter initially and continued to have strong feelings for him. However, over the past three or four months she had begun to realize that they had very different life goals and that perhaps Peter was not going to be her choice for a long-term partner. These feelings were only magnified when Peter began pursuing the idea of their immediate marriage to legitimize the pregnancy. Although she was christened in the United Church as an infant, Ann's family had not been active participants over the years and she had not attended church since going to college. She had never pictured herself having an abortion, yet she did not have strong negative feelings about those who chose to have one. She had really never given it much thought until now. Ann's parents had been married right after high school and neither of them had the opportunity to have any post-secondary education. Ann had been born only a year after their marriage and her brother eighteen months later. Ann reflected that her mother had a rather difficult life raising two children and working full-time at relatively low wages and she felt that her parents had always taught their children to want more from life. Ann was very angry with her parents' response to her fears of being pregnant. She felt that once again her parents were telling her what to do and not giving her the credit to make the best decision for herself.

Utilizing the social worker's assistance, Ann determined that her options were: to marry Peter and raise their child; to remain single and raise their child on her own or with Peter's and/or her parents' assistance; to remain single, carry the pregnancy but place the child for adoption or to terminate the pregnancy, and remain with Peter or end the relationship with him.

Ann worked through these options by addressing her own priority and belief system. This process revealed that

1) she felt that she was not ready emotionally to be responsible for a dependent child;
2) she felt that she was not ready for the commitment or responsibility of marriage;
3) she was uncertain of the future of her relationship with Peter;
4) she felt that she could not ask her parents to take on responsibility of her child;
5) she felt strong negative feelings toward single parenting;
6) she refused to consider accepting public financial assistance;
7) her education and future career opportunity were primary priorities at this time;
8) she experienced no strong moral or ethical conflicts in regard to pregnancy termination and
9) she felt that she could not follow through with placing an infant for adoption after carrying and delivering.

Ann went home to her parents after the interview with the social worker, far clearer about her own belief system and armed with factually correct information. She had been offered an opportunity to address her most personal desires and plans and to examine her own strengths, weaknesses, hopes and fears in a safe, supportive, non-judgmental therapeutic relationship.

In this case, Ann chose to terminate her pregnancy. The lengthy process of working through the issues was crucial to Ann's ownership of her decision and her future responsibility for consequences both positive and negative resultant from her decision. It was essential for Ann to realize that this was her decision, based upon her own beliefs and acceptance of herself as an individual, quite separate from what her parents or her boyfriend had wanted her to do for their own reasons. Ann was encouraged and supported by the social worker to present this information both to Peter and her parents prior to undergoing her abortion, and she did this with very positive results.

At a follow-up interview, one month after her abortion, Ann reviewed the process of the difficult weeks before her procedure and described her own evaluation of her experience.

In her discussion with her parents and boyfriend, Ann

addressed her need to make her own decisions and to take responsibility for the consequences as a young, independent adult. She felt her parents had a new respect for her ability to discuss these issues on a more mature level. Ann hoped that this crisis, although emotionally painful, had opened the pathway for generally improved communication between herself and her parents. Although Peter had told her that he understood her decision, Ann was not sure about the future of their relationship. Even though this saddened her, she did not regret her decision. Ann reflected that she had learned things about herself that she previously hadn't had reason to address. She believed that she had acquired new personal skills and strengths from which she would be able to draw when confronted with other major issues in her life. Further, Ann clearly recognized that this pregnancy and voluntary termination would not be forgotten, as if it had never occurred, as she had once thought would be possible, but she knew that she had made the right decision for herself and felt that she had the strength to look ahead, in a positive direction to her future.

References

Berger, C. (1984). *Abortion: A Counsellor's Guide.* Ottawa: Canadian Public Health Association.

Birnbaum, J. (1979). *Cry Anger.* Toronto: Paperjack.

Gardner, J. (1985). *Abortion – a Personal Approach.* Seattle: Snohomish Publishing Co.

Hatcher, R., Josephs, N., Stewart, F., Guest, F., Stewart, G. & Kowal, D. (1982). *It's Your Choice.* New York: Irvington Publishers.

Ooms, T. (Ed.) (1981). *Teenage Pregnancy in a Family Context.* Philadelphia: Temple University Press.

Pipes, M. (1986). *Understanding Abortion.* London: The Women's Press Ltd.

Stein, R. A. (1983). *Personal Strategies For Living With Less Stress.* New York: John Gallagher Communications Ltd.

Chapter 13

SOCIAL WORK PRACTICE WITH DOMESTIC VIOLENCE IN HOSPITAL SETTINGS

Don Ebert, MSW
Shan Landry, MSW

Abstract

It is a medical problem which brings the patient to hospital, however, it is the interrelationship of the social and emotional factors of domestic violence which demand social work involvement. Social workers must take leadership, not only in the delivery of direct patient services, but also in the development of domestic violence intervention protocols and programs, and the teaching of other health care professionals. It is the social worker's unique training in treating the patient as a whole person and interacting within a social and familial context that gives shape and focus to his/her role in domestic violence.

SOCIAL WORK PRACTICE WITH DOMESTIC VIOLENCE IN HOSPITAL SETTINGS

Social workers in health settings must have knowledge about varied and numerous social problems and issues. Every day, hospitals treat hundreds of people whose illnesses and injuries are directly or indirectly related to social and/or emotional trauma. Alcoholism, poverty and prostitution are examples of social ills that may result in an individual seeking or receiving medical treatment. One social problem that has been overlooked for many years, and is still often ignored, is a problem that affects many Canadian lives: domestic violence. Every year, thousands of Canadian families experience the anger, frustration, stress, poor impulse control and low self-esteem that leads to interpersonal violence and to victimization of children, women and the elderly. To work effectively in a health care setting, most notably a hospital, social work practitioners must be fully cognizant of and conversant with the etiology and reality of domestic violence, and with their own personal value system, which impacts on this knowledge. They must also be able to apply their knowledge and practice skills to work with both the client system and their professional colleagues on a multi-disciplinary team.

Social workers in a hospital are secondary not primary caregivers. They are often dependent on others in the hospital to identify and refer clients as, usually, patients do not come to the hospital seeking social work assistance. Someone else, most often another health care professional, must make the connection between the medical problem and the social problem. In the case of domestic violence, the client and the medical caregiver often form a relationship that impedes the referral to medical social work in that the client and medical personnel collude to treat the medical problem while ignoring the social and emotional aspects of the social and familial problem.

Examples of this "blocking" phenomenon related to domestic violence referrals came from a limited survey completed in one urban Canadian hospital emergency department by the Saskatchewan Interhospital Domestic Violence Committee. For example, over a two month period, researchers examined medical charts of all women over 16 years of age seen in the Emergency department. They found 20 cases where the precipitating cause for the emergency visit was clearly stated on the chart as domestic violence (spousal abuse). None of those 20 women received a referral to the social work department. Ten of the women received medical treatment only, and the other 10 received psychiatric consultation in conjunction with medical treatment. Psychiatric consultation appeared to result from recorded evidence of the client's previous psychiatric problems rather than the reported violence. This could be interpreted to mean that the reported violence was perceived by the health caregiver as a psychiatric problem of the victim rather than an interpersonal relationship problem between the partners. For those 10 women without a psychiatric history, the system completely failed to address the social problem of domestic violence (Saskatchewan Health, 1986).

For the purposes of this discussion, examples of domestic violence are confined specifically to spousal abuse. While each form of domestic violence—child, spousal, and elder abuse—has its unique issues in the assessment, treatment and discharge process, many of the basic principles associated with cause and symptoms are identical and the multiple roles of the social worker as policy maker, educator, advocate, problem-solver, consultant and counsellor are synonymous.

THE CLIENTELE

Spousal abuse involves victims and perpetrators (abusers) and is present in all levels of society. Therefore, the issues of who is the client and where the client might be found in the health care setting must be addressed first.

Spousal abuse is most commonly recognized in its physical form. Women who have bruises, broken limbs, lacerations and other injuries are likely, if identified at all as victims, to be most easily recognized. But abuse can take other forms. Women may be sexually abused with no outward signs of the violence that has been perpetrated against them. Further, women may be emotionally and/or verbally abused; told they are worthless, have their behaviour controlled and find themselves humiliated and psychologically scarred. Or, women may suffer the acute emotional pain associated with the destruction of something that one loves, by seeing their valued possessions damaged or watching their pets harmed or killed.

Social workers must be aware that whatever the form abuse takes, victims may seek medical assistance for only the obvious physical injury. At other times, they may outwardly seek assistance for the physical injury while attempting, sometimes unsuccessfully, to also address and draw attention to the less obvious psychological trauma.

In our current North American society, it is well accepted that the answer to pain is "taking a pill," and the administration of medication becomes the desired analgesic prescription. Domestic violence creates pain — the pain of emotional hurt, severely diminished self-esteem, humiliation and degradation, together with physical pain. In seeking to avoid pain, it is not unusual, therefore, to see both the patient and the helping professional use medication as a panacea; thus a collusion results in that the patient's anticipated solution for the pain coincides with the prescribed treatment.

I. Victims in the Emergency Room

Domestic violence victims may be found anywhere in a hospital from employees in administrative offices to the patients arriving at out-patient clinics. In the emergency room, patients may present with multiple bruises, fractures and other physical injuries that frequently do not correspond directly with the explanation given by the patient herself. It is also known that there may be a time lapse of anywhere from a few hours to two days after the violent incident before the client seeks treatment in the hospital (Roy, 1982). The victims of violence who seek medical treatment but delay arriving at the hospital for that treatment often deal with fear, guilt, denial and a wish to mask any symptoms that would point directly to violence. Many women are also reluctant to seek treatment because they are known to emergency room personnel as having been treated previously for similar complaints. It is crucial to recognize that the eventual arrival at the emergency department may be indicative of the patient's need for more than medical treatment and might be a silent "cry for help." A North American study has revealed that 21% of adult women who seek treatment in emergency rooms are there as a direct or indirect result of domestic violence (Ghent, Da Sylva & Farren, 1985).

The severity of the injuries that result from physical violence, on the other hand, may lead to an immediate in-patient admission. In these situations, the medical staff are, and must be initially, focussed on the specific medical treatment. The precipitating factors and a consideration of their implications necessarily become secondary. However, after the required medical treatment, or in those situations where the injury is not severe enough to require extensive treatment, the patient/client may openly share information about the cause of injury without the hospital staff responding to this newly revealed information. An example of this follows.

> During a dressing change for a severe burn, Rose, 25 years old, mentioned to the nurse that her boyfriend had thrown scalding water at her. This comment was recorded on the chart by the nurse, but no affirmative action was taken to investigate or resolve a definite domestic violence situation.

Another problem that arises in the emergency room treatment process is that staff may see the same patients on a repeating basis for a variety of injuries. This pattern of repeat visits may reinforce the myth that some women enjoy violence and even provoke it. "Blaming the victim" is not unusual, and it is known that some women may seek community assistance (leave their husbands and move to shelters, etc.) several times before they permanently sever a relationship (MacLeod, 1987). Women may also return to an abusive relationship if professionals have not provided them with sufficient information to gain strength and make informed decisions and take action (Ghent, Da Sylva & Farren, 1985).

II. Victims on Inpatient Wards

As mentioned above, the most obvious form of domestic violence is physical abuse. However, patients receiving treatment may be suffering from other less obvious but equally damaging forms of violence. For instance, some victims report that emotional abuse is infinitely more painful than physical abuse. In many situations, the physical pain heals faster than emotional scars.

Some patients present diagnostic problems in their reluctance or inability to articulate the pathological factors in their environments. This frequently results in misdiagnosis and a negative labelling of clients that has implications for future health care services.

> Jane, 38 years old and a Chartered Accountant, had a series of admissions to hospital for severe abdominal pains. Each medical investigation revealed no organic basis for the

complaints. Jane was labelled and it was written in her chart that she was "over fastidious and inappropriately anxious about her health." Six months after her fifth admission, a new internist seeing her in the emergency room of the hospital and with no prior knowledge of the patient's history, discovered through compassionate questioning that Jane's husband was being sexually abusive to her.

Although social workers cannot assume that every patient admitted to a hospital has an underlying problem associated with domestic violence, the possibility must always be considered in a thorough psychosocial assessment. Social workers must be aware that patients recover faster, leave hospital sooner and return less often if they are treated as whole persons with accompanying social and emotional dimensions. Patients admitted for surgery, or investigation and treatment of an illness which may be totally unrelated to abuse may nevertheless be experiencing abuse in their relationship. A woman admitted for routine gallbladder surgery may find excuses to stay in a hospital several days longer if she is frightened to return home to an abusive and angry spouse who will expect her to resume heavy housekeeping chores immediately.

III. Victims in Outpatient Clinics

In the recognition of abuse one cannot limit oneself to the emergency room and in-patient wards, but must also broaden the scope of parameters to include the multitude of medical out-patient clinics. One high-risk group of patients attending out-patient clinics are those dealing with long-term chronic illnesses. Often the stresses associated with these illnesses create fertile ground for tension culminating in violence within the family. These clients may be most reluctant to identify the abuse because they already feel vulnerable in their relationships as a result of their illness. This is often compounded by the realization that their illness has made them dependent upon their spouse both financially and physically.

Margaret, age 51, has been wheelchair dependent for the last 10 years due to progressive symptoms of Multiple Sclerosis. In a review of her medical situation at the outpatient MS clinic, Margaret stated her embarrassment over recently developed bladder incontinence. Her husband, bringing her in for treatment was overheard talking to her in baby talk and cruelly teasing her about wearing diapers. Margaret refused to let staff talk to her husband as she stated "I'm grateful for him keeping me at home and out of a nursing home for the last 10 years. If he got angry at me where could I go but to an institution? Please don't upset him."

IV. Victims on Psychiatry Units

The hospital staff caring for psychiatric patients must also be well versed in the symptomatology and identification of domestic violence, as a large number of female psychiatric patients have been victims of such abusive relationships. For instance, patients may be admitted to acute psychiatry for depression, substance abuse and psychoses. These diagnoses may well be appropriate, but may also be symptoms of violence. In fact, statistics show that one out of every four suicide attempts by adult women is attributable to battering (Ghent, Da Sylva & Farren, 1985).

V. The Abuser

Domestic violence is not a single-person phenomenon. Abuse requires that there are at least two people involved in the occurrence. Therefore, it is important for the social worker to see her/his clientele as not always, or only, the victims of abuse. The perpetrator of the violence, often guilty, afraid, remorseful or even still angry, is an integral part of the client system. The social worker must recognize that rather than being a "bad" person, the perpetrator has frequently come from an abusive upbringing and learned to deal with frustrations in relationships through violent methods (Roy, 1982). The etiology of the abusive personality, the abuser's anger and poor impulse control, his desire or need to control others, extreme stress and low self-esteem must also be addressed by the health professional for the benefit of both the victim and the abuser.

Counselling specifically for abusive men, often in a group context is a relatively new phenomenon in Canadian cities (Currie 1988). Either sentenced by a court or seeking help voluntarily (quite rare) the abusive man is assisted in learning methods of anger control and impulse control. Violence is a learned behaviour as over 81% of men who abuse their wives are reported to have been victims themselves as children, or lived in households where they observed violence (Roy, 1982).

Since we now understand and are ready to treat the situation of the abuser, hospitals must also be prepared to assess male patients in the area of domestic violence as readily as they would women.

VI. Victims in the Health Professions

A recent statistic from the National Clearing House on Family Violence in Ottawa indicated that one out of ten Canadian women are victims of abuse (MacLeod, 1987). Therefore, social workers in health care settings must recognize that some of their health care colleagues will also be the victims/perpetrators of abuse, or may have witnessed abuse in their childhood. It is unique to the health care field that social workers are recognized to be both a colleague and a service resource to other professionals looking for a resolution of personal problems. The situation is not just a "we, they" concept.

> Susan, 28 years old and a head nurse in the emergency department, worked with a social worker to develop a pamphlet on child abuse. During the course of their discussions and work, Susan confided that her husband had been abused as a child and was showing some of the symptoms mentioned in the pamphlet. The social worker and Susan investigated possible resources in the community for Susan's husband.

PRACTICE ROLES AND RESPONSIBILITIES

The practice responsibilities for the social worker in the abuse situation begin long before the face to face contact with the client. The social worker must take **leadership** in establishing an environment within the hospital where recognition of the responsibility to treat the whole person is one of the primary considerations of care.

There is an identifiable role and process for the social worker that must be accomplished long before the assessment and treatment of the actual client system. Due to the inter-relatedness of social, emotional and medical factors and social work expertise in these areas, it is important that the Social Work Department identify the need for, and participate in the drafting of policies and protocols related to the identification, assessment, and intervention process specific to domestic violence. Much work is involved in the process of enlisting the co-operation and support of social work colleagues, other professionals (including hospital administrators), and ultimately the Medical Advisory Committee and hospital Board.

Hospitals are responsible for delivering multiple services that reflect a continuum of care embracing medical, social and emotional concerns. The social worker's continuing presence and practice in a health setting reinforces the necessity and capacity to facilitate the connection for the client and fellow professionals between the medical, social and emotional aspects of the illness and injury. Social work practice must, as stated previously, commence with raising the institution's consciousness level about domestic violence. The social worker must not assume that other health care professionals are aware of, and/or understand the facts related to domestic violence. In fact, many professionals believe the myths commonly held by the lay-public. For example, many hospital staff erroneously believe that abuse takes place only in lower socio-economic families; therefore, they often fail to recognize the signs and symptoms of domestic violence in patients who are well-off, or appear educated and well-dressed (MacLeod, 1987). The social worker assists others to recognize and understand that the cause of the violence must be treated in addition to the acute symptoms.

Once identification of the problem occurs, the social worker must continue to provide leadership. For example, a health care professional's identification of a domestic violence situation may demand involvement with a family thath has a history of long-standing problems. This may be overwhelming and frustrating if the professional is not experienced in working with chronic, and/or multi-problem family dynamics. It is the social worker, skilled at dealing with such situations, who must provide leadership in assessment and treatment. One matter that inhibits health professionals (including social work) from responding appropriately is the possibility of being subpoenaed to appear in court to provide testimony in a case. The possibility of a court action is never a legitimate excuse for not becoming involved. Rather, it may be a reality and, as a result, all health care staff must be meticulous and conscientious in recording events on the client chart. Clear, concise records facilitate accurate court review and presentation of violence.

The issue of documentation (recording or charting) itself in domestic violence cases is a hotly debated topic in a hospital setting. For example, many professionals are reluctant to record the fact that abuse has been confirmed because they believe in the myth that violence is a private family matter and/or because they fear that the patient will be stigmatized. This pseudo-concern for confidentiality is often rationalized as protective of the patient [the victim] when in fact, it is the abuser who is being protected. A woman who admits that she has been abused is unlikely to have concerns about documentation of the abuse that harmed her (Ghent, Da Sylva & Farren 1985).

This highlights again the notion that domestic violence is not a neutral problem. It evokes strong personal and emotional responses that may cloud clear decision making and the development of responsible policies on the part of all who must make those policies.

Of course, like other social problems, the victim or client system is also vulnerable and often unlikely to be willing or able to demand a responsive institution. A woman who has been emotionally and verbally abused by her husband and repeatedly told she is "no good" and/or "stupid" is hardly likely to be assertive and demand compassion and acceptance and protective involvement from the health care staff who treat her. In a similar manner, an abuser suffering fear and remorse is unlikely to insist that any hospital staff refer him for help.

Social workers must be skilled **problem solvers** who can balance both the affective and cognitive components of the controversial domestic violence subject. One of the concepts that social workers employ in problem-solving is that they cannot do things for or to other people. A client who presents with a domestic violence problem cannot simply be given a behaviourial prescription as to how to solve her problem. It is not unusual to hear well-intended professionals give strong advice to the patient as a "cure" for the problem. Advice such as, "leave that terrible man immediately," or "take him to court for assault and he will learn he can't do this to you," do not truly help her solve her problem and may even exacerbate it. There are many reasons why she cannot leave: no money, fear of reprisals, no place to go, lack of self-confidence, a sense of humiliation, lack of friends and supportive family, a hope that life will improve, strong feelings of love or utter overwhelming discouragement (e.g., what's the use?). These same issues may further prevent her from taking steps to affirmatively and productively stop the violence. A prescription for solution gives no credence to the client as a complex individual with inner resources.

The social worker's job as a problem-solver involves developing a relationship with the client and working with her to achieve a sense of self-competence and the skills and knowledge to make decisions and take action. The social worker must never choose the solution and push the client in that direction. The social worker assists the client in clearly delineating the problem, reviewing options and resources and also potential consequences of each action. When the client ultimately makes her own decision, the social worker must accept that decision.

In the role as **counsellor**, the social worker acts not only in a supportive role but also as a catalyst for change with the victim and at times the victimizer/abuser. As noted, skilled counsellors recognize that imposing a solution removes responsibility and forces a value set upon the client that may impede change. As defined by the nature of the setting, social work intervention usually requires short-term counselling and referral to the appropriate community agency for follow-up.

> Called by the emergency nurse, the social worker spent two hours in emergency with Bernice who was being treated for lacerations and bruises. During their time together, the social worker helped Bernice recognize the increasing frequency of violent episodes between her and her husband. The social worker also pointed out the potential danger to both Bernice and her three children and the need for respite. Bernice decided to go to a women's shelter and the social worker arranged a referral for the family.

In addition to problem-solving skills, the social worker as a counsellor needs specifically to

1. understand medical symptomatology;
2. understand and put into perspective her own personal values and beliefs;
3. respond to the client with a non-judgmental attitude;
4. have a working knowledge of the community resources both informal and formal and
5. be capable of interpreting for other health professionals the system dynamics and ultimate disposition of each case.

While the social worker may assist others in the hospital to prepare the groundwork for policies, her role as **educator** becomes paramount after a protocol (a step-by-step procedure) is established. The focus with the health care professionals is to provide them with knowledge of the cycle of violence, the potential escalation of anger and the severity and frequency of violence. The social worker must expunge myths surrounding violence and promote and teach an awareness of available resources in the community. In addition, the social worker assists in the application of knowledge to develop intervention skills and techniques. The social worker's ability at interviewing, assessment, crisis intervention and problem-solving are all available to be shared with others. If the social worker in a hospital attempts to be protective and secretive of her skills, if she expects others only to identify domestic violence situations and then turn over the "case" to her, she is defeating the very uniqueness and importance of social work practice in health care. As Wax (1968) pointed out, power and strength in practice come from sharing knowledge and teaching skills to others who work with us. A social worker who manages to teach an emergency room physician the skills of crisis counselling in domestic violence beyond the medical has, albeit indirectly, assisted the client in dealing with the problem. Social workers need to view and promote themselves as teachers in this process.

Analogously, the worker in her role as an educator with the client, shares knowledge about violence and enables her, once she has achieved an understanding of the situation, to make informed choices based upon sound knowledge and a review of the consequences related to each potential decision for action.

The social worker must **advocate** on behalf of the client within the hospital to ensure the client's needs are met. Externally, the social worker must be able to identify gaps in service and to advocate for the development of new resources. The hospital is not an isolated practice setting and the social worker's responsibility is to connect the hospital to the community of which it is a part.

A social worker assigned to a psychiatry in-patient department saw a number of clients and identified amongst them a pattern of inadequate day care and marital stress culminating in physical abuse. Forming an *ad hoc* committee with representatives from the YWCA and the Family Service Bureau, the social worker assisted in the development of a community crisis nursery.

One of the responsibilities of the social work profession is the sharing of psycho-social knowledge with other health care professionals. In the role of a **consultant**, the social worker gives guid-

227

ance, direction, encouragement and/or support to the activities of other health care professionals on the team. Frequently, the social worker is called upon to help other team members deal with the stress that comes from emotional involvement in individual care situations. As noted, domestic violence creates strong personal and emotional response that has the potential to erode professional objectivity. Like other social problems and value dilemmas, domestic violence may demand an involvement level from the professional far beyond that of dispassionate hands-on treatment.

POTENTIAL FOR ROLE DEVELOPMENT

As social workers, our ability to understand human behaviour and to perceive the client as an individual within a social context, and our skills in community development, afford great opportunities for many unique roles, some of which are described herein.

I. Community Development

Hospitals are becoming increasingly aware of the need for a "continuum of care" with the consequence that they perceive value in community involvement. Social work as a profession has an extended history in the process of linking systems together. The wider vision of hospital administrators and the current mission statements of many hospitals provide legitimacy for the social work role. As a result, it is most appropriate that health care workers become actively involved on boards of transition houses and with inter-agency committees assisting in the development of community resources to meet the needs of domestic violence victims and abusers, and to identify new and additional intervention and prevention resources.

II. Teaching

Health science colleges (in particular medicine and nursing) are beginning to recognize the interrelationship between the social, emotional and physical factors in health care. This provides social workers with new roles in teaching and participating in the design of human growth and development curricula for these colleges. It is important that social work move into these areas with confidence, recognizing its expertise in the social and emotional aspects of health service. The profession must guard against territorialism and find useful methods to encourage other professions to achieve understanding of the "whole person."

III. Administration and Management

Historically, social workers in psychiatric settings have been recognized for their clinical and administrative skills. It is not uncommon, therefore, to find senior social workers appointed as co-ordinators of intake programs, adolescent teams, clinical outpatient teams, etc. In other than mental health settings, though, this recognition of skills has not developed as quickly as one would have expected. As social workers manage caseloads of clients, so are they able, quite effectively, to manage teams of co-workers and professionals. Social workers must first recognize their own skills in human resource management before they promote their abilities to hospital administration and medical staff.

IV. Team-Builder

The developing awareness of domestic violence may result in social workers providing leadership in the establishment of domestic violence teams (family crisis teams) that would deal with abuse cases as they present to the hospital. The development of such a team, involving many different professionals, provides a natural opportunity for social workers to assume the role of co-ordinator or overall case manager.

V. Research

Social workers must recognize and assume responsibility for clinical and epidemiological studies in domestic violence. The value of research cannot be underestimated in specifically giving direction to the role as advocate. Practitioners are already aware that accurate delineation of the form and incidence of abuse through research and evaluation has resulted in increased resources for victims (MacLeod, 1987).

CONCLUDING REMARKS

It is clear that the social worker plays a multitude of roles and works with a wide range of clientele in health care settings, in particular, hospitals. In cases of domestic violence, the practice approach must be designed comprehensively. The key for effective assessment and intervention lies in a multi-disciplinary team process. Team membership requires that the social worker has a commitment to collaborative and cooperative problem-solving both with fellow professionals and the clientele.

As a member of the professional team, the social worker brings to the problem psycho-social knowledge and a comprehensive understanding of health that includes more than medical or physiological well-being. The social worker must develop the ability to know when to act as a team leader and team resource facilitator, and when to assert herself as a case manager. The social worker must also be willing to promote other health care professionals as team members and direct service providers.

The case examples and references included here have focussed specifically on spousal abuse and its particular dynamics; however, all forms of domestic violence (child, spousal and elder abuse) share certain common characteristics including pain and personal turmoil for the victim. While victims may differ in age, they all share a vulnerability and sense of entrapment. The definitions and forms of abuse vary only slightly.

There are some legal protections in place especially for victims of abuse. In Canada, all provinces have laws that make it mandatory for people to report to authorities situations where children may be "at-risk" and in need of protection. These laws should make it somewhat easier for social workers in hospitals to insist on multi-disciplinary team programs for accurate identification and treatment of abused children. However, despite these laws and increasing public awareness, there remain thousands of children who are physically and sexually abused and neglected every year. Similar to cases of spousal abuse, health care professionals need education in order to dispel their misconceptions and take responsibility for action in preventing abuse. Much work remains to be done in this area.

To date, the laws pertaining to elder abuse are at the most elementary level. This form of violence has only recently begun to be identified and researched. Only one Canadian province (Nova

Scotia) has legislation that directly protects the frail, vulnerable, incapacitated elderly from caregivers who mistreat them. The elderly are frequent users of the health care system (CMA, 1987). Therefore, social workers have a pioneer role in work with elder abuse victims and their social network.

Research has demonstrated that the cycle of violence is common to all forms of abuse in that there is a pattern wherein families repeatedly experience the tension build-up, the explosions of violence and the caring respite phases. Newer research shows that the cyclical pattern may have a secondary application of a generational cycle where children, adults and the elderly take turns, in various life stages, in the roles of victims and abusers. The elderly person who is abused may well now be the victim of the adult whom he once abused.

The actual and potential roles for social workers in health care settings are similar whatever the form of domestic violence. Breaking the cycle of violence becomes the goal no matter who the client is.

Social workers have a responsibility to promote the right of women, children and the elderly to live a life free of violence, and to fulfil their purpose as change agents in the treatment and prevention of domestic violence. To do this, we must achieve for ourselves practice skills that enable and produce change in others. Practitioners must seek to develop and structure a caring environment where victims and perpetrators of abuse are assisted to make changes towards more rewarding, positive social relationships and to promote the achievement of total health.

CASE EXAMPLE

The social worker in a large general hospital was called to the emergency department one evening to speak to Mrs. M, a married woman with three daughters aged eight, six and four.

The social worker learned from the physician and nurse in emergency that Mrs. M had four previous visits to the department in the last four months. On each occasion, the doctor and nurse were concerned that Mrs. M's explanation as to the cause of her injuries did not fit well with the nature of injuries she presented. On every visit, Mrs. M was adamant that she is "just a clumsy person." Mr. M was in the waiting room and appeared to be oversolicitous with his wife and agitated about the length of time emergency staff were taking to deal with her injury. He made repetitious requests for information about his wife. The nurse, who called the social worker, explained that all of these factors had led to a query about possible spousal abuse.

The social worker introduced herself to Mrs. M in the examining room and Mrs. M immediately responded that she did not need social work services. The social worker ignored Mrs. M's comment and expressed a concern about the accident and Mrs. M's clumsiness. Unthreatened, Mrs. M described to the social worker her painful shoulder, her concern that it might be broken and that she might have to miss work. Upon inquiry, Mrs. M indicated the she had returned to work as an executive secretary four months ago because the family was having financial concerns. Mrs. M added that child care arrangements had been quite difficult.

The social worker asked where the accident had occurred. Mrs. M said that she had rushed and fallen down the stairs. The social worker asked what Mrs. M had been doing at the time. Mrs. M stated that she and her husband had been talking in the kitchen. "What were you talking about?" Mrs. M replied, "Finances." The social worker wondered aloud if Mrs. M's return to work had solved financial problems. Mrs. M stated that her husband "doesn't understand the expenses involved in my going back to work. I have been out of the work force for almost ten years and a housewife wardrobe isn't suitable for a career woman." The social worker suggested that this tension must cause extra pressure. Mrs. M concurred and stated that they argued every time they got on to the subject of her return to work. The social worker inquired as to how Mrs. M handled the arguments. Mrs. M explained that she usually tried to get away from her husband when he became loud and angry.

"What happened when you tried to get away tonight?" Refusing to make eye contact, Mrs. M looked down at her hands and stated quietly that she had just been clumsy as usual and fallen down the stairs. "But you were trying to get away from your husband?" It was apparent that tears were building up in Mrs. M's eyes.

The social worker gently touched Mrs. M's arm and again asked, "What happened when you tried to get away from your husband during the argument?" Mrs. M began crying at this point stating that while she was trying to run down the stairs her husband had pushed and kicked her. The worker questioned other injuries that brought Mrs. M to emergency previously and asked if they had been a result of similar incidents. Mrs. M responded that this was "the worst" but everything was going to be much better now because Mr. M had been so upset when he realized he had injured his wife. He had promised her repeatedly that it would never happen again.

The social worker assured Mrs. M that her husband was undoubtedly sincere in his promise, but it appeared the situation was more and more out of control. Mrs. M protested saying that the worker obviously had the wrong impression of her husband. She stated that Mr. M was a good provider, adored his three daughters and was very upset about the consequences of their arguments. She also said, "This fight was as much my fault as his."

The social worker assured Mrs. M that she did not perceive Mr. M as a "bad man." The worker went on to explain that Mr. M was perhaps a man who had difficulty in handling his anger in a constructive manner. Despite his best intentions, he would sometimes lose control. Mrs. M agreed that her husband did not like to get angry because he did not want to be "like his father." Mrs. M told the worker that Mr. M's father had been physically violent with his mother when Mr. M was growing up.

The worker suggested that Mr. M was obviously very troubled by his angry feelings in view of his earlier childhood experiences. The worker mentioned that counselling might be useful for Mr. M to overcome these feelings and resolve some of his bad memories. Mrs. M vehemently stated that her husband would never agree to such an idea and attempted to elicit a promise from the worker that she would not tell Mr. M what had been divulged.

The worker reviewed the various episodes that had brought Mrs. M to the hospital four times in four months and identified that each incident had been more serious in spite of Mr. M's promises to the contrary. The worker explained the cycle of violence and the tendency for violence to escalate. The worker assured Mrs. M that she was not responsible for her husband's behaviour and that both of them had a right to life without violence.

In addition, the worker shared information with Mrs. M about a transition home for women in the community. Mrs. M was surprised to think that women of her "position" might use such a resource as it had been her perception that only women on welfare required that kind of assistance and housing. Mrs. M took a pamphlet about the transition home, but was very definite that she had no fear of returning home with her husband and that he had given her every reassurance that everything was going to be fine. The worker accepted Mrs. M's decision, but reminded her that these assurances had been given before. The social worker then role-played briefly with Mrs. M as to how she might go about approaching her husband to discuss the possibility of seeing a counsellor.

The social worker contracted with Mrs. M and promised to call in two days' time while Mr. M was away at work. She also gave Mrs. M her card and phone number in the event that Mrs. M would want to call for help before that time. Finally, they reviewed a safety plan that Mrs. M might use in the future if it appeared that more violence was imminent.

After Mrs. M's departure from the emergency ward accompanied by her husband, the social worker spent time with the physician and nurse discussing the referral and process that had just taken place. The social worker noted on Mrs. M's chart the interview and disposition. After her further contact with Mrs. M two days hence, the worker would make a final note in the chart to prepare other hospital staff with information and guidance should Mrs. M return again for further treatment as a result of domestic violence.

References

Currie, D. (1988). *The Abusive Husband — An Approach to Interventions*. Toronto: Clarke Institute of Psychiatry.

Canadian Association of Social Work Administrators in Health Facilities (1986). *Domestic Violence Protocol Manual: For Social Workers in Health Facilities*. Ottawa: National Clearing House on Family Violence.

Canadian Medical Association (1987). *Health Care For The Elderly*. Ottawa: Department of Communications and Government Relations.

Ghent, W., Da Sylva, N. & Farren, M. (1985). Family violence: guidelines for recognition and management. *Canadian Medical Association Journal, 132*, 541-549.

Jones, A. (1988). *Women Who Kill*. Toronto: Random House.

MacLeod, L. (1987). *Battered But Not Beaten*. Ottawa: Canadian Advisory Council on the Status of Women.

Pressman, B. (1984). *Family Violence Origins and Treatment*. Ontario: University of Guelph.

Roy, M. (Ed.) (1982). *The Abusive Partner: An Analysis of Domestic Battering*. New York: Van Nostrand Reinhold Co.

Saskatchewan Interhospital Domestic Violence Committee (1986). Unpublished committee research.

Sinclair, D. (1985). *Understanding Wife Assault; A Training Manual For Counsellors and Advocates*. Toronto: Ontario Government Bookstore, Publication Services Section.

Swanson, R. (1984). Battered wife syndrome. *Canadian Medical Association Journal, 30*, 709-712.

Wax, J. (1968). Developing social work power in a medical organization. *Social Work 13*.

Wax, J. (1971). Power theory and institutional change. *Social Service Review, 45*(3).

Chapter 14

SOCIAL WORK PRACTICE IN A BLACK COMMUNITY-BASED TEACHING HOSPITAL

Marvin D. Feit, PhD
Sheila D. Miller, DSW

Abstract

Social work services appear to be overutilized in a black adminis-tered and operated community teaching hospital; however, the ser-vices they provide have a different emphasis from traditional medi-cal social work. Concrete services and patient advocacy with health and medical care personnel are provided first, followed by individu-al and family counselling. Indeed, environmental factors are the greatest source of stress. The effects of racism, disproportionate poverty and the lack of adequate community resources serving black patients all continually complicate treatment plans, while the strength and resiliency of the black family continues to be a source of support for patients and their recovery.

SOCIAL WORK PRACTICE IN A BLACK COMMUNITY-BASED TEACHING HOSPITAL

This chapter describes the role of a social worker in an urban, community-based hospital that is administered and operated by blacks. Medical social work has had a long history and a rich tradition in the profession. Yet, there is little information related to the practice of medical social workers in hospitals that are minority controlled, are located in minority communities and serve mostly minority clients.

THE CLIENTELE

The Norfolk Community Hospital is fully licensed to operate 210 beds by the Commonwealth of Virginia State Board of Health. It is also nationally accredited by the Joint Commission on Accrediting of Hospitals. According to its Annual Report (1985), it provides medical training to minorities in the fields of nursing, medicine, podiatry and health care administration. It has affiliations with Howard University Medical School, Ohio College of Podiatric Medicine and Eastern Virginia Medical School for training medical students; with Hampton University, Norfolk State University and Norfolk Vocational Technical School for training nursing students and with Norfolk State University for training social work students.

The hospital is located in a predominately minority section of the city of Norfolk and is adjacent to Norfolk State University. The immediate community is a mixture of poor and middle class individuals and families, with a movement toward optimism and an enhanced community. Evidence of this optimism is the construction of a new housing development, adjacent to the hospital, which will have approximately 280 single family homes averaging about $100,000 per unit.

The hospital provides a wide range of services consistent with an urban facility. Some of these services include 24-hour emergency care, outpatient medical services, outpatient surgery, nuclear medicine, ultrasound, breast cancer detection, obstetrics and gynecology, diabetic and hypertension classes, cardio-pulmonary function lab, social service, physical therapy services and skilled nursing care services. In 1985, 3,728 people were admitted, staying a total 29,555 days with an average length of stay of 7.9 days. The hospital continues to operate with an excess of revenue over expenses.

I. The Patient Profile

The patients in this hospital are black, about 35% live alone, 20% reside in boarding homes, 13% live with their children and 14% live with non-relatives. Approximately two-thirds are female and one-third are male. The age range is 16 to 83, with the average patient age being 53 years old. Most of the patients are single, either never married, separated or widowed. Almost half have less than an eighth grade education, and almost 75% report that they have less than $3,000 in income each year.

This demographic profile has remained fairly constant over the past several years, when it was first systematically studied (Miller, 1986). There are a number of medical conditions that confront this population and are treated constantly at the hospital. For example, patients when admitted to the hospital tend to be sicker, have multiple illnesses and suffer multiple and serious consequences.

Most of the patients have a primary diagnosis of hypertension, followed by diabetes mellitus, and a small number have seizure disorders. Patients with other diagnoses usually had a secondary diagnosis of hypertension. While most needed medication to control their chronic condition, almost twenty percent did need some assistance to function adequately in the community; e.g., shoe braces, canes and walkers.

There is a high percentage of patients with a functional disability, which is consistent with national statistics indicating that black adults have a higher proportion of disability then do white adults (Department of Education, 1984). In this context, the definition of disability according to the World Health Organization (*Perspectives on Aging*, 1988) is used:

> An impairment is a loss or abnormality of an anatomic structure of physiological or psychological function. Disability occurs when the person loses the ability to perform an activity. Handicap arises when societal or environmental conditions make it difficult or impossible to overcome a

disability....(basically), a disability limits the type or amount of activities that a person would otherwise be expected to perform. (p. 7)

In this regard, all of the black patients were considered to be disabled. The black disabled patients have a diagnosis of hypertension, cancer and other illnesses that may be associated with their low economic status and the poor health conditions associated with the kinds of jobs that they are likely to hold. Diet, poor housing and the additional stress of racism that prohibit opportunities for successful adjustment in personal, family, social and vocational categories have been among the top of the list of complaints by this group.

Further, these patients usually vividly describe their feelings of frustration, alienation and hostility when trying to use services established to assist disabled persons in their adjustment process. They often find social service agencies and health facilities just as unresponsive to their needs, as all other systems seem to be.

One outcome of the generally negative response to the needs of the black disabled is a mistrust or scepticism of people in the helping professions. While over two-thirds of the patients have an eligibility worker at a social service department out of necessity, most tended not to pursue other available community resources and were hesitant to use the services of the hospital's social work department. Only a handful of patients (usually around five percent) tend to have social workers assigned to them.

II. Presenting Needs

The majority of the patients are considered "moderately disabled" although they have symptoms that prevent them from functioning. These symptoms are not always constant and on some days a patient may not perform well in her/his daily living activities. On other days, symptoms such as dizziness, weakness, blackouts, pain, etc., may prohibit functioning completely. This pattern of temporary dysfunctioning is typical of many patients and is impossible to adequately measure at times. For instance, the large number of patients who exhibit this pattern, which may exist for their remaining years, presents a rather unique and difficult challenge for social workers.

Further, patients have difficulties with trying to provide for themselves and maintaining a standard of living comparable to what they had when they were working. This is equally troubling when they have difficulty finding and maintaining employment due to health conditions. If employed, the struggle of when and how to tell a potential employer about their illness is prevalent. The sympathetic rather than empathetic attitudes of vocational workers and potential employees further tests the disabled person's self-concept and self-esteem. Many, therefore, tend to view household chores, babysitting, gardening, church and community work and volunteer efforts as their main employment.

Patients complain about the costs of health insurance and medication, especially when such medications/prescriptions cost as much as $50-$150 or more a month. Those that have insurance that helps defray the cost of prescriptions often have to add a small amount of money which competes with the need for food in the household.

Patients, at times, complain about the existence of so-called "new racism," even when they perceived it was unintentional. Specifically, racist attitudes and behaviours influence their utilization of available services despite the obvious and apparent needs in the population. As well, they generally perceive they are deliberately kept uninformed of services they felt they were entitled to, or should have been made informed of services they could use, as an example.

PRACTICE ROLES AND RESPONSIBILITIES

Social workers serve this (hospital) population by providing concrete services, discharge planning and, when possible, a range of individual, family or group services. As well, they often do advocacy work on behalf of the patients by providing assessments, assisting in patient and family adjustment, working in team meetings and educating other professionals in other meetings where they present the patient's case.

Concrete services are one of the more important aspects of practice because social workers must work to overcome any scepticism presented by patients and to establish a solid base for providing additional needed services where trust and concern are necessary. Concrete services, therefore, form a base from which opportunities for intervention in personal, family, work and other institutional agencies are made possible. For example, such services include helping to secure needed equipment or health related appliances, helping the patient to obtain funds from the state human resources department, accompanying patients to referral agencies or treatment locations, or helping them to understand letters, medical procedures and so forth.

Discharge planning has become a critical component of hospital care as a result of the diagnostic related groups (DRG's) federally initiated financial reimbursement plan. Social work, in this hospital, is responsible for achieving this function. Thus, interfacing with the community becomes another way for social workers to implement their responsibilities.

Discharge planning often starts in a multi-disciplinary team approach. Meeting regularly with patients, physicians, nurses and other health care professionals, a social worker assists in developing realistic treatment plans. Social workers can and do provide useful information regarding case and family histories and other data, which allows for patient assessment. They also help to keep formal or informal communication contacts open with the team, which allows for early identification and resolution of new concerns that develop throughout hospitalization. Further, it is not unusual for the social worker to assist the health team in identifying and understanding their unique concerns regarding their own abilities to provide effective treatment. Support is, and has been found, extremely helpful to those team members who face daily a crisis of success and failure while trying to deliver concrete, comprehensive services.

Another aspect of discharge planning is developing community-based resources. Social workers maintain collaborative contacts with people in other agencies, which usually help facilitate the referral process. Support networks between service agencies assist in developing a continuity of care between the hospital and referral agencies.

An additional and serious problem facing social workers in this setting is the effect racism has on both patients and service providers. For example, a patient's history of constantly dealing with racism, the effects of the previously mentioned "new racism" and the consequent "unintentional" remarks take their toll most directly in this phase of providing services. Please accept the sweeping generalization that arranging for community services for a predominately black and poor population is often met with second rate service provision or no services at all. Further, quality care seems to lie with those who can pay or who are non-black; i.e., "just out of the reach" of these patients. Often, services in the community are not available. If they are, being on a waiting list is the expected norm.

When possible, provision is made for counselling with patients and their families and in groups. Such services are based on the available time of the social worker, the interest of the patient and/or the family and whether there has been some previous contact where a sense of trust and a helping relationship has developed. In this regard, the usual medical care services are provided with the understanding that they are time-limited. Thus, social workers are constantly assessing the short-term nature of problems, as long term resolutions require the assistance of other agencies.

In addition, social workers realize that serving the disabled group often goes beyond their own hospital's capability. The advocacy role extends to educational and professional groups and others in the community through participation in professional organizations, memberships on boards and participation in conferences in other health areas, such as allied health, rehabilitation, psychology, etc.

POTENTIAL FOR ROLE DEVELOPMENT

Research is one area where social work practice may be developed. It is important to note that assessment devices or scales measuring family support are generally not adequate in identifying families that are indeed supportive, despite having limited resources and living long distances from each other. Also, unique communication patterns significant to a family may measure as conflict rather than cohesiveness, resulting in misperception or misunderstanding. This is important since a patient's perception is that health providers' attitudes and actions are usually dependent on their understanding of family support. Developing more accurate assessment measures and continuing to educate health providers seems appropriate in this regard.

Research efforts need to be included as recognition that black patients, particularly the disabled, have benefited very little from available research efforts. Their concerns are the same as white patients, yet as indicated in this chapter, are compounded by the presence of intentional and unintentional racism, prejudice and/or discrimination. Thus, their responses are indeed different.

One of the difficulties with studies conducted with black subjects is that they seem to need white subjects as a comparison group to validate their worthiness for research efforts. What may appear insignificant to one cultural or racial group may, in fact, be very significant to the black disabled recognizing their uniqueness as a group. This area has been neglected in the literature.

It seems plausible to assume that if more social workers, especially minority social workers, expressed greater concern, there could be instruments designed to collect data that would reflect richer, more realistic experiences of black hospitalized patients, their families and needs.

Another area for role development is working directly with the patient and the family on problems related to disability adjustment, the pressures produced by hospitalization and other changes in life situation resulting from an illness. Presently, this is the least developed service and is done usually after other services are provided. Adequate funding for social work departments, allowing for more than one or two social workers, would be beneficial to achieve this end.

CONCLUDING REMARKS

Society has a history of having negative attitudes toward deformity and disability. People are living longer, and thus the possibility of disability is distinctly high. The needs of the black patient group, particularly its disabled, need to be continued to be addressed on all governmental levels (Barker, 1953).

The black disabled recognize that they have additional concerns and problems imposed on them because of race. They are living or feel forced to live, with disability in a hostile environment, which greatly influences their adjustment capabilities. The additional presence of managing stress, anxiety andemotions, having proper diets and maintaining adequate shelter greatly hinder disability status. Indeed, these conditions usually exacerbate existing or chronic disability conditions such as hypertension, diabetes, seizure disorders, cancer and so forth (Gary, 1978).

Counselling has been identified as being extremely helpful to the patient and the family. The availability of appropriate services and resources can help develop the coping skills of both patient and family (Johnson, 1962; Kaplan, Cassell, & Gore, 1979). Still, the black community continues to function with whatever support one's family, friends and community facilities can provide. Although they perceive that the majority of society is disinterested, the black disabled maintain strength and courage as they strive to be responsible members (Goldenberg, 1980; Wakabayaski, 1977).

There is much support within the black community and among family members for the black disabled patient. Miller (1986) identified expressiveness as the most important variable one can use to measure black family support. Family members, particularly those who were disabled, were encouraged to express themselves. The disabled black group in her study reported that their families were very supportive, despite having enormous financial and health problems, myths and fears and other difficulties facing them. Since employment was not likely, these patients viewed housekeeping, yard work and church work as their forms of "employment," and were encouraged to continue in these efforts by their families. It is this form of internal support provided within the black family that is often not well understood by social workers.

The fact that many patients are ineligible for services and training opportunities because of prescribed disability definitions, and the nature of the patient's symptoms, means the broadening of the disability definition needs to be addressed (Smith, 1978). Indeed, patients acknowledge that they need to become more advocating for themselves and that social workers could assist by encouraging them to be a part of the planning and decision making of appropriate organizations and the activities that are available to them.

One of the more salient observations about social work in this setting, and working with this population, is that the pressures are produced mainly from external or environmental sources. There is nothing unusual about practice when working directly with clients and their families. Yet, having to constantly battle the effects of racism, the grinding poverty, the lack of adequate community resources serving black patients and their families, the need for the continual education of health and medical personnel as to patient need and an understanding of behaviour and the lack of measurement scales that adequately assess the black disabled patient are realities that are inherent to this population. Indeed, one of the most satisfying aspects of practising social work in this

context is that one learns to appreciate the resiliency and support-
iveness black families give to their members.

CASE EXAMPLE

The following case contains several issues one can explore. There
is the possibility of misdiagnosis by private physicians; however,
the emphasis is on the women's interaction with a social worker.
The case illustrates the very difficult decision social workers must
make when they are overwhelmed and cannot meet everyone's
expectations. This is less likely to be the case in a teaching hospital, which usually treats white people and is financially secure and
can afford the "luxury" of hiring social workers.

In this case the only social worker in the hospital made a decision based on the perception that the client had financial and family supports not usually possessed by most patients, that concrete
services could be obtained by the patient and her family and that
the client did not require immediate attention. Indeed, this client
could have benefited from social work services, particularly in
helping her to get into a cancer support group, to overcome her
hesitancy to engage other health care professionals, to make use of
available community resources and to seek counselling for herself
and her family in regard to her disease and its effect on the family.

Medical Situation:

Ms. N. was diagnosed in 1985 as an inpatient with malignant
breast nodules—breast cancer that had spread to the bone. Prior
to this hospitalization, Ms. N. was seen by two internal medicine
physicians with complaints of chronic backache. She was diagnosed as having muscle problems and treated for such problems
for two years. She continued to complain about her pain, and had
a mammogram done that showed nothing. She continued to
receive treatment for muscle pain and was confined to bed rest.
She was hospitalized, after collapsing on the floor at home, and
diagnosed by a different physician at the hospital after a number
of tests and scans were done.

Ms. N. received chemotherapy every three weeks, an annual
chest x-ray and a bone scan every 3 or 4 months. Her medication
included Nolvadex tablets from 1985-1988 and since 1988, Magace
tablets. Her prognosis is terminal.

Family Situation:

Ms. N. is a 37-year-old black female. She was married in 1974 and widowed in 1977. Her husband, a Vietnam veteran, collapsed and died at home following a long medical history of lung illness. Three days prior to her husband's death, Ms. N. had a miscarriage.

Ms. N. is the second oldest of four children. Her parents and siblings are in reasonably good health. Her parents are over 60 and take medication for hypertension. There is a history of heart disease and cancer in the family.

Ms. N's mother is a retired registered nurse. Her father is a retired x-ray film processor, one brother is a medical doctor, one sister is a medical social worker and another brother is a factory worker with many years of seniority.

Social Situation:

Ms. N. built a nice home in 1978, after the death of her husband. She continues to live in the home, which has been adapted to the changes necessitated by her physical and ambulatory conditions. The house has 3 bedrooms, 1 1/2 baths, utility room, kitchen, screened back porch, storage house outside and driveway. Ms. N. owned a 1976 Cordoba Chrysler, which she sold to a friend while recuperating. She currently owns a 1982 Mercedes Benz.

Shortly after her hospitalization and diagnosis, her 40-year-old boyfriend ended the relationship because he could not cope with the changes in her appearance produced by her cancer therapy. However, she has been fortunate in the last three years because she has enjoyed a warm and supportive relationship with a 32-year-old man, who lives with her and assists her during her relapses. He works in a hospital as a transportation/dispatch worker with an annual income of $10,000 per year. He aspires to be a musician and plays guitar for two bands, from which he does not earn much additional money.

Education/Vocational History:

Ms. N. completed high school in 1969. She graduated from a Business College in 1971 and received a B.S. degree from an Ivy League University with a major in paralegal studies. She has earned 15 hours towards a masters degree in criminal justice.

Ms. N. was employed from 1971 to the time of her hospitalization in 1985. She worked as secretary and as an administrative assistant in a city school system. She volunteered in many school and criminal justice programs, and is a member of the American Business Women's Association.

Ms. N., prior to her hospitalization in 1985, made entrepreneurial attempts as a travel agent and as a provider of typing services. While she retains office space downtown, these attempts did not succeed due to her inability to be as available as necessary.

Financial Situation:

Her financial situation appears stable, but is vulnerable due to her condition. She receives US Government checks of $583 monthly, a VA retirement check of $446 monthly and a Social Security check of $501 monthly. She has an active saving account of $3,000, a checking account, no charge cards and a variable annuity program of $3,000.

Fortunately, Ms. N. is covered by health insurance. She has Blue Cross Blue Shield, a U.S. government medical service plan for active duty personnel, medicare health insurance and belongs to a drug benefit program.

Social Worker's Assessment:

The social worker had one contact with Ms. N. while hospitalized. Ms. N's perception was that the social worker was unable to assist her and attributed it to "inexperience" or being overwhelmed by her diagnosis. She was not certain as to the social worker's purpose, although she did ask lots of questions.

As already noted, the social worker had assessed this case in relation to her priorities in this setting. This patient, who clearly had more visible resources than others, fell into the lower end of the social worker's priorities despite indicating some needed attention.

Ms. N. has adjusted well considering the changes in her personal, medical, social, vocational and social situation. She attributes her ability to accept and adjust to her illness and disability to the supportive and positive attitude of the health team that has been encouraging her throughout this ordeal.

Included in this team are a physical therapist, nurses, blood technicians, an occupational therapist, an oncologist, a radiation specialist and two internal medicine physicians. Ms. N. also discussed the significance of family support throughout her hospitalization and while at home. She believes that her family's health backgrounds and ability to explain and support her treatment plan are also contributing to her adjustment.

Ms. N. has had difficulty, however, adjusting to physical changes and the need for a walker and/or cane during periods of relapse. She is depressed, at times, about the excessive weight gain due to the medication. Her medical team, family and boyfriend try to be realistic and yet encouraging about her physical appearance. Changing her style of dress has helped in her outlook.

Ms. N. could benefit from cancer support groups, but is hesitant to become involved. Understanding its importance would be of benefit to Ms. N. While the patient talks about the death and dying phase, she is resistant to writing her will though she has followed through with power of attorney to a family member.

References

Barker, R. (1953). *Adjustment to Physical Handicap and Illness: A Survey of the Social Psychology of Physical Disability.* New York: Social Science Research Council.

Department of Education (1084). Who is rehabilitation serving. *Rehab Brief, 7*(3), pp. 1-4.

Gary, L. E. (1978). *Mental Health: A Challenge to the Black Community.* Philadelphia: Dorrance and Company 1978.

Goldenberg, S. (1980). *Family Therapy: An Overview.* California; Brooks.

Johnson, W. R. (1962). *Health Concepts.* New York: The Ronald Press, Co.

Kaplan, B. H., Cassell, J. C. & Gore, S. (1979). Social support and health. In G. Jaco, (Ed.). *Patients, Physicians, and Illness* (pp. 102-116). N.Y.: Collier Macmillan Publishers.

Miller, S. (1986). Patients' perceptions of their adjustment of disability and social support in a community based teaching hospital. *Equal To the Challenge.* Bureau of Educational Research, School of Education, Howard University, Washington, D.C., p. 22.

Norfolk Community Hospital (1985). *Annual Report, 1985.* Norfolk, VA: Norfolk Community Hospital.

Disability: Facts and definitions. *Perspectives on Aging* (September/October, 1988). *17*(5), p. 7.

Smith, L. (1978). Social work with epileptic patients. *Health and Social Work, 3*(2), pp. 160-173.

Wakaboyaski, R. (1977). Unique problems of handicapped minorities. The White House Conference on Handicapped Individuals, Volume One: Awareness Papers. Washington, D.C.

Chapter 15

SOCIAL WORK PRACTICE IN HOSPITAL–BASED CRISIS INTERVENTION

Robert J. Todd, RN
Mary Webb, BSW, CSW

Abstract

The authors practise within a multidisciplinary crisis intervention team in a largely rural area. This unique practice is described focussing on clientele, staff roles, positive and negative aspects of the job and methods used to cope with stress. This work requires a combination of individual advocacy and the ability to negotiate compromises. Rapid decision making, flexibility of thinking and an eclectic approach to intervention are necessary to resolve the broad range of emergencies which present.

SOCIAL WORK PRACTICE IN HOSPITAL–BASED CRISIS INTERVENTION

In Ontario, Canada, deinstitutionalization of psychiatric patients, increasing demands on our health care system and limited availability of physicians is pushing us toward more cost effective and expeditious handling of mental health problems.

Crisis intervention, as an effective, and even essential component in the delivery of mental health services, is increasingly being recognized (and more importantly funded by the Ontario Ministry of Health) as an effective intervention. As recently as 1983, Dr. G. F. Heseltine, FRCP(C) noted in a discussion paper for the Ministry of Health that "of all gatekeeper activities, perhaps the most in need of immediate improvement is that of psychiatric emergency or crisis services....The first contact an individual has with mental health services is often when he or she suffers from a psychiatric crisis involving disturbing behaviour and immediate action is required" (Heseltine, 1983, p.60). The paper goes on to recommend that:

> within the treatment component, resolving the issue of psychiatric crisis should be a major priority. An adequate crisis service is characterized by: accessibility 24-hours a day, seven days a week; medical and psychiatric staff available at all times; a safely-kept unit or special observation room; and the capability to maintain the patient for a short period—up to 72 hours—during which time the patient's condition can be stabilized, a psychiatric, and if necessary a full medical, assessment carried out and a decision made regarding the most appropriate treatment and care plan (Heseltine, 1983, p.223).

The Ministry of Health responded by augmenting existing programs and funding new programs. As an example, funding for crisis programming doubled from 1985/86 to 1986/87 (Graham, 1988, p.IV-3). Despite this influx of money, again in 1988, "crisis services were identified as a major deficit in the province" (Graham, 1988, p. 35). "These services should provide diagnostic evaluation, supportive counselling and psychotherapy, medication management and crisis assistance" (Graham, 1988, p.45).

In the last six months of 1988, two new teams were funded in Ontario. Both as a treatment modality and an area of specialization for social work, crisis intervention will continue to grow into the 1990s.

THE CLIENTELE

A crisis team serves all people. Whether a problem is a crisis is defined by the client. Any person who believes that the issue facing them is distressing enough to require immediate resolution, s/he should have access to the crisis worker 24 hours a day through the hospital emergency room. The Canadian Mental Health Association estimates that 34% of the population suffer from a diagnosable mental disorder.

The focus for many mental health professionals is on the "walking well." Our speculation is that clinicians in these roles have neither the training nor the time to deal with emergencies during an already hectic, over-booked schedule.

During a program's initial two years, the team works at establishing credibility with those clients who have previously been served by the institution. Predominant in this group are those with major mental illnesses (depression, schizophrenia and manic depressive illnesses). The experience of the crisis team suggests that those from lower socio-economic groups have difficulty understanding and utilizing referral and treatment systems often designed by middle-class professionals.

As a program gains credibility with hospital staff it becomes attractive to persons with more acute problems. Many of these acute issues had not been addressed by the institution which focussed largely on hospitalization for treatment.

After the initial start-up phase, the client population stabilizes into three major groups:

I. Major Mental Illness

Approximately 40% of the individuals assessed have a diagnosis that fits into a readily identifiable psychiatric category. For many of these individuals, "psychiatric emergency" might more closely define their presentation.

II. Impaired Community Functioning

Approximately 20% of the people worked with need help to resolve life crises that are due to their impaired ability to solve problems or to a lack of available resources. Developmental delay, intellectual impairment, poverty, and illiteracy are examples of *handicaps* that make dealing with what most of us consider minor changes in life insurmountable emergencies. A somewhat extreme example is the young male who presents with suicidal ideation asking for hospitalization. His precipitant is the failure of the postal system to deliver his welfare assistance on the expected day. He has no money to eat, no friends or relatives to borrow from and lacks the skills to utilize (or manipulate) the social/health system to get funds to tied him over.

III. Well-Adapted Functional People With Unexpected Life Crises

This group represents approximately 40% of the caseload and is as variable as the general population. All of us cope with an increasing pace of life and frequent complicated life decisions. Who amongst us has not had a time when too many things went wrong at the same time and we felt unable to cope?

Even these three broad groupings cannot clearly separate the population because individuals frequently cross boundaries and present multiple inter-linked issues. For instance, the schizophrenic suffers grief after the loss of a parent, and a bankrupt business man has no knowledge of the methods used to have his health care insurance subsidized.

Figure 1 presents a general idea of the types of presenting problems identified by our clientele. Keep in mind that people sometimes identify one complaint, while assessment reveals a quite different problem.

257

FIGURE 1
Presenting Problem
January - June, 1987
N = 742

Description	% of Total
1. Bizarre or inappropriate behaviour or speech	15.1
2. Depression	37.4
3. Request hospitalization	5.2
4. Request O/P psychiatry treatment (including all disciplines)	2.6
5. Suicidal/homicidal	25.8
6. Medications	9.2
7. Alcohol	18.7
8. Drugs other than alcohol	5.3
9. Marriage - relationship	22.7
10. Parent - child	11.1
11. Anxiety/agitation	19.8
12. Antisocial/problems getting along with others (exclude family)	2.7
13. Mental retardation	3.1
14. Finances — social problems — placement	17.5
15. Problem with someone else	3.1
16. Physical problem	10.2
17. No psychiatric complaint	1.7
20. Unknown/other	1.6

Total number of clients does not equal number of complaints because more than one complaint may be reported (average 2.1 complaints per person).

Figure 2 represents diagnoses documented after assessment by clinicians. While presenting problems and diagnoses appear to be closely linked (37.4% identified depression as a presenting problem, and 36.1% were diagnosed as being in a major depression), these figures are not related to each other. The clients presenting with depression are frequently not those who receive the diagnosis.

FIGURE 2
Diagnosis
January - June, 1987
N = 742

Description	% of Total
1. Schizophrenia	8.6
2. Depression	36.1
3. Manic-depressive illness	3.1
4. Psychosis	6.7
5. Suicide attempt	11.3
6. Chronic organic brain syndrome	1.1
7. Acute organic brain syndrome	1.2
8. Alcoholism	8.8
9. Alcohol abuse	15.7
10. Other drug abuse	5.9
11. Marital problem — relationship	20.7
12. Parent — child problem	14.3
13. Anxiety/panic disorder	6.8
14. Personality disorder	19.9
15. Mental retardation	6.6
16. Social problem (placement, finances, etc.)	24.3
17. Adjustment disorder	17.8
18. Physical problem	31.9
19. No diagnosis	0.7
20. Unknown/other	2.6

Total number of clients does not equal number of diagnoses because more than one diagnosis may be reported (average 2.4 diagnoses per client).

Perhaps most notable in Figure 2 is that 31.9% of the clientele have a physical problem that is having an effect on their ability to handle the current crisis. This points out the need for availability of medical assessment for the crisis clientele.

Crisis team services are used almost equally by men and women. Ages have ranged from 9 years (overdose secondary to school phobia), to 101 years (grief over death of 87 year old nephew who was last remaining relative).

Statistics show an increasing number of child abuse cases, sexual assault and general family violence. Staff who have worked in the field for some time attribute this to increased awareness in both professionals and the general public, and social acceptance of reporting, rather than an increase in actual occurrences (Ellman, 1983).

Our clientele present with the widest variety of problems imaginable. If you tried to make up an outlandish case history and told it to a crisis worker, they might well be able to tell you the person's name (but wouldn't because of confidentiality issues).

This diverse population presents when they are highly distressed and needing immediate relief. The crisis worker must be able to assist the client to accurately pinpoint the cause of the distress, problem solve regarding potential solutions and arrange treatment to diffuse the emergency. Treatment may be with the crisis team, elsewhere in the hospital or in the community. Predominant at the time of assessment is the goal of helping the client gain understanding of the problem and a feeling of being back in control.

PRACTICE ROLES AND RESPONSIBILITIES

I. Emergency Room Assessments

Using about 40% of available time, this is the major point of intervention. The team serves as the major entry point to all mental health services for emergency cases. Almost 90% of clients come to seek help voluntarily and crisis teams use a "customer approach to patienthood" (Lazare, et al., 1975).

Within a one to two hour time frame, the worker gathers a social history and helps the client identify the cause of distress. Rather than a full life history, the focus is on the "here and now" problems. Basic questions include why are you here, why now, has this happened before and what did you do then?

During the initial phase of assessment, clients are often anxious, confused and feel overwhelmed by the state of crisis. While maintaining an awareness of how the client is making the worker feel, the worker must present a calm, controlled exterior. The client uses the worker as a role model and will frequently become less anxious because he can see that his problems have not overwhelmed the therapist.

Part of the assessment includes a thorough mental status and history of previous illness. If possible, the history is collaborated with family or agencies involved. It is not uncommon in interviewing significant others (family or professionals) to discover a state of crisis in those affected by the identified client.

Once the history is gathered, the worker and client try to reach some consensus as to the variety of options available. Combining what the patient wants with what the worker feels is needed, a *practical* plan of action is worked out.

People faced with difficult life decisions (e.g., the need for marital separation) frequently procrastinate in order to avoid the inevitable emotional pain involved. Many people end up in crisis because procrastination has led to incapacitation.

Unlike many other modalities, crisis work takes a "directive approach" to treatment. While the client must make the final choice, workers make strong recommendations, accompanied with facts, to support the conclusion.

In all emergency assessments, the basic question of "in or out" must be considered. Should the patient be brought into hospital for treatment in a protected, structured environment, or arrangements made for them to return home with follow-up by an appropriate outpatient agency?

An evaluation of the person's ability to care for himself and understand the consequences of his actions is essential. The individual's strengths, weaknesses, home environment and support network are also relevant factors. Crisis workers have the strong belief that if safe to do so, people should remain in the community and receive treatment. In order to realize this, workers often spend longer time arranging follow-up than it took to do the assessment.

Figure 3 provides a general picture of the range of resources referred to from the emergency room. The "other" category is a compilation of referrals to numerous agencies where the number of referrals is too small to be statistically significant.

FIGURE 3
Disposition
January - June, 1987
N = 742

Description	% of Total
1. Admit Crisis/Psychiatry	24.7
2. Admit other	11.0
3. O/P Psychiatrist	16.4
4. O/P Social Worker	4.7
5. O/P Psychologist	3.7
6. O/P Registered Nurse	9.3
7. O/P Crisis Worker	11.7
8. O/P Alcohol Services	7.2
9. General Practitioner	7.1
10. Bruce Grey Children's Services	2.6
11. Children's Aid Society - Catholic Children's Aid Society	1.9
12. Adult Protective Services/Association for the Mentally Retarded	2.4
13. Public Health	1.3
14. Women's Centre	3.9
15. Probation/Parole	1.1
16. Police/Jail	2.0
17. Family and Social Services	4.7
18. Community and Social Services	1.1
19. Bruce Shoreline Family Centre	2.2
20. Church	3.7
21. Home, no follow-up	4.8
22. Other	19.9

More than one referral may be made (average 1.4 referrals per client).

II. Telephone Counselling

Problems with distance, transprtation and finances mean that assessment and consultation by telephone use about 30% of available time. Often first time clients wishing anonymit, telephone, and out of town physicians and therapists call to consult on cases they believe are emergencies. Fewer than 50% of these calls result in the team doing a "face to face" assessment.

Clients in treatment with other agencies and hospital programs use the crisis team as an emergency resource because it is frequently the only mental health service for children or adults available 24 hours per day, 7 days a week. Other "after hours" helping professionals, such as police officers, Children's Aid

Society workers, ministers, family and social service workers, and even Bell Canada operators route emergency work to the crisis team. [*Please remember that this is rural Ontario*]

III. Outpatient Crisis Treatment

Some 15% of the clients assessed in the emergency room return for outpatient visits with a worker on the team. Compliance is high because clients quickly establish a therapeutic alliance with a professional who has helped in a time of crisis. The focus is short (2 - 8 visits), fast (2 - 6 weeks) and aimed at implementing concrete practical solutions.

At times, clients are followed for less than ideal reasons, such as lengthy waiting lists for programs, or problems which do not fit other programs' criteria. Occasionally, the crisis team works with a patient because no one else will get involved. These are usually more chronic, non-compliant individuals who have "burned their bridges" throughout the mental health system.

In order to preserve a sense of balance, each member of the team treats, when possible, an "ideal patient." An "ideal patient" is bright, able to verbalize and abstract and motivated to change. These clients generally respond well to crisis treatment and recover quickly.

IV. Teaching

All helping professionals encounter various degrees of crisis with their clientele (e.g. most adolescents experience crisis as they move from child to adult). A crisis team devotes 15% of its available time for public speaking (recognizing depression, dealing with stress, As, Bs and Cs of assessment, dealing with suicide) to charitable groups, other agencies and schools. Crisis teams also teach assessment of suicide risk, basic crisis intervention and systems manipulation to other mental health professionals.

Included in all aspects of the assessment, consultation, treatment and referral of clients is the crisis worker's role of negotiation and compromise. Staff are seen variously as part of the Emergency Department, part of the out-patient mental health services, the admitting officers for in-patient psychiatry and part of the network of community social and mental health agencies. They work with the Police Department, Ambulance, Children's

Aid Society, Family and Social Services, local churches, self-help groups, detox centres, schools, Justices of the Peace, Probation and Parole and all segments of mental health services. Any service that exists in the community can make referrals to the crisis team and receive referrals back.

While each of the programs and agencies have the common goal of providing service, rarely do they agree on mandates, admission criteria and types of problems treated. In most geographical areas, services have more clients than they can manage. Because crisis clients are highly distressed, need immediate treatment and sometimes have previously failed in therapy, agencies do not always view them with favour.

Up-to-date information on waiting lists, types of treatment offered and who to contact is essential. As pointed out earlier, workers often spend more time negotiating follow-up treatment than doing the actual assessment. Rarely are all parties (patient, family, emergency room, psychiatrists, inpatient units and agencies) satisfied with the completed arrangements. Choices for treatment are often the "best immediately available" type rather than "best for the problem."

Further, all programs refer to crisis. They expect immediate assessment and prompt resolution when they refer. As cases come in, so must they go out. Because the acuity level of crisis clients is high and resolution must be expedited, waiting lists can be bypassed, admission criteria stretched and co-operation, particularly with hospital staff and physicians, stressed. Simply put, the co-operation required to work in the context of "crisis intervention" is a major concern for the social workers in the program and a critical reason for its success.

The team operates 24 hours per day, 7 days per week, 365 days per year. Staff work a combination of 8 and 12 hour shifts, and 8 hour on-call periods at home from midnight to 8:00 A.M. While these are non-traditional hours for social workers, staff enjoy frequent days off, flexibility of scheduling and a large degree of independence in their day-to-day practice. Night cases are infrequent, but usually of a most urgent nature. Staff take phone calls from home and respond to the emergency room when needed.

Every 24 hours, all cases and telephone calls are reviewed by team members with the psychiatric consultant. Day-to-day casework is done with the physician covering the emergency room, but staff also have a psychiatrist on-call available.

The Team Manager maintains an "open-door policy" for

supervision and consultation and is available 24 hours per day by pager. Staff work with confidence, knowing their decisions will be backed up administratively and help is "only a call away."

POTENTIAL FOR ROLE DEVELOPMENT

Crisis teams, because they require a varied group of professionals to work closely together, and because they cross traditional boundaries between inpatient units, emergency rooms and community agencies, are in an ideal position to break down the traditional barriers. The administrative structure provides a Director of Social Work for consultation and supervision around professional issues, and a Crisis Team Manager for supervision of clinical functioning and program operation. This matrix management system further encourages breakdown of traditional roles and creates a blurring of responsibilities across disciplines within the team. While this blurring of responsibility boundaries can be disconcerting to the uninitiated, its positive effects allow social workers to perform in areas normally "off limits" to them. It's an essential ingredient of the crisis team. The Director of Social Work and Team Manager together ensure that tasks are performed within professional standards of practice.

The traditional role of the social worker is challenged by the nature and function of the crisis team. The hours of operation, acuity and diversity of clientele, plus the wide spectrum of resources utilized, provide a wealth of experience and innovative practice to any clinician.

Crisis work requires social workers to see patients not only from a social perspective, but also from a medical, psychological and behaviourial context. Knowledge of medical and psychiatric terminology, diagnosis and the ability to work with physicians as peers are essential tools in the eclectic and ever-changing role of a social worker on a crisis team. Social work training brings particular expertise to bear in several areas. While nursing and medicine tend to focus "inward," that is within the institution, social workers balance this with emphasis toward the community. Frequently staff must act as advocates for individual clients in seeking services. Social work plays a major role in representing such clients.

When agencies and institutions offer services for particular problems, clients are referred and treated. When no services exist for specific groups of clients, these people are more likely to be seen in crisis (adolescents from age 16 - 19 and the homeless are two examples of over-represented groups in crisis).

Social work has the opportunity to advocate for the under-serviced in planning new and expanded programming. Nowhere else is such a small group (teams usually have 3 - 7 staff) so influential in both individual assessment and systems organization.

CONCLUDING REMARKS

An essential ingredient for success in crisis intervention work is the people on the team. Basically, people who do crisis work must be flexible; they should enjoy working with the unpredictable with no schedule for events. Crisis workers must remain calm under pressure and utilize their own life experiences seasoned with a strong dose of common sense. They should enjoy stress and be able to deal with alternating quiet times and periods of frantic activity. They must be able to "debrief" quickly and be able to perform again. They must be willing to deal daily with high levels of frustration and criticism. In practice, they are, without exception, outspoken individuals strongly committed to immediate short term intervention. Perhaps most importantly they are individuals with a strong sense of humour. They must be able to laugh, both at themselves and the absurdities of life. Crisis workers see clients gain immediate relief, get control of their lives, and grow interpersonally. They work after "business hours" in a context of professional independence and responsibility.

However, all the factors that people find enticing in this work are also the pitfalls. Stress, high activity and unpredictability can lead to burnout and callousness. In this job, it's easy to forget what "normal" is.

At times, frustration is experienced because clients cannot be followed for longer periods and/or they are not seen through to recovery. On a good day, staff feel that "the buck stops here" because the crisis team is the only resource that knows how to resolve the problem. On a bad day, it can seem that the clientele are those whom no one else wants to work with.

Team members develop a strong "esprit de corp" and try always to stay in tune with each other. They consult, support, critique and survive together as a team unit.

In terms of expanding this "esprit," the Crisis Workers

Association of Ontario was established in 1984 by a group of professionals working in crisis intervention programs to provide a network of support and education.

As the network expanded and professionals met at the annual conference, it became apparent that despite administrative, organizational and demographic differences, the teams had much in common. With a membership of over 150 professionals working in crisis intervention, the association continues to grow and provide a variety of services, from consultation on writing proposals to fund teams, to clinical workshops for crisis team secretaries.

CASE EXAMPLE

Presenting Problem:

Mrs. Smith was brought to the Emergency Department by ambulance after an overdose of an "over-the-counter" sleeping medication. After she received medical treatment in the Emergency Department, she was referred by the family doctor for a crisis assessment.

Assessment:

Mrs. Smith presented as a tired-looking 43-year-old woman, who appeared older than her stated age. She was slightly obese and quite tearful during the interview. Mr. and Mrs. Smith have been married for 20 years and have 2 children, ages 16 and 13 years. She explained that she and her husband had been having marital problems for the past 8 months and are no longer able to communicate with each other.

Mrs. Smith described her feelings and perceptions that her family would be "better off" if she no longer existed. Mrs. Smith stated that for the past 3 months, she had been experiencing fleeting suicidal thoughts, but no intent to act on them. For the past 2 days, she had been thinking of suicide as a reasonable method to solve her problem. She took the overdose in the bathroom and went to bed, but within 1/2 hour she became frightened of dying and told her husband who called the ambulance. She denied any previous attempts and spontaneously stated "I feel foolish now. It's no answer."

Mental status examination revealed that Mrs. Smith was having difficulty functioning in many aspects of daily life. Her sleeping pattern had become quite disturbed in the past two months. She was having problems falling asleep (initial insomnia) and early morning awakening (terminal insomnia) after only 3 - 4 hours of sleep. Mrs. Smith complained of feeling depressed, tired all the time and restless. As well, she was having problems concentrating at work and tended to "day dream" most of the day. She explained her energy level had decreased significantly and she no longer participated in what had been a quite active social and recreational life style. In the past three months, she had gained 20 pounds. The crisis worker noted that Mrs. Smith had difficulty concentrating during the interview, as several questions had to be repeated. Her eye contact was quite poor. She did not appear to be responding to auditory and visual hallucinations, and denied the same when questioned about this.

Mrs. Smith explained that she and her husband had been receiving marital counselling for the past four months at a local family counselling centre. At the present time, she did not feel there had been any significant improvement in their relationship and now worried that her husband would request a separation. She denied any previous inpatient or outpatient psychiatric history. A brief exploration of Mrs. Smith's family of origin revealed that her mother had received inpatient treatment for depression several years earlier.

With Mrs. Smith's permission, the crisis worker requested to speak with her husband. Mr. Smith described what he perceived as a very happy and stable marriage until eight months ago when he began to notice gradual changes in his wife's functioning. Previously his wife had been a perfectionist who devoted herself to child rearing, managing the home and working part-time as a bookkeeper. In the past eight months she had increasingly become argumentative with her husband and the children and less interested in the children's activities. Mr. Smith explained he tried to assist his wife in managing her home responsibilities, but "everything I did was wrong." Although he stated he loves his wife, he recently considered separation as he no longer felt Mrs. Smith was committed to the marriage. "I don't know what happened. This is not like her to be like this."

After interviewing the patient and her husband, the crisis worker discussed the diagnosis and potential treatment plan with the emergency physician who referred Mrs. Smith for assessment.

Because the Crisis Intervention Team is a multidisciplinary team, a standardized diagnostic reference is required, commonly known as DSM-III R (*Diagnostic and Statistical Manual of Mental Disorders*, Third Ed., Revised, 1987).

Using the DSM-III R as a guideline, the diagnoses were as follows:

Axis I	(Clinical syndromes)	Major depression, single episode
Axis II	(Personality disorders)	No diagnosis on Axis II
Axis III	(Physical disorders and conditions)	No physical problems were reported except for an occasional headache
Axis IV	(Severity of psychosocial stressors)	Moderate - marital discord
Axis V	(Global assessment of functioning)	Serious - level 50 (based on a scale of 0 - 100)

Treatment Plan:

1. Mrs. Smith was assessed by a psychiatrist who started her on an antidepressant medication.
2. The crisis worker discussed the diagnosis of major depression with the patient and her husband and gave information about the diagnosis, including material to take home.
3. The patient's family physician was informed of the assessment and agreed to monitor the antidepressant medication prescribed.
4. The crisis worker arranged for a crisis outpatient follow-up appointment the next day (and subsequent appointments to continue over a six week period).
5. With the patient's signed consent, the crisis worker discussed the assessment and treatment plan with the local agency counsellor who agreed to continue the marital counselling after the crisis follow-up.

Discussion:

A critical aspect of the crisis assessment is to decide if a patient requires inpatient treatment or if outpatient treatment would better meet the needs of the patient. Although Mrs. Smith attempted suicide by overdosing, the emergency physician assessed the patient as being in no physical danger. The overdose was not of a life threatening nature and Mrs. Smith sought help by informing her husband of her suicide attempt.

The crisis worker also needed to consider if the patient was able to care for herself. Realizing that the patient's suicidal thoughts could return and that the patient could not expect the antidepressant medication to improve her vegetative signs of depression for at least two to three weeks, it was important to consider if sufficient supports were available to her. As Mrs. Smith denied any active suicidal ideation or intent, and her husband was supportive and willing to monitor her symptoms, it was decided she could be treated in the community.

It was difficult to determine if Mrs. Smith would comply with the treatment plan as she had no previous psychiatric history to refer to. Because the patient had expressed hope that her condition would improve and responded to the educational material given about the treatment of depression, crisis outpatient follow-up was considered appropriate. The crisis worker was able to engage the patient in a therapeutic alliance and was comfortable with the patient returning home.

Predominant in her symptoms at the time were the "vegetative symptoms" of depression (poor sleep, low energy, loss of interest, decrease in ability to concentrate, etc.). Her confusion about what was happening and her hopelessness related to a lack of understanding of her illness. For this reason, tricyclic antidepressants (to relieve the biological symptoms) and supportive psychotherapy and education about depression were needed immediately.

At this point the precipitant or initial cause of her depression and marital problems was unknown. Mrs. Smith's lack of response to marital counselling was directly related to the vegetative symptoms she was having and not to the marital counselling received. After her depressive symptoms improve, she may be better able to actively participate and benefit from marital counselling. This information will be shared with the marital counsellor so that the counsellor does not see Mrs. Smith as unmotivated, or his intervention as unsuccessful. Mrs. Smith's prognosis for a complete recovery is excellent.

References

Diagnostic and Statistical Manual of Mental Disorders (third edition) revised. (1987). Washington, D.C.: American Psychiatric Association.

Ellman, J. P. (1983). Emergencies in medicine North America: Psychiatric emergencies. *MEDICINE North America, 34.*

Graham, R. (1988). *Building Community Support for People: A Plan for Mental Health in Ontario.* Ontario: Provincial Community Mental Health Committee.

Heseltine, G. F. (1983). *Towards a Blueprint for Change: A Mental Health Policy and Program Perspective.* Government Printing Services, Queen's Park, Toronto, Ontario.

Lazare, A., Eisenthal, S. & Wasserman, L. (1975). The customer approach to patienthood: attending to patient requests in a walk-in clinic. *Archives of General Psychiatry, 32,* 553-558.

Chapter 16

SOCIAL WORK PRACTICE IN CRITICAL CARE AND TRAUMA UNITS

IRENE TIEGS, BSc, MSW

Abstract

Patients in critical care and trauma units suffer from a variety of critical illnesses and/or injuries. They may experience anxiety, anger, guilt and/or depression in response to their trauma and potentially death and dying issues. They are also susceptible to suffering from the ICU syndrome or psychosis as a result of the environmental consequences of sensory deprivation, sensory overload, immobility and sleep deprivation. The social worker may be requested to address not only their acute emotional and psychological responses but also the potential long-term post-traumatic stress disorders. The social worker's assessment, crisis intervention and grief counselling skills are used in meeting the needs of families or significant others who may experience similar emotions as a result of the usually sudden onset of the trauma. As a member of a health care team, the social worker may also be requested to provide in-service training and support groups for the staff and to participate in decision-making processes when physicians have exhausted their resources.

SOCIAL WORK PRACTICE IN CRITICAL CARE AND TRAUMA UNITS

A critical care unit, which may be called an intensive care unit in some health care facilities, with its massive doses of human suffering, is a setting that challenges the crisis intervention skills of even experienced social workers. The environment itself with its array of technical equipment and critically ill patients, who may be physically disfigured from their trauma or infections, may initially be visually overwhelming for some social workers.

THE CLIENTELE

Patients in a critical care setting may be suffering from life threatening illnesses such as meningitis, multiple organ failure, heart failure, Guillain Barre Syndrome, Legionnaire's disease, brain hemorrhages, severe asthmatic attacks, severe stroke drug overdose, or they may be suffering from multiple trauma as a result of a suicide attempt or an infliction such as a stabbing or a gunshot wound. Patients in this unit may also be victims of a fire or an explosion, or a farming, industrial or a motor vehicle accident. Their trauma may include burns, head injury, organ damage, fractures or spinal chord injury. Their injuries may cause only acute or short-term problems, or they may result in long-term deficits and disfigurement or may be potentially lethal. Other individuals may be admitted to a critical care unit following major surgery, such as coronary artery bypass grafting or an esophagectomy. This latter group may require only a short stay in the unit and, unless they suffer with post-operative complications or anxiety, social work intervention with this group of patients is generally not indicated.

Many patients who are critically ill from a life threatening illness or trauma may present in an unconscious or confused state. Thus, social work intervention is not feasible with these patients; however, their families or significant others will likely benefit from counselling during this stressful period.

The vast majority of patients in this unit are ventilator-dependent, which involves a tube that is inserted through either their nose or mouth into their windpipe. This tube restricts the movement of their vocal chords and retards the lucid patient's ability to vocalize. Consequently, these patients experience difficulty communicating unless they are able to write. Unfortunately, many critically ill patients are either too weak or physically impaired to the extent that they are unable to handle a pen. Others may be illiterate, mentally handicapped or on massive doses of medication, which may distort their handwriting or their ability to write legibly. Thus, many of these patients are dependent on staff and their relatives to lip read or interpret their non-verbal gestures. If they are orally intubated (i.e., the ventilator tube is inserted in their mouth), it may be particularly difficult for these patients to form words effectively, which makes lip reading more frustrating.

Since these patients are attached to machines such as ventilators and heart monitors and also intravenous lines and catheters, they are immobile. Thus, intervention must take place at the bedside of a room, which is usually occupied by three other patients and potentially numerous health care professionals. Consequently, privacy for purposes of intervention is generally not practical.

To awaken in a critical care unit, amid an array of technical equipment and unable to vocalize, may be anxiety provoking for some patients. They may lack an appreciation of their condition and may be fearful of their unknown prognosis. Some may fear death, loss of ability or disfigurement while others may fear prolonged suffering. Accident victims may express a need for information regarding other victims in their accident. Others may be concerned how their loved ones are coping, especially those who may be dependent on them. Other patients may share financial and/or legal concerns.

A social worker may assist anxious patients by orienting them to their surroundings and by clarifying information that the medical team may present to them. Traumatized patients, especially those receiving massive doses of pain medication may experience short term memory loss and may benefit from reiteration of pertinent information. The social worker may also serve these patients by providing an opportunity for them to ventilate their fears and concerns and, when appropriate, provide reassurance.

Patients in a critical care unit may become depressed if their stay is prolonged or if they evidence a lack of improvement or a deterioration in their condition. Depressive symptoms may also present in patients who become frustrated with their loss of autonomy and dependency on others. Those grieving the loss of ability, such as victims who suffer with permanent paralysis or loss of a limb, may withdraw from social interaction with their loved ones and/or staff. These patients would also benefit from verbal ventilation. A social worker may be supportive in encouraging these patients to share their frustrations. The worker may also liaise with staff and express the patient's need to be given some control. This may involve giving the patient some choices such as when they would like to be bathed or which direction they would prefer to be turned to first. The patient should also be given control over visitation when feasible.

Some patients may have a need to ventilate their anger, which is a common response of those who feel victimized. Since patients are not usually clothed in the unit, some may be angered by their perceived loss of dignity. Patients experiencing guilt may misdirect their personal anger towards staff. Some may feel responsible for their present condition and others may experience guilt for the pain and suffering they may have caused others. Patients who have attempted suicide may be angry that their efforts were futile while others may feel guilty for emotional suffering they have caused for their loved ones by their actions. Some patients have expressed remorse for failing to seek medical attention when early symptoms appeared. Many traumatized patients have no appreciation of their source of anger and may require professional intervention to gain insight. The social worker may be effective in assisting the angry or guilt-ridden patient to reframe their assessment of their situation and thus deal more appropriately with their anger and, usually, unwarranted guilt.

Lucid patients who spend prolonged periods of time in a critical care setting are susceptible to suffering from the ICU Syndrome or ICU Psychosis. This syndrome is a result of a lack of sleep, immobility, sensory deprivation and simultaneous sensory overload. One Australian physician compared critical care units to KGB spy camps as patients are subjected to painful stimuli, variant levels of lighting and noises, medical jargon (which is like a foreign language and consequently may be misinterpreted), a loss of autonomy and denial of oral consumption. Some units lack windows and thus patients may be disoriented to day and night. When the brain is not continuously stimulated, dream-like states, fantasies and hallucinations may transpire to maintain arousal. Patients may struggle to make sense of their environment and consequently suffer with distorted perceptions. Many patients have suggested that they are being tortured and some have expressed fears that they may be killed. Thus, their confusion may result in paranoia and potentially even psychosis.

Sleep deprivation is a common problem in the critical care setting where patients need to be monitored regularly. These assessments may be intrusive and may require continuous lighting that disturbs their sleep patterns. This problem is of particular concern as sleep is essential in the healing process.

Since patients are attached to ventilators, intravenous lines and other technical monitors, immobility is a consequence. Psychological experiments have evidenced that immobilized healthy individuals may experience changes in body image, psychosomatic aches and pains, depersonalization and impairment in intellectual, cognitive and psychomotor functioning.

Patients in a critical care unit are visually deprived as there is generally a lack of stimulation. The colour scheme of the unadorned walls, ceiling and technical equipment are usually muted tones in this sterile environment. Patients' taste and smell may be affected by their nasogastric tubes, which are inserted for purposes of either feeding or suctioning their stomachs. There is also an absence of familiar voices and sounds. Simultaneously, patients may be exposed to an intolerable noise level of monitoring equipment, including loud alarms and the medical and personal discussions of staff.

Social workers working in the critical care setting should be aware of this syndrome so that they may interpret their patients' experiences and counsel family members, who may be distressed by their observations of the patients' disorientation and psychotic states. Some patients when alerted to the likelihood that they are hallucinating are sometimes able to differentiate between reality and their dream-like states and thus become better oriented to their surroundings. This may be particularly beneficial during their recovery period on a medical floor, after leaving the unit. Social workers may also be productive in bringing about change in the environment by encouraging other members of the health care team to be cognizant of factors that contribute to this syndrome. These symptoms generally subside after a few days on a medical floor if the patient obtains sufficient sleep.

Patients who are traumatized and/or spend lengthy periods in the critical care setting, are susceptible to suffering from post-traumatic stress disorders, which may include anxiety attacks, psychological flashbacks, sleep disorders, phobias, depression, difficulty with memory and/or concentration and loss of interest in previously enjoyed activities. Early intervention is pertinent in minimizing the effects of these stress disorders. Thus, social workers should be consulted as soon as the patient is lucid and able to benefit from therapy.

Anxiety attacks usually present with a sudden onset and may occur during restful periods when the individual is not consciously thinking about their trauma. Consequently, it is usually difficult for the victim to associate this event with their trauma. These attacks may involve rapid heart palpitations, profuse sweating, laboured breathing, nausea, trembling and/or tightness in the chest. Many feel they are having a "heart attack" as these symptoms are also indicative of cardiac problems.

Sleep disorders are common following a trauma. Some individuals experience difficulty falling asleep as they are preoccupied with their overwhelming experience, while others, who may be fatigued, may fall asleep and awaken four hours later and be unable to fall asleep again. Others may experience sleep disturbances such as violent or disturbing dreams. These latter individuals usually awaken emotionally and physically exhausted. Some victims of trauma experience hypersomnia. They sleep for lengthy periods of time as they find sleep a secure state and an escape from their disturbing thoughts.

Psychological flashbacks generally occur when individuals experience a trauma that they are able to vividly recall, and their recollection of the event is visually distressing for them. These images usually occur during periods when they are fatigued or resting.

Individuals who are traumatized may suffer from phobias especially if the event is perceived as a threat to their security. Certain premorbid personalities are more prone to developing agora-phobias. These individuals experience difficulty socially and suffer with fears of losing control or fainting.

Victims of trauma or a critical illness may also suffer from depressive symptoms following their recovery. These may include poor self-esteem, loss of appetite, insomnia, physical weakness, psychomatic complaints, apathy and irritability. Some experience feelings of hopelessness and/or helplessness. They feel no one really appreciates what they have experienced and thus they frequently withdraw socially from family and/or friends. Some may even experience suicidal thoughts.

Many traumatized individuals have evidenced difficulties with their memory and/or their ability to concentrate. They are frequently preoccupied with their negative experience and are unable to absorb events or activities that lack a strong emotional component. Some have expressed difficulty retaining information that they read and others have shared their difficulties in following plots of stories they watch on television. These individuals need support and encouragement to write down pertinent information as their short term memory loss may be very frustrating and distressing for them.

Following a critical illness or injury, individuals may lose interest in previously enjoyed activities, which may include a loss of libido or their sexual drive. They may not only be unable to show affection but may also experience difficulty responding when they are shown affection. They may suffer from anhedonia, which is the inability to experience pleasure. These individuals usually withdraw socially and refrain from engaging in the leisure activities they premorbidly enjoyed. These symptoms may be particularly stressful for the spouse of the victim and consequently marital discord is a concern. Spouses of traumatized victims generally describe them as "self-centred" or "preoccupied."

Social workers should be attuned to these stress disorders so that they will be able to identify symptoms when shared by traumatized patients. When patients are reassured that these disorders are common after experiencing a critical injury or illness, they seem to cope more effectively.

These post-traumatic stress disorders are usually addressed in follow-up interventions after the patient has left the unit. During the patient's stay in the unit, their acute psychological responses need to be addressed. However, as previously mentioned, most critically ill patients are unable to benefit from social work intervention as they are either comatose or too confused to appreciate their interactions. Others, who may seem lucid, may benefit at the time; however, due to short term memory impairment, they may not retain or recall previous involvement. Thus, most social work referrals in this unit are requests for supportive or grief counselling for their families or significant others who are usually overwhelmed by the sudden onset of their loved one's critical state. Families confronted with a crisis may experience disequilibrium, disorganization and role changes (Hodovanic et al., 1984).

When the family initially attends in the unit, the medical team is usually occupied with either assessing or stabilizing the patient and thus the family may have to wait for a substantial period of time before it may be feasible for them to see the patient. During this period their fantasies and fears may be very distressing and thus a social worker, utilizing crisis skills, may be very supportive. The family's need, at this initial stage, is to see the patient and to obtain information about the patient's condition. Prior to meeting with the family, the social worker should attempt to acquire some basic information from the medical team to relay to the family, if a physician is not immediately available. This information may include what events led to the patient's admission to the unit; the patient's present state of consciousness, i.e., conscious or unconscious; whether the patient is on a ventilator or other support machines; the general presenting appearance of the patient, especially if the patient has facial lacerations, burns or disfigurement, which may be potentially upsetting for their significant others to view and an explanation of why they are presently unable to visit and how long it will be before they will be able to see their loved one. The social worker may also reassure the family that a physician will inform them of the patient's injuries or illness as soon as s/he has completed their initial assessment. In the interim, the social worker may secure an office or some privacy for the family to share their concerns and ask questions. The social worker may also commence her/his assessment of the family composition, their coping skills and ascertain who will be the designated family spokesperson. The family may have additional information about the trauma that may be helpful for the team in understanding the patient's and family's reaction to the event. This initial assessment should be shared with the medical team as soon as it is appropriate. Thus, in the initial stage the social worker liaises between the family and the medical team and provides the primary professional support to the family. If the significant other attends alone, the social worker may be helpful in assisting the individual to contact other family members or friends to provide additional support during this difficult period. The social worker may offer to contact a member of the clergy, if desired by the family.

If feasible, the social worker should attend the initial interview between the family and the attending physician to gain an appreciation of what the family is experiencing. Observation of the family's reactions and interpretation of the medical information is pertinent in the assessment of the family's coping mechanisms. If the social worker perceives that the family has misinterpreted the medical information, the physician should be asked to re-address the family for clarification. Individuals experiencing a crisis frequently experience difficulty absorbing or retaining information and thus the social worker may be instrumental in reiterating information for the family. The social worker may also be helpful by writing down the names of the specialists attending to their loved one.

After the family is oriented to the unit and adequately prepared for what to expect, the social worker, when possible, should accompany the family and provide support during the family's initial visit. Following the visit, the family may have additional questions that may need to be addressed. If the family is visiting from out of town, they may require assistance with accommodations. Some units have information pamphlets about the unit and pertinent information for families from out of town. Relatives, who are distressed, may experience a loss of appetite and insomnia and hence they should be encouraged to address their own needs during this crisis period. In studies to assess the needs of relatives of patients in intensive care, conducted by Molter (1979) and Stillwell (1984), they found that the greatest need was "to visit the patient frequently." They may also feel that they should remain in the waiting room for extensive periods and thus they may need "permission to leave." They may require reassurance that a nurse or a physician will contact them if the patient's condition changes. The family should be given the unit's number and encouraged to call through the night if they are concerned about the patient.

The patient's significant others may experience similar emotional responses to the trauma. They may also suffer from anxiety, guilt, anger and depression and may require intervention to ventilate their fears and concerns. Many family members fear that their loved one may die or be permanently disabled or disfigured. Some may express feelings of helplessness as they are unable to physically care for their loved ones. Others may be angry with the patient who may have failed to seek medical attention when symptoms initially appeared or they may feel that the individual's carelessness or alcohol abuse may have contributed to their present state. Some may have a need to express warranted or unwarranted guilt as they may feel some responsibility for the patient's condition. Another source of guilt may be premorbid marital or familial discord. Some individuals experiencing guilt may misdirect their personal anger toward staff and become very demanding. The social worker may act as a support to staff in assisting them to appreciate the family dynamics that may be responsible for their inappropriate display of anger. The worker may also be instrumental in helping the guilt-ridden family member to ventilate their guilt.

In spite of the efforts of the medical team, some individuals do not survive. Although it is not the social worker's role to inform the family of their loved one's death, they are requested to attend with the physician to inform the family of the death and provide grief counselling. The family may choose to view the deceased and the social worker may be helpful in preparing them for this visit and also providing support during their visit. Some family members may have a need to see the body to accept the loss while others may wish to maintain their previous memories. The social worker can be supportive in showing respect for each individual's decision and by suggesting that it is a personal choice so that each family member will feel comfortable with their decision. Family members may also need encouragement to grieve overtly and reminisce as these expressions facilitate the grieving process.

When it becomes apparent that the patient's condition is irreversible, the medical team may decide to divert their efforts from aggressive to compassionate care. A physician meets with the significant others to share the team's decision and gain the family's support for their decision. The social worker should be involved in this process to assist the family in accepting the inevitable. Some family members who agree with the decision may express guilt for their initial feelings of relief. With families who experience mixed emotions, the social worker can be supportive in assisting the family to appreciate that we grieve on two levels. On the intellectual level, they appreciate that continued medical treatment will not reverse their loved one's condition; however, on the emotional level, it is difficult to accept the loss of a loved one. Some individuals who have not had an opportunity to deal with their guilt may insist that physicians continue to be aggressive in spite of the patient's premorbid wishes. These individuals may need intervention to deal with their guilt in order to reframe their assessment of the situation. As Sherlock and Dingus (1985) suggest: "the family does not have the right to subject the patient to weeks or months of pointless suffering especially when the course of action chosen by the family does not reflect some special values or beliefs held by the patient when he or she was competent." Thus, it is the health care team's responsibility to act as the patient's advocate. Family members involved in this decision-making process may require bereavement follow-up to assess them for unwarranted guilt.

PRACTICE ROLES AND RESPONSIBILITIES

In the critical care setting, the social worker is a member of a health care team. The social worker's major role is to address the psychological and emotional responses and needs of the critically ill patients and/or their relatives and significant others. This clinical role includes a psychosocial assessment, crisis intervention, resource brokerage, grief counselling and bereavement follow-up.

In obtaining a psychosocial assessment the social worker assesses the patient's and/or family's premorbid and present coping skills; their presenting needs; the family's composition as only relatives and identified significant others may visit in the unit; the patient and/or family's supports and which family members may require continued intervention. In providing crisis intervention, the social worker attends to the family's initial questions and orients them to the unit. The social worker also takes on the task of preparing the family to view the patient and provides the initial support when visiting at the bedside. Additional roles include setting up interviews with physicians; clarifying misconceptions; reiterating pertinent information; providing concrete direction and encouragment to family members to maintain their own health and assisting the patients and their families in adjusting to the realization that the trauma may result in a permanent disability or disfigurement.

The social worker may act in the capacity of a resource broker by providing assistance with financial concerns; income benefits they may be entitled to during their illness; child care resources they can access during their hospitalization and other pertinent community resources that may be available to reduce their stress during this difficult period. Clergy or pastoral care services may be accessed if desired by the patients and/or their relatives. If the patient dies suddenly or if it becomes apparent that the patient will not survive, the role of the social worker would entail providing grief counselling; encouraging relatives to utilize their support systems and providing concrete information regarding family responsibilities following a death. If the patient is considered to be brain dead, and s/he is a candidate for being an organ donor, the social worker may be asked to assess the family's receptivity to a discussion of this issue. The actual request for organs is the responsibility of the attending physician; however, the social worker may be helpful in preparing the family, offering feedback to the physician and attending this interview with the physician to address any emotional responses that may arise. When a patient dies suddenly, when organs are requested or when the family does not seem to be coping effectively at the time of death, the social worker should initiate a bereavement follow-up contact to assess how the family is coping and to encourage the utilization of professional intervention, if indicated. If the patient does survive and continued intervention is indicated, during their rehabilitation on a medical floor, the social worker is responsible to either continue with the patient and or her/his family or appropriately transfer this case to another social worker for follow-up.

As a member of the critical care team, the social worker has a responsibility to relay pertinent information from her/his assessment to other members of the team, both verbally and in the form of a written consultation, on the patient's medical chart. The worker should continue to update the chart by providing any additional relevant information throughout the patient's stay in the unit. When feasible, the social worker should attend team rounds to keep informed of the patient's status in order to maintain a current appreciation of what they are experiencing and also to offer input and ongoing consultation to the team. In this role, the social worker functions as one of the primary liaisons between the team and the family.

The social worker may also be asked to provide in-service training to staff on either an ongoing or intermittent basis. In a teaching facility this role is inevitable. It may be the social worker's responsibility to provide orientation lectures to new staff members and provide weekly social work rounds to address ongoing patient/family concerns for nursing staff. Due to the stressful nature of working in such an intense environment, the social worker who possesses groupwork skills may be requested to provide ongoing support groups for staff. The social worker may also be asked to organize or contribute to ethics rounds, which are generally held on a monthly basis in teaching facilities.

POTENTIAL FOR ROLE DEVELOPMENT

In an attempt to set up a social work service in a critical care unit, the social worker should request to meet with the medical co-ordinator of the unit and the head nurse and initiate a discussion of the type of patients and/or families they may encounter on a daily basis. They may suggest that the majority of their patients are either confused or comatose and hence would not likely benefit from intervention. Thus, the social worker may have to convince them of the needs of the family members who spend lengthy periods of time in the waiting area. It may be helpful to empathize with them and express an appreciation of the need for their efforts to be directed toward the physical care of the critically ill patient, which may leave little time to address their emotional concerns or the needs of their relatives or significant others.

Most critical care units have patient rounds on a daily basis. The social worker may ask to attend rounds. Following rounds, the social worker could share with the team what skills s/he may have to offer the team in meeting the emotional and psychological needs of the patients and/or their families.

Another approach to initiating social work services in such a unit may be to provide an in-service lecture to the team on the potential role of a social worker in a critical care setting. It is particularly helpful if the social worker is able to cite a previous critical care case that was referred after the patient was transferred to a medical floor. The social worker should try to demonstrate how early intervention may have prevented or reduced the effects of a post-traumatic stress disorder, experienced by either the patient or a family member.

Once the team is convinced of the potential role for a social worker in the unit, the worker should attend daily rounds and establish an avenue for receiving consultation requests. Referrals may be made either during rounds or the worker may set up a daily meeting with the head nurse or charge nurse to discuss any new admissions to ascertain if social work intervention is indicated. It is also helpful to have referral forms available for staff to make referrals in writing when a need is identified. The social worker should provide in-service lectures, during this initial stage of development, to assist the staff in determining what cases would be appropriate to refer. The social worker can often be initially overwhelmed by the response and may find it necessary to prioritize cases, as potentially every patient admitted to a critical care unit, or her/his family, could benefit from intervention. The worker should be realistic in regards to the size of a caseload that is feasible to handle in such a setting. The social worker should also be cognizant of the immediate need to provide an assessment to the team.

When the social worker is established with a caseload, s/he may commence other roles such as providing support groups and ongoing in-service or weekly rounds. Frequently, the social worker finds it necessary to convince the physicians of the need to involve the worker in interviews with the family so that their emotional responses may be addressed. To create privacy for intervening with families, the social worker should request access to an office or an interviewing room in close proximity to the unit.

CONCLUDING REMARKS

With scientific and technological advances in medicine, individuals, who would have previously died of critical illnesses and multiple traumatic injuries are being maintained on life support drugs and machines in specialized critical care and trauma units. The line between life and death has become finer and at times blurred, and physicians are faced with ethical issues and daily decisions to either continue with their aggressive efforts or to divert their efforts to providing compassionate care and allow nature to take its course. Families and lucid patients are being involved in this decision-making process which may be guilt-producing, if their needs and concerns are not adequately addressed at the time. Brain dead patients, who previously died in emergency rooms, are now being maintained on life support machines as potential organ donors. Their families, who initially may have derived false hopes, are being approached to make difficult decisions while grieving the sudden loss of a loved one.

Social workers, who are equipped with interviewing skills, assessment skills, crisis intervention skills, an understanding of family dynamics and an appreciation of the grieving process, have an essential role to play in this setting. The social worker can be instrumental in assisting the patient and her/his family to maximize their coping skills and minimize the psychological effects of their trauma while simultaneously bringing relief for the other health care professionals, who need to focus their efforts on providing optimal physical care for the critically ill patient. Thus, social workers have a unique and valuable contribution to bring to this technically oriented environment.

The critical care setting offers the social worker daily challenges as the roles are multiple and the presenting diagnoses, and needs of their clients, are variant. However, this environment may be demanding and at times stressful as the worker is continuously confronted with critical events such as death and complex ethical issues as a member of the health care team. The workload is usually overwhelming and hence being well-organized and prioritizing work schedules are imperative for professional survival.

CASE EXAMPLE

Mr. B. was critically injured when the vehicle he was driving was struck head-on. His passenger suffered a lacerated liver and the occupants of the other vehicle were all killed. Mr. B.'s injuries included multiple facial fractures and lacerations; a fractured ulna (forearm); a fractured patella (knee); a fractured right femur (thigh bone); a chest injury and a head injury. When he presented in Emergency, the charge nurse requested social work intervention for his significant others who were apparently en route.

Since Mr. B. was intubated (ventilator-dependent), it was apparent that he would be admitted to CCTC (Critical Care Trauma Centre) and thus, to provide consistency, the Emergency social worker requested that the CCTC social worker be involved from the onset.

Since Mr. B.'s family had not yet arrived in Emergency, there was ample opportunity to see the patient and speak with physicians to gain an appreciation of his injuries and what the family would be confronting. Mr. B.'s wife eventually arrived with one of Mr. B.'s colleagues. She appeared very distressed and very anxious to gain information about her husband's condition. The physicians were still assessing Mr. B.'s injuries and thus they were initially unable to speak with her and suggested that the worker offer her some basic information in the interim. Mrs. B. was advised that her husband was awake and obeying commands upon his arrival in Emergency. She was also informed that he was having multiple X-Rays to ascertain the extent of his injuries and she was reassured that physicians were aware of her presence and a doctor would speak with her as soon as possible.

During this period, an attempt was made to address her concerns and assess who composed her family and support system. Within ten minutes, an Emergency Room physician attended to inform her of her husband's suspected injuries. He suggested that it would likely take an hour and a half to complete the required X-Rays and scans. He also alerted her to the fact that he was intubated and would require an admission to the (CCTC). As time progressed, Mrs. B. became more anxious and consequently the worker contacted the X-Ray suite to inquire if it would be feasible for Mrs. B. to see her spouse between X-Rays. With the surgeon's agreement, Mrs. B. was prepared for what to expect and provided with emotional support during her visit. After viewing her spouse, Mrs. B. seemed to cope more effectively and was able to share her fears, concerns and what information she had received about the accident. She also expressed concern about how to inform their 5- and 8-year-old daughters. She was advised to share some of his injuries with them; however, it was suggested that they not visit at this time as his multiple facial injuries would likely be very upsetting for the children to view. Mrs. B. was encouraged to bring in pictures of the children to attach to his intravenous poles and any drawings the children may wish to make for their father.

Mrs. B. was oriented to CCTC and given a pamphlet describing the unit, the technical equipment and the staff that would be involved in her husband's care. She was also accompanied during her first visit in the unit. When surgeons informed her of his required surgery, the worker attended the sessions and addressed her emotional responses and questions following the interviews. Since Mrs. B. had spoken with four physicians from different services, the worker wrote their names and specialties on her unit pamphlet for future reference. Physicians were asked to re-address the family on two occasions to clarify medical information.

Mr. B. suffered minor complications and thus continued emotional support was provided for his family during his stay in the unit. Mrs. B. was encouraged to make a cassette tape with her children to provide additional stimulation for her spouse. Mr. B. was seen regularly for emotional support and an attempt was made to orient him to his surroundings.

When his parents visited from out of town, they requested a letter to verify their son's critical state in order to cancel their vacation tickets. A letter was written to their travel agency and co-signed by a physician.

Mrs. B. was also advised that this would likely be an insurance and Workmen's Compensation claim as he was on company business when the accident occurred and thus she was encouraged to document any expenses.

When Mr. B.'s condition improved, he was transferred to a medical floor. Although Mr. B. was awake and alert during his stay in the unit, when followed on the ward he had no recollection of his stay in the unit. He requested information to fill in the two week void in his life and thus an attempt was made to outline events during his stay. Mr. B. grieved overtly as he expressed his gratitude that he survived the trauma and his sympathy for the victims' families. He was also encouraged to share any flashbacks or disturbing dreams that he may experience as a result of his accident.

Although Mr. B. was advised by physicians to attend the rehabilitation unit, he was anxious to return home and receive physiotherapy via the home care program. When Mr. B. goes home, follow-up contact will be provided by the worker. Also, Mr. B. will be encouraged to visit the unit prior to leaving the facility and his spouse will be encouraged to contact the worker if a need arises after his discharge.

References

Civetta, J.M. (1981). Beyond technology: Intensive care in the 1980's. *Critical Care Medicine, 9*(11), pp. 763 - 767.

Danis, M., Patrick, D.L., Southerland, L.I. & Green, M.L. (1988). Patients' and families' preferences for medical intensive care. *Journal of American Medical Association, 260*(6), pp. 797 - 802.

Hodovanic, B.H., Reardon, D., Reese, W. & Hedges, B. (1984). Family crisis intervention program in the medical intensive care unit. *Heart and Lung, 13*(3), pp. 243 - 249.

Kwasnicki (Tiegs), I.P. (1986). Ethical concerns in the critical care environment. *Medicine North America, 3*, pp. 588-595.

Luce, J. M. & Raffin, T. A. Withholding and withdrawal of life supports from critically ill patients. *Chest, 9*(3), pp. 621 - 626.

Molter, N.C. (1979). Needs of relatives of critically ill patients: A descriptive study. *Heart and Lung, 8*, p. 332.

Moonilal, J.M. (1982). Trauma centers: A new dimension for hospital social work. *Social Work in Health Care, 7*(4), pp. 15 - 25.

Parker, M. M., Schubert, W., Shelhamer, J. H. & Parrillo, J. E. (1984). Perceptions of a critically ill patient experiencing therapeutic paralysis in ICU. *Critical Care Medicine, 12*(1), pp. 69 - 71.

Sherlock, R. & Dingus, M. (1985). Families and the gravely ill: Roles, rules and rights. *Journal of the American Geriatrics Society, 33*(2), pp. 121 - 124.

Stillwell, S. B. (1984). Importance of visiting needs as perceived by family members of patients in the intensive care unit. *Heart and Lung, 13*(3), pp. 238 - 242.

Tiegs, I. P. (1988). Emotional concerns and ethical issues in critical care. In W.J. Sibbald (Ed.), *Synopsis of Critical Care* (3rd ed.). (p. 288 - 295). Baltimore, MD: Williams & Wilkins.

Chapter 17

SOCIAL WORK PRACTICE WITH PLASTIC SURGERY/BURN PATIENTS

CLIFFORD H. LEVY, BA, MSW

Abstract

For the social work practitioner on a burn unit/plastic surgery floor, the issues of patient stress, loss of function, independence and family distress must be dealt with in a context of a view of the treatment team that includes both patient and family members. The roles and functions of a social worker with burn patients and their families can vary from the traditional provider of moral support and legal assistance, to the provision of psychotherapy or cognitive behaviourial interventions (e.g., pain and stress management). Of particular interest to the practitioner is the stress level of the burn unit staff themselves, in addition to the ongoing and long-term follow-up of discharged burn patients and their families. Frequently, with the guidance, support and monitoring of the social worker, ex-burn patients can return to provide support to other patients and their families. Future directions for social work include a further integration of the network of supports possible for patients and a source of public education.

SOCIAL WORK PRACTICE WITH PLASTIC SURGERY/BURN PATIENTS

The Burn Unit/Plastic Surgery Floor in our setting is located in an older part of the hospital, which used to be called the isolation floor. As such, it is cut off from the rest of the hospital and, as the issue of isolation is still a prime one, most rooms are set up for private occupancy, with only one or two set aside for optional semiprivate use. Patients come to the Burn Unit, predominantly, following a traumatic burn situation and having come through the hospital emergency department or the emergency of their local hospital (if they are from out of town). Both patients and family members are distraught and exhibit all of the characteristics of high stress and anxiety. Upon admission, all major burns are bathed in one of the specially designed tubs on the unit. This bathing process, referred to as "tubbing" is a daily affair and includes the cleaning of the wound bed (debriding), which is a thorough cleaning and removal of dead skin to allow healthy tissue re-growth. Following the initial tubbing, the most common treatment regime is the application of burn dressings and their subsequent removal and reapplication twice more during the day. Also, a medicinal cream is applied with each dressing, which helps fight infection and with the process of sloughing the dead skin. Therefore, the average daily treatment includes one major tubbing and three dressing changes. Throughout this process, the patient is medicated. However, there is still a fairly high degree of anxiety and discomfort. These stressors may interact and create a complex situation whereby the pain and the emotional responses need to be acknowledged and treated accordingly.

THE CLIENTELE

An approximate breakdown of the demographics of burn patients[1] is as follows: About 65% - 70% are males. The main causes, in descending order of incidence, are flame or ignited gasoline, hot grease contact, propane, electrical and chemical burns. Almost a third of the patients seen are six years old or younger, and most of these children have been scalded by hot tea, coffee or water. Approximately 70% of adults are burned in and around their homes, with a little under 20% at industrial locations. Approximately 30% of burns occur when a person is alone and, for adults, 23% happened when other people were around. Surprisingly, at least half of the children burned were with their parents at the time. From anecdotal reports, most parents were within "touching distance" when the actual accident took place.

Both children and adults alike come to the burn experience with very little awareness of what to expect. They are quickly awakened to the realities of burn care and healing. Obvious problems that burn accidents bring forth include the exaggeration of existing financial, emotional and social difficulties, together with overwhelming pain and stress, and interference with ongoing roles or job functioning. For burn patients who are parents, they can no longer share in the care of their children and maintenance of their homes. For most, school, employment and most social relationships have to come to a temporary halt as the initial part of the burn healing process includes fairly strict isolation procedures. Both staff and visitors are seen wearing masks and isolation gowns. The patient's room and tub room are the two main areas of activity for periods ranging from several days to several weeks or sometimes even months. With more serious and debilitating burns, the patient must deal with the added problems of adjusting to loss of appearance and function and struggling through the sometimes lengthy rehabilitation process. While family members of burn patients share, to some extent, in most of these problem areas, they also have their own unique set of problems, including extreme feelings of guilt, anxiety, frustration and helplessness related to the injury and the painful treatment process. For instance, family members will often feel so helpless that they will project these feelings onto each other, occasionally onto the patients, and onto the hospital staff in the unit. With serious burns and those of medium severity, patients often go through a period of confusion or reduced awareness, usually in the early part of their admission. Family members have to cope with this state (i.e., the patient seems unaware and apparently unresponsive) while it lasts, and have no real sense how long this phase will last, how serious the injuries are or the level of disfigurement.

A preliminary inventory of psychosocial needs (for the patient) would include reassurance; an explanation of procedures; an introduction to normality as soon as feasible, including contact with non-medical staff and friends and family and ongoing support with the pain and stress of the treatment procedures. As the healing and rehabilitation becomes noticeable to the patient, other areas of concern usually arise. For example, financial and practical considerations will begin to become more important, and anxiety will usually begin to increase around discharge and possible subsequent rehabilitation. For the most part, family members exhibit similar needs from their own particular perspectives and, like a majority of patients, will tend to underestimate the impact of discharge on physical and emotional energy. This issue certainly has implications for ongoing follow-up and post-discharge, which shall be addressed later.

I. Meeting Patient Needs

In order to meet the basic needs of the patients and their family members, social work intervention needs to begin as soon as possible. Sometimes, this may be accomplished at the "admission to emergency" stage, while patients are still conscious. In this process, when emergency room physicians and/or plastic surgeons have been able to make their initial assessment and pass this information on to patients and family members, it is most helpful to have a social worker present so that they in turn can repeat and clarify information that has initially been provided. No new information is added at this time but it is understood that patients and family members alike will not necessarily hear or understand everything that they are told. This "availability" of a social worker is also the first step in developing the therapeutic relationship that is important throughout the various difficult phases of the treatment process. Once the social worker has been able to establish a defined relationship with patients and/or family members, subsequent difficulties can be dealt with, ideally, in a more humane and economical fashion.

Practical considerations may also be facilitated by the social worker, including accommodation for out of town family members or facilitating communication with an interested and involved employer. As well, nursing staff carry out the integral day-to-day treatment processes and monitor the patient's reaction to the treatment process and healing. In this regard, the social worker also pays particular attention to both a patient's reactions and those of family members. For example, where difficulties arise around pain management, stress management or, in general, inappropriate reactions to some of the situations, social work interventions can be made in a variety of ways. Often, there are misunderstandings on the part of the patient or family member and occasionally on the part of the staff. Usually, patients require extra support and assistance in developing new skills in coping with the stress and pain of burn care. Social work intervention can include one or all of the following modalities: traditional psychotherapy (including ego-supportive interventions, ventilation, problem-solving approaches); cognitive behaviourial interventions (cognitive restructuring, relaxation training and other stress inoculation techniques) and the provision of concrete assistance to patient or family (help in securing a T.V. for the patient, accommodation for a family member, liaison with a community agency to meet other related needs).

In completing the treatment process and preparing for discharge, and/or transfer to a rehabilitation floor, the issues of separation from the burn unit and fear of failure are common and need to be identified and dealt with. That is, the social worker can help both patients and family members anticipate these concerns and begin to struggle with them in a healthy way while still an inpatient.

PRACTICE ROLES AND RESPONSIBILITIES

As previously indicated, the social worker may become involved as early as the hospital admission to an emergency department. In general, the social worker's function then becomes an ongoing monitoring of psychosocial needs for both the patient and family members and an "initiator" and "organizer" of how the treatment team can best meet those needs. Along with the doctors, nurses, physiotherapists, nutritionists and other hospital support staff, the social worker also attempts to include the patient and family members in a healthy, co-operative venture, so that all parties can feel they are participating on a "treatment team," which is working toward the same ends (i.e., getting the patient and family through the treatment process as painlessly and as economically as possible). This strategy, while used in other areas of the hospital, is of particular benefit in a high stress setting such as the burn unit. For instance, encouraging active participation from patients and their families in the treatment process can be very helpful, especially in restoring a sense of "normality" to a painful and usually demoralizing situation. However, care must always be taken in identifying the larger share of responsibility of the medical staff on the treatment team. Thus, "balancing" the roles becomes part of the social worker's responsibility.

As a general guideline, patients and their families are told that the social worker is there to help with non-medical concerns, although there are some areas of overlap (i.e., working with patients during dressing changes in dealing with stress and pain management). In addition to facilitating communication between the various members of the treatment team, the social worker usually takes the responsibility for co-ordinating discharge plans, particularly where there are difficulties involved (i.e., limited resources, family out of town or in conflict, arranging extra support services from the community). When patients exhibit difficulties such as manipulative behaviour, non-compliance, avoidance or resistance to treatment, denial of their condition or the need to make plans for the future, the social worker is then expected to help assess the situation and participate actively in the overall treatment approach directed at resolving some of these difficulties or issues.

A brief overview of the **what, why** and **how** of the social work role in the burn unit is described in Figure 1, which is a handout often used in the orientation package to new staff and also in presentations to interested groups and the public. Reference has been made in this figure (under WHAT in the fifth section) to making informal connections between family members of different patients. Since drawing this figure, however, a patient and family support group has been started, and is seen by both ex-patients and burn unit staff as an important function for the patients and their families

Figure 1.
The What, Why and How of the Role of Social Work on the Burn Unit

WHAT	WHY	HOW
Automatic Social Work referrals on all burn patients.	Most burns are a devastating injury, to both the patient & the family.	talking, observing, answering their questions.#
Assess & support the coping skills of the patient & the family	They are in a crisis – encourage their strengths, supplement weak areas.	Read chart, consult with staff, try to be present when staff are talking to patients & families.
Repeat (when asked) what patient & family have been told by medical staff.	Under stress, patients & families do not hear and/or understand what they have been told.	Observe, consult with staff, less frequent contacts.
Monitor physical and emotional progress.		CAREFULLY, in the waiting room, halls, etc...wherever possible.
Connect (informally) family members of different patients and, when possible, patients themselves.	As their needs decrease, so does my involvement.	
	For mutual support.	Provide information, make phone calls, write letters, help with forms.
Practical assistance –liaison with community agencies & services.	To ensure that patients & families secure all the assistance & services for which they are eligible.	Out-Patient clinics, phone calls, home & office visits.
Follow-up	For continuity, an ongoing source of support (& assessment).	
	Referral usually filled out on intake.*	
	Spend time with them,	

Sometimes from Emergency or Critical Care Trauma Centre if a transfer to the Burn Unit is imminent.
Can spend longer more relaxed time with patients than is possible for medical staff.

It should be noted, however, that other types of patients who go through the plastic surgery floor are not involved in any ongoing support activity of which this author is aware.

The last item in Figure 1, **"follow-up"** can often be the longest phase of social work involvement with burn patients and their families. If a patient is in the hospital for one month, follow-up can be required for days, weeks, months or even years following discharge. The long-term view that social work can bring to this area of need is very crucial. While the physical healing can be primarily concluded within a few weeks or months of discharge, emotional healing continues, and the social work practitioner who has been able to establish a positive long-term relationship with a patient and their family is able to be available for any new crises as they occur. In the current climate of fiscal restraint, this practice can contribute, to a significant degree, to the consumption of time and money, and for the social worker, be a potential stress.

POTENTIAL FOR ROLE DEVELOPMENT

The issue of practitioners' stress is a consideration which cannot be ignored in terms of the overall burn unit staff and their day-to-day functioning, with patients in pain and family members working through their own anger, suffering, rage and feelings of helplessness. It is this author's view that, if a potentially high-stress, high-pain, dynamic and absolutely necessary service such as a burn unit is to continue and grow, the pain, stress and anxieties of the staff cannot be ignored. Ideally, the social work practitioner can assist with staff stress in at least two major ways. First, by providing practical and emotional support to patients and families as part of the treatment team, thereby helping us to share the load of providing service to a very needy client population. A second more indirect way of assisting staff is to monitor their interactions with patients and with each other, and encourage peer support by both modelling and in-service education. Specifically, some of the stress inoculation techniques such as cognitive restructuring and relaxation training are interventions carried out predominantly by social work and sometimes other clinicians; however, as suggested in some literature (Warnick, 1983), there is no reason why other burn unit staff cannot be trained to use some of these interventions. In addition to resulting in a reduced stress level on the patient's part, there would also be a significant increase in the amount of control perceived by staff. The issue of perceived control is just as important for staff as it is for patients and, within realistic limits, the increase of options will be beneficial to both staff andpatients.

Another area where the social work practitioner could further develop is the area of networking and prevention. The network of support systems presently includes the patient family, close friends, the in-patient staff and the out-patient clinic follow-up team. Another element of this support network that could be explored by the social worker, is the population of fire fighters who are regularly delivering burn patients to burn units. Specifically, there is a potential for fire fighters to provide and receive some added support from the social work practitioner plus the in-patient staff and the patient and family support group. Fire fighters as a rule have to be very strong and single-minded physically and emotionally. By including those fire fighters who are willing in this support network, there could be a two-way benefit (both to them and from them). Thus, in either the individual or group context, social work could provide an added support to fire fighters and include those fire fighters in providing support in an ongoing way to burn patients and their families, together with assisting the support group in their educational efforts in the community. It should be acknowledged that both the fire fighters in this hospital's community and the burn unit staff are already aggressively involved in educational and preventative programs. Further, by facilitating some support relationships that are not otherwise there, this network could be enlarged and strengthened, and be more beneficial to the participants andthe general public.

CONCLUDING REMARKS

Ideally, a succinct analysis of role definition should include a few distinct categories of role function and allow for most social work activities to fall within these "steps" of intervention. Retrospectively, looking at work in the burn unit, these steps might include four major categories of activity. These would be:

1) problem identification (what are the emotional, physical relationship needs of the client/patient?);
2) role clarification (how can I help?);
3) co-ordinating/encouraging commitment of resources (family, friends, outside agencies, fellow staff) and

4) redefining a healed or healthier patient/client (encouraging or re-labelling a healthier level of function).

By generalizing most of the burn unit social work activities in one of these categories, it becomes clear that a general job description is possible and generalizable. Also, this "sequence" or "category of functions" may be used as a guide to ongoing re-assessment. As new problems arise, or old ones manifest differently, these four basic steps can be re-applied. However, a more specific description of role function follows in the case example.

CASE EXAMPLE

It has been almost a year since Mrs. V., a 60-year-old widow, had been admitted to the burn unit in pain, confusion and total bewilderment. Apparently, she had passed out while over a hot sink of water and incurred full thickness scald burns to both her hands and wrists. Thus, almost every square millimetre of skin, which was affected, needed to be grafted in order to allow healing in a reasonable amount of time. As medical tests progressed in her initial stay on the burn unit, it became evident that Mrs. V. did indeed suffer from a form of seizure that had been previously undetected. Consequently, social work intervention began with the identification of two broad problem areas:

1) loss of independence and
2) adjustment to illness and injury (seizures and burns). [Problem identification]

Mrs. V. has been living on her own for over 20 years and has two married children in their thirties, one of whom lives just outside the city and another who lives about an hour's drive away. Over the years, contact with her family has been sporadic as Mrs. V. likes her independence and does not like to be a "burden" on any family members. This low level of contact within this family had been forced, by the accident, to change drastically for a period of time. For instance, both children tried to make extra time available to visit their mother in the hospital and later, while she was recuperating at home, some extra contact was also needed. An already close relationship with an only grandchild did not change markedly, either during or after treatment. Mrs. V.'s main source of income was through Health and Welfare Canada in the form of a spouse's allowance and a small additional support from Department of Veterans Affairs.

Mrs. V.'s initial tasks in the early weeks of hospitalization included dealing with her loss of independence, the extreme discomfort of dressing changes, the emotional loss of control (the original blackout and injury) and future prospects of limited function around her scarred and healing hands. Social work involvement provided emotional support for the immediate stress of day-to-day coping. Also, Mrs. V.'s children were contacted during the normal process of their hospital visits and encouraged to help their mother and become involved in the treatment process as much as practically possible. [Role clarification]

As referred to in the first paragraph of this chapter, the issue of anxiety and discomfort can be a very complex matter. Mrs. V.'s perception of pain and discomfort during dressing changes and physiotherapy sessions was quite high in comparison to the actual tissue damage that still remained. However, in the context of her severe sense of loss and fear for her future, the overall suffering that she experienced was very real and much higher than that accounted for by the pain of her healing hands alone. As such, Mrs. V. was a prime candidate for some cognitive behaviourial interventions, which included examining her perceptions of the accident, her future and the treatment process in a very realistic manner. Also, stress reduction techniques such as relaxation and imagery were used. While none of these techniques were seen as "magic answers," in conjunction with compassionate nursing care and the use of medication, they can help reduce the overall level of suffering significantly. Mrs. V. did indeed report an improvement in her pain level and a slight improvement in her sense of control.

Mrs. V. was eventually discharged following several weeks of slow and stressful healing. Prior to discharge, social work involvement also included the securing of some funds from the Department of Veterans Affairs in assisting Mrs. V.'s purchase of pressure garments. [This, along with the day-to-day team functioning on the unit, may be seen as part of the co-ordinating role]. Pressure garments are those individually measured and made items for exerting pressure on the healing scars on her hands and wrists. Since they are individually measured and made, they are extremely expensive. Following her discharge, Mrs. V. came to the Out-Patient Burn Clinic on a regular basis to see the plastic surgeon and out-patient physiotherapist, and was also seen by myself for further contacts to continue her relaxation training. This was eventually reduced to contact only at the Out-Patient Clinic as her functional and emotional healing demonstrated quite clear improvements. [Redefining a healthier patient]

Now, almost a year following her discharge, Mrs. V. is ready for some corrective procedures in the areas of her hands where scar tissue has not responded to the ongoing treatment of pressure garments and natural healing. At this time, Mrs. V. is much more confident in her day-to-day functioning, and her pattern of behaviour and interaction with her family has reverted to its old style and frequency (i.e., on a lower key and less frequent). Although she does anticipate some mild anxiety around the normal stress of an operative procedure, it is entirely within reason and she has, in effect, benefited from the learning and healing that she has already experienced. In turn, Mrs. V. is now potentially ready to assist other burn patients in their adjustment process, and the social work role is to allow and encourage this sort of outreach and sharing of strength and experience. Specifically, when a social work practitioner can assist a supposed "victim" in their own physical and emotional healing and help them return to aid other "victims," then the sense of job satisfaction and the social worker's identity is indeed very positive. More importantly, Mrs. V. herself can feel that there is and will be positive outcomes to her burn experience.

References

Buchanan, K. (1981). The impact of critical illness on the family: Stresses and responses. In D. S. Freeman & B. Trute (Eds.), *Treating Families with Special Needs* (pp. 207 - 217). Ottawa: Alberta Association of Social Workers & Canadian Association of Social Workers.

Ellis, A. & Greiger, R. (1977). *Handbook of Rational Emotive Therapy.* New York: Springer.

Gazzinger, M. S. (1988). *Mind Matters* (Chaps 1, 11, 12). Boston: Houghton Mifflin.

Kendall, P. C. (1983). Stressful medical procedures. In D. Meichenbaum & M. E. Jaremko (Eds.), *Stress Reduction and Prevention* (pp. 159 - 190). New York: Plenum Press.

Pearsal, P. (1988). *Super Immunity* (pp. 233 - 243). New York: Ballantine.

Wernick, R. L. (1983). Stress inoculation in the management of clinical pain: Applications to burn pain. In D. Meichenbaum & M. E. Jaremko (Eds.), *Stress Reduction and*

Prevention (pp. 191- 217). New York: Plenum Press.

Endnotes

[1] For purposes of this chapter, burn patients will be used as the focal point; however, other plastic surgery patients are seen and often display similar needs and require similar social work interventions.

Chapter 18

SOCIAL WORK PRACTICE IN A PSYCHIATRIC AMBULATORY CARE SETTING

Sherrill Hershberg, MSW, RSW
Craig M. Posner, MSW, RSW

Abstract

This chapter describes the practice roles and responsibilities of two ambulatory care psychiatric social workers at the Health Sciences Centre, Winnipeg, Manitoba. The clientele served are described in terms of psychiatric problems, family, social, housing, socioeconomic and vocational needs. It emphasizes the importance of a psychiatric knowledge base and describes the day-to-day clinical functions of the authors. The ways in which a psychiatric social worker applies this knowledge to clinical practice are discussed and demonstrated through a case illustration.

SOCIAL WORK PRACTICE IN A PSYCHIATRIC AMBULATORY CARE SETTING

The field of Psychiatry in the twentieth century has witnessed the development of psychotherapeutic and psychopharmacological approaches to the treatment of mental illness. The more primitive approaches to mental disorders have given way to a complex set of assessment and treatment tools, and social work has played an important role in the development of these tools. The perspective of looking at the psychosocial aspects of patient care was pioneered by Ida Cannon and Dr. Richard Cabot at the Massachusetts General Hospital. Cabot was concerned that his patients' individual and family problems were interfering with the completion of their medical treatment (Bartlett, 1975). In 1905 he hired Ida Cannon and brought the first social workers into the Outpatient Department of the hospital. They went on to develop the field of medical social work and influenced health care centres throughout North America. The Winnipeg General Hospital (re-named the Health Sciences Centre in 1973) was one of the institutions influenced by Cabot and Cannon's initiative. A Social Services Department was established in 1920 and has since grown to its present complement of 41 social workers.

The Department of Psychiatry at the Winnipeg General Hospital was established after World War II, and social work was involved from its inception. Today there are 13 social workers involved with Child, Adolescent and Adult Psychiatry. This chapter will focus on the adult outpatient psychiatric population within the ambulatory care psychiatric services of the Health Sciences Centre.

Ambulatory care psychiatric services at this hospital are provided through different programs and clinics established to meet the needs of a diverse population. The service originated with what is now called the Psychiatric Outpatients Department where, on the average, patients and families were seen in therapy for one-hour weekly appointments. Two additional outpatient programs have evolved in the past decade in order to meet the growing need for specialized short-term crisis oriented care together with extended care for the chronic mentally ill. While functionally the ambulatory programs are separate, the role of the psychiatric social worker in each of these programs is more similar than different.

This chapter will focus on the functional aspects of the social work role in a hospital's outpatient setting. The authors have drawn from their clinical experience in order to demonstrate how psychiatric social work's theoretical concepts are practically applied.

THE CLIENTELE

Most patients come to see an ambulatory care social worker following initial assessment and treatment on an inpatient psychiatric service. The types of problems referred are primarily major mental disorders, including schizophrenia, mood disorders, mood personality disorders and eating disorders as described in the *Diagnostic and Statistical Manual of Mental Disorders* (American Psychiatric Association, 1987). While the majority of clinical work is done with this population, patients and families presenting life crisis issues, such as adolescent separation and death of a spouse, are also seen.

In this ambulatory care setting the frequency of patient visits to their social worker may range from as often as once per day, as would be indicated when monitoring an acutely suicidal outpatient, to as infrequently as once per month when the patient situation is very stable.

Depending on the treatment plan, patients are interviewed in an office setting, either individually or with their families, and in groups with other patients. The length and degree of the treatment structure must be sensitively geared to the patient's tolerance level. For example, a newly discharged patient with a diagnosis of schizophrenia generally is very sensitive to the stress of clinical interviews (Anderson, 1986), and brief interviews focussing on concrete issues work best.

When describing the patients seen by the social worker one should address the following psychiatric and psychosocial features:

1. Psychiatric problems
2. Family and social relationships
3. Housing needs

4. Socioeconomic needs
5. Vocational needs

I. Psychiatric Problems

In the 1960s with the advent of de-institutionalization, long-term hospital beds were significantly reduced. As a consequence, some patients who would have received extended hospitalization then are now discharged into the community prematurely, before their treatment is completed (Talbott, 1988). Patients with active psychiatric symptoms are now managed in the ambulatory care programs. Most of these patients, who have a diagnosis of schizophrenia, frequently experience auditory and visual hallucinations, delusions and paranoid ideation (American Psychiatric Association, 1987). Once these symptoms are under control, many patients are left with residual problems such as lack of energy, amotivation, difficulty forming and maintaining relationships and a poor tolerance for stress.

Patients with a diagnosis of schizophrenia will in almost all cases be treated with psychiatric medication. These medications help control the symptoms described earlier and help a patient reintegrate her/his thinking. Unfortunately, psychiatric medications do not remove the residual problems such as motivation and do produce side effects, the most prominent being dry mouth, blurred vision, muscle stiffness and drowsiness. Most of the side effects can be managed with special medication for this problem. However, side effects can be difficult for some patients already struggling with a disorder that impairs their thinking (Andreasen, 1984), and they often need much encouragement and education about the importance of tolerating these side effects and taking medication as prescribed.

Another problematic area for such patients is managing the residual symptoms of their disorder. While medication may control or erradicate hallucinations in some patients, excessive anxiety may remain, and the patient will have difficulty assuming various day-to-day tasks such as leaving home to do grocery shopping, riding buses or even coming to hospital for appointments. One of the ways a social worker can help the patient is by breaking the tasks down into manageable components.

Many psychiatric patients experience lowered self-esteem and the assumption of the patient role often results in "...introspection and questioning Who am I? Why do I suffer so? What am I to make of my life? How can I ever feel worthwhile again?" (Hatfield, 1987, p.69). The social worker helps the patient to deal with these issues through a supportive and nurturing relationship.

II. Family and Social Relationships

Family relationships are significantly disrupted by the presence of a family member with a major mental disorder. Furthermore, patients and families experience guilt, anger, frustration and isolation (Posner, 1987). It is important for patients, families and therapists to address disrupted family and social relationships often brought on by the presence of a psychiatric disorder. Terkelson (1987) has noted that "the appearance of mental illness in a family member is invariably a disaster for the whole family, a disaster in which all are victims of the event and its sequelae" (p.128). Since everyone in the family is affected by the presence of a mentally disordered family member, the patient may experience severe changes in family responsibilities and roles. The family now must assume the roles the patient once carried out and as a result they become even more burdened. "Families who feel burdened may in turn be less able to provide support and thus further deplete clients' support systems. Lack of social support then can lead to clients' readmission to hospital" (Crotty, 1986, p.186).

III. Housing Needs

Psychiatric patients require different types of housing depending on their level of functioning (Talbot, 1988), and most patients find that their level of functioning declines with the onset of a major mental disorder (Lefley, 1987). Patient requirements may range from highly supervised settings with 24-hour professional supervision, to independent living programs. The psychiatric social worker, having completed a psychosocial assessment of the patient, helps identify what type of residential setting best accommodates the patient's needs.

IV. Socioeconomic Needs

Most psychiatric patients are not self-supporting because of the debilitating effects of the disorder (Lefley, 1987). As the rehabilitation period is lengthy, they become reliant upon family and the social welfare system. This includes public and private disability insurance policies, unemployment insurance (UIC), and social assistance. The social worker can help by providing practical support in this area and linking the patient with appropriate community agencies.

V. Vocational Needs

Psychiatric patients have great difficulty maintaining regular employment, even if they were employed prior to hospitalization. Some patients who become psychiatrically disabled in adolescence have never had the opportunity to develop vocational skills and therefore might require the social worker's help in setting vocational goals. Many of our patients are referred to Vocational Rehabilitation Services, which is a comprehensive community program aimed exclusively at the vocational needs of the physically, mentally and psychiatrically handicapped.

PRACTICE ROLES AND RESPONSIBILITIES

Ambulatory care social work in a psychiatric setting can be quite demanding. The social worker operates as a member of a multi-disciplinary team consisting of a psychiatrist, psychiatric nurse, psychologist, occupational therapist and recreational therapist. Each discipline brings its own expertise to the team and it is essential that each has a clear perspective of its own unique contribution. The social worker on the team brings a special systemic understanding of the patient's needs and, in addition to all the generic tasks she or he performs, this understanding is the basis of all planning and treatment strategies. The following case example from our practice demonstrates how a social worker functions on a multi-disciplinary team.

A 37-year-old, depressed male patient who had been attending the Day Hospital Program, taking medications regularly, and who was thought to have a low-stress living situation, continued to be depressed. When the social worker on the team suggested that his social situation be further evaluated, it was discovered that the patient was attempting to take care of an ailing elderly parent, and also a sister with a diagnosis of schizophrenia. Helping the patient to apply for homemaker services for his family relieved his burden, and he quickly improved.

In order to competently practise psychiatric social work in any psychiatric setting, a social worker must have knowledge and understanding of psychiatric disorders, their symptomatology and known treatments in addition to social work knowledge and training. DSMIII-R is an essential reference for all practitioners in the mental health field. It is a diagnostic manual categorizing psychiatric illness in a descriptive manner, without consideration of causality.

The practice responsibilities of a psychiatric social worker in an ambulatory setting are many and diverse. They are as follows:

I. Social and Psychiatric Assessment

In this setting the social worker completes a psychosocial assessment on a patient. This involves a comprehensive analysis of the individual within his social and psychological environment. In addition, the social worker in consultation with the psychiatrist participates in the psychiatric assessment of the patient.

II. The Case Manager Role

In addition to being a member of a multi-disciplinary team, psychiatric social workers in ambulatory care often function as case managers.

Defining what is meant by case manager is a difficult task, and in fact the concept has been characterized as a Roschach in which individuals project whatever definitions they desire (Kurtz,1984). Generally, the case managerial concept has encompassed assessment, planning for the patient, linking with community resources, monitoring patient functioning and advocating on the patient's behalf.

In addition to these linking tasks, the social worker in our setting is expected to provide psychotherapeutic services to patients and families.

III. Interventions

Individual, group, marital and family therapies are all part of the social worker's practice in this setting, and the social worker is the facilitator for network therapy when this is required. The latter refers to bringing the various components of a patient's social network together for the purposes of clarification and planning.

Psychoeducational therapy is an essential part of our practice with patients and families of the mentally ill. Goldman (1988) defines it as follows:

> The education or training of a person with a psychiatric disorder in subject areas that serve the goals of treatments and rehabilitation, for example, enhancing the person's acceptance of his illness, promoting active cooperation with treatment and rehabilitation and strengthening the coping skills that compensate for deficiencies caused by the disorder (p. 667).

IV. Consultation and Referral

A psychiatric social worker in this setting should recognize the importance of utilizing the best resources available to her/his patient. Clearly none of us can provide all the services required by our patients, and learning to consult colleagues both within our own department and the broader agency network is an extremely important part of our work.

V. Education and Research

The expectation of this setting is for the social workers to provide clinical supervision to others on the team, make academic presentations, attend conferences, keep up with current psychiatric and social work literature and carry out clinical research when time permits.

POTENTIAL FOR ROLE DEVELOPMENT

Often the clinical demands of the job limit opportunities for role development. However, if we are to develop professionally in a way that best serves our patients, attentiveness to this area is a necessity. As a result, we do our utmost to reach beyond the daily tasks of our job. We have identified three areas from our clinical practice that lend themselves to role development.These are Research, Lobbying and Education.

I. Research

Social work will increase its legitimacy in the health care field, and ambulatory care psychiatry specifically, if it looks at what is being done already and what can be done in the future. This requires research. Above all, "psychiatric research requires that staff possess very specialized knowledge, " (Boronow, 1988, p. 233) and social work must acquire that knowledge so it can be self reliant, rather than dependent on others to direct professional practice. A hospital's psychiatric outpatient department is a natural setting in which to conduct research. Currently, a family group psychoeducational research project is being administered by one of the authors (Posner). This project is a two-year, controlled study involving families with a schizophrenic member. The goal is to determine if an 8-week psychoeducational program will help reduce re-hospitalization rates.

II. Lobbying

This is an age of lobbying and pressure groups. If one does not publicly push for the needs of particular interest groups, they are often ignored. This principle applies to those with a diagnosis of a major mental disorder. Social work can make a difference by examining, documenting and informing the public and government of where to direct its resources.

Those with major mental disorders have specialized needs, and while much has been documented in the literature, the ambulatory care social worker is constantly identifying new needs as they arise. Being sensitive to these, keeping track of them and then lobbying when appropriate is an important area for role development.

The nature of a psychiatric illness is such that patients are often not capable of being strong advocates for their own positions. As a consequence, the psychiatric social worker in the ambulatory care setting should assume the responsibility of lobbying for their patients' needs. In our clinical setting, some of the needs we have identified are adequate financial assistance as a basic right; the special needs of the mentally disordered female patient (Anderson, 1989) and the need for more specialized housing and recreational outlets.

III. Education in the Hospital Milieu

Social work should be prepared to share its knowledge and expertise with other professionals on the multi-disciplinary team. This can be done through teaching rounds, case consultation, research, publications and workshop presentations.

CONCLUDING REMARKS

Social work can make a positive difference in the care of the psychiatric outpatient. We have shown that knowledge about psychiatric disorders is one integral part of the psychiatric social worker's professional role. What also distinguishes this role from other disciplines on the hospital's multi-disciplinary team is the social worker's ability to assess the patient within his social context. This provides other dimensions to the care of the patient and also to his family, and the possibilities for treatment and preventive interventions are greatly expanded. Many new treatment concepts are being developed, and this ultimately will lead to better prognosis for the patient, and may even help to prevent patients' children from becoming psychiatric patients themselves.

CASE EXAMPLE

The patient is a 36-year-old, married caucasian female who has two adopted children ages 8 and 10. The patient, whom we will call Karen A., was diagnosed as suffering from schizophrenia and was hospitalized nine times over a period of 10 years. When she was acutely psychotic, she experienced auditory hallucinations of a command nature telling her to kill herself, together with delusional beliefs that the world was going to end and that she and her children would be killed because they had broken the holy grail. Before discharge from hospital to the ambulatory care services, the patient reintegrated gradually, after having been treated with medications and supportive therapy. After each admission, the patient, who previously functioned as a school teacher, could not carry out the most basic of homemaking tasks. This type of deterioration is not at all uncommon with a schizophrenic disorder. Fortunately, her marriage was reasonably stable and the patient's husband, Bill A., competently took care of the children while she was in hospital.

The focus of Karen's hospitalizations were to help relieve her of the symptomatology she was experiencing. As a result, the effects of the disorder on her husband and children, and also on Karen's role in the family, were not addressed in depth. When Karen was discharged from hospital after her 8th admission and returned home, she felt guilty about her disorder and her inability to resume her previous responsibilities as wife and mother. She attempted to do all the things she had done prior to her illness onset, but was simply unable to and became very anxious. This excessive anxiety contributed to her re-hospitalization four weeks later.

During the course of this 9th hospitalization, one of the authors completed a psychosocial assessment on Karen when she was referred to the Adult Partial Hospitalization Day Treatment Program. It became clear through this assessment process that, in addition to the debilitating effects of her illness, this patient was faced with an extremely difficult home situation. Her son was recovering from leukemia and was hyperactive, and her daughter was hearing impaired. Both required extensive medical care, and her husband was struggling to manage all the responsibilities at home and at a full-time job. It was apparent to the social worker that a pattern had ensued in which the patient would become stressed at home, symptomatic and require re-admission to hospital. The social worker identified this pattern to the inpatient hospital team and recommended that a full-time homemaker be placed in the home in conjunction with the patient attending the Adult Partial Hospitalization Day Treatment Program. This is a multi-disciplinary ambulatory care program addressing the social, vocational and recreational needs of the mentally ill through daily activities.

Four weeks later Karen was discharged. She began attending the Adult Partial Hospitalization Day Treatment Program and was assigned a social worker as her case manager.

Karen's individual therapy sessions with her social worker initially focussed on her feelings about having a psychiatric illness. She expressed fear, anger and guilt and eventually was able to work through her denial of the illness. When Karen began to accept her disorder, her ability to manage it increased. Through the psychoeducational process she recognized the importance of complying with her medication treatment and she also became aware of the need to limit stressful situations as much as possible. She also learned to identify the signs and symptoms that forecast the return of her illness.

As Karen's situation stabilized, homemaking services were cut back and then terminated as she was able to take over this role herself. She moved from being a woman who spent hours in bed unable to cope, to a fully self-sufficient homemaker. In fact, she came to a therapy session one year into treatment and proudly announced to her social worker, "I had ten people over for dinner this past weekend and it went very well."

In her individual sessions, Karen expressed the concern that her psychiatric disorder was placing pressure on her husband and children because she was not consistently available to help out at home. As a result, Karen and Bill were referred to a social worker colleague in the outpatient department for family therapy while her individual therapy continued.

The following issues were identified and dealt with. They were commitment to the marriage, discipline of the children and management of the home.

Karen was concerned that after nine hospitalizations her husband Bill would give up and end the marriage. He had been forced to take over more of her roles in order to compensate for her decline in functioning. After each hospitalization her increasing dependency on Bill made it harder for Karen to resume previous social roles. She stated she was unhappy placing such a load on her husband. Bill supportively understood and agreed that Karen, when ready, should resume her past activities and roles. He made it clear in the family sessions that he was totally committed to their marriage and reassured his wife directly about this. This was a pivotal event in the course of the therapy and helped Karen open up with her husband. Resolving the issue of commitment helped the A's focus on their relationship. The A's were next able to work out new ways of sharing parental responsibilities such as discipline, and they reported positive change over time as tasks discussed in the therapy were carried out. These tasks applied to issues such as organizing school work, bed time and managing public behaviour.

It should be noted that it was very important to Karen to resume traditional roles in the home. As a result, Karen began to prepare meals, clean the home, shop and entertain, and performing these tasks made her feel much better about herself. Bill confirmed that her competence had significantly increased and he felt very positive about the results. He felt the burden he had been under had lifted. Their relationship was now achieving a level of increased balance.

Now one and one-half years after this comprehensive treatment plan was implemented, Karen has not required admission to hospital and remains symptom free. Homemaker services have ended and she manages the home on her own. The family therapy sessions were terminated as the marital relationship stabilized and the childrens' functioning improved in the family context. Karen now is working as a teacher's aid in a local school. Her need to attend the day treatment program has diminished and a discharge date has been established.

This case succeeded when multiple systems interactions, i.e., medication management, homemaking services support and individual and family therapy, were utilized. The key to success was co-ordination of these services by the social worker in day treatment who was sensitive to Karen's changing needs over time.

References

American Psychiatric Association (1987). *Diagnostic and Statistical Manual of Mental Disorders* (3rd ed. revised). Washington, DC: Author.

Anderson, C. M., Reiss, D. J. & Hogarty, G. E. (1986). *Schizophrenia and the Family: A Practitioner's Guide to Psychoeducation and Management.* New York: The Guildford Press.

Anderson, C. M. & Holder, D. P. (1989). Women and serious mental disorders. In M. McGoldrick, C. M. Anderson & F. Walsh (Eds.), *Women in Families: A Framework for Family Therapy* (pp. 381-405). New York: W.W. Norton and Company.

Andreasen, N. (1984). *The Broken Brain: The Biological Revolution in Psychiatry.* New York: Harper and Row.

Bartlett, H. M. (1975). Pioneer in medical social work. *Social Service Review, 49*(2), 208 - 229.

Berg, W. E. & Wallace, M. (1987). Effects of treatment setting on social workers' knowledge of psycho-tropic drugs. *Health and Social Work, 12*(2), 144 - 152.

Boronow, J. J. (1988). Inpatient psychiatric research units. In J. R. Lion, W. N. Adler & W. L. Webb (Eds.), *Modern Hospital Psychiatry* (228-250). New York: W. W. Norton.

Crotty, P. & Kulys, R. (1986). Are schizo-phrenics a burden to their families? Significant others' views. *Health and Social Work, 11*(3), 173 - 188.

DeChillo, N., Matorin, S. & Hallahan, C. (1987). Children of psychiatric patients: Rarely seen or heard. *Health and Social Work, 12*(4), 296 - 302.

Goldman, C. R. (1988). Toward a definition of psychoeducation. *Hospital and Community Psychiatry, 39*(6), 666 - 667.

Hatfield, A. B. (1987). Coping and adaptation: A conceptual framework for understanding families. In A. B. Hatfield & H. P. LeFley, (Eds.), *Families of the Mentally Ill: Coping and Adaptation* (pp. 60-84). New York: The Guildford Press.

Kruzich, J. M. (1986). The chronically mentally ill in nursing homes: Issues in policy and practice. *Health and Social Work, 11*(1), 5-14.

Kurtz, L. F., Bagarozzi, D. A. & Pollane, L. P. (1984). Case management in mental health. *Health and Social Work, 9*(3), 201 - 211.

Land, H. M. (1986). Lifestress and ecological status: Predictors of symptoms in schizophrenic veterans. *Health and Social Work, 11*(4), 254 - 264.

LeFley, H. P. (1987). Behavioural manifestations of mental illness. In A. B. Hatfield & H. P. LeFley, (Eds.), *Families of the Mentally Ill: Coping and Adaptation* (pp. 107-127) . New York: The Guildford Press.

Posner, C. M. & Smith, S. (1987, May). Schizophrenia and the family: A psychoeducational approach. Paper presented at the Western Canadian Conference on Family Practice, Banff, Alberta.

Talbott, J. & Glick, I. (1988). The inpatient care of the chronic mentally ill. In J. R. Lion, W. N. Adler & W. L. Webb (Eds.), *Modern Hospital Psychiatry* (352-370). New York: W. W. Norton.

Terkelson, K. G. (1987). The meaning of mental illness to the family. In A. B. Hatfield & H. P. LeFley, (Eds.), *Families of the Mentally Ill: Coping and Adaptation* (128-150). New York: The Guildford Press.

Chapter 19

SOCIAL WORK PRACTICE WITH INSTITUTIONALIZED FRAIL ELDERLY

Len Fabiano, BA, RN
Ron Martyn, MA

Abstract

The dramatic increase in the number of older people in recent years and on into the next century has heightened awareness of the need for increased and improved institutional services for the elderly. The field of social work has changed and will continue to change to meet the new demands placed by the system and by the older frail clients. This chapter focusses attention on the changes and expectations of social workers in response to the special needs of the frail elderly in both generic and age-specific institutions. The skills required of the social worker for this specialized area are presented, along with strategies for future development in the field.

SOCIAL WORK PRACTICE WITH INSTITUTIONALIZED FRAIL ELDERLY

THE CLIENTELE

I. The Numbers

In recent years, the dramatic increase in the number and percentage of people over 65 years of age in Canada and North America has been a major focal point for demographers and service providers alike. Expectations of an ever increasing cohort of senior adults has heightened concern for the demands that will follow in the health care sector. The reality is that the percentage shift of elderly persons has already begun. The number over 65 years of age will peak to over 20% of the total population (as compared to an average of 11% in 1986) by the year 2020 (Marshall, 1987).

The institutionalized frail elderly account for between 3% of the population over 65 years (e.g., United States) and 8% of the population over 65 years (Canada, Sweden) (Berg, Branch, Doyle & Sundstrom, 1988; McPherson, 1983). This major variation in percentage terms reflects a combination of several factors. Where there are insufficient affordable institutional services, the rate of institutionalization is lower. Similarly, where there is an availability of extensive home support services, the rate of institutionalization will be decreased. Conversely, where there are limited home supports, combined with affordable available institutional services, the percentage of institutionalized frail elderly will be increased.

A further consideration is that the major increase in this age group falls into the category of the "old-old" — those over the age of 85 years. This age group is the fastest growing segment of the older population and represents the largest portion of the institutionalized frail elderly (Atchley, 1980).

The implications for the future are obvious. Not only will the numbers of older persons increase significantly, but the number of "old-old" (and consequently, the frail institutionalized elderly) will increase even more dramatically. This shift has already resulted in changes to the health care delivery system, and it will force even more dramatic changes over the next thirty years.

II. Profile of Institutional Care Settings

The institutionalized frail elderly are found in both general population or generic health care settings and age specific facilities.
General or generic settings include acute care hospitals, psychiatric facilities and special treatment centres. Age specific settings
include nursing homes, homes for the aged and, to some extent,
retirement facilities. The roles and functions of social workers in
relation to the frail elderly will be examined relative to both types
of settings.

III. General Population (Generic) Care Institutions

By their very nature, general population institutions were never
specifically geared to a particular age group. The intent of such
service agencies has been to provide care to all regardless of age.
However, as a result of the recent surge in the numbers of older
adults, such institutions have increasingly recognized that this
segment of the population constitutes a disproportionately high
number of the total clients being served.

The impact of an increasingly older client has presented new
challenges for the generic facilities. Not only do the special needs
of this clientele place special demands, but there are also increased
operational pressures on the system that impact the entire organization. Older clients require longer recovery times for most treatments and, as a result, the turn-around time from admission to
discharge increases significantly (Novak, 1985). Generic settings
today are finding that their costs are increasing as more and more
clients become long-term in nature — not only is there added cost
for the longer treatment program, but there is added pressure for
more bed capacity to resolve the shortage of bed space for those
awaiting admission. To increase the bed capacity puts added pressure on an already financially taxed system.

Social workers are employed in most generic settings. They
provide services to the broad range of clients within such institutions, but they too feel the impact of encountering more older
clients. The need for more time to serve these long term stay
patients adds pressure to the job that was not there until recent
years. Likewise, this segment of the population requires from the
professional new skills and knowledge to effectively deal with
their complex problems.

Some generic facilities have responded accordingly by providing an increased psychogeriatric perspective in treatment plans, upgrading staff and hiring gerontological specialists within each discipline area (Becker & Kaufman, 1988).

IV. Age-Specific Care Institutions

Until the early 1970s, few social workers were employed in age-specific care institutions. The focus of care in such settings was quite limited. Further, programming, supports and resources were at a minimum. The average age of resident populations was typically mid-to late-70s, and although the clientele were frail, they were provided few supports.

In the late 1980s, a different resident profile has emerged. The average age of the resident population is now late 80s, with a new mandate for care that employs concepts such as quality of life, individualized care and home-like environments (Singer & Lyons, 1985).

There now exists two distinct groups of long-term care facilities. There are those that are preparing for the next decade. These are facilities that have clear and progressive focusses in their philosophy, programming, staff supports and resources. Looking toward the next decade, they have become the forerunners in establishing innovative ideas for the service industry.

The other group of long term care facilities are those that are still trying to figure out how to get into the 1980s. This group fits the stereotypes of such settings. They have been delinquent in keeping up with the knowledge, trends and expectations within this specialized area. Such facilities are struggling to continue functioning, let alone provide quality of life for unique clientele (Grossman & Weiner, 1988).

Long-term care is very diverse, not only in its progressiveness, but in its configuration. For example, working in a 600 bed facility creates different demands than working in a 60 bed facility. A facility located in a major urban setting is quite different from one located in a remote rural setting. Likewise, the configuration of the resident population within any one facility can vary dramatically. Many facilities have three distinct groups: those clients who are cognitively and physically well; those who are cognitively well but physically disabled and those who are mentally impaired.

Furthermore, one cannot guarantee a homogeneous age group even in what are usually considered age-specific institutions. Some facilities in some regions have individuals as young as 14 mixed with others as old as 105, all under the same roof. Some even have a mixture of seniors with long time institutionalized mentally handicapped individuals of a variety of ages.

When one speaks of becoming involved in age-specific long-term care institutions, there are many options from which to choose. Without national guidelines, there are no guaranteed standards of services and supports within any long-term care facility across the country. Direct-care staff in most long-term care facilities consist mostly of nurse's aids, with registered nursing staff generally assuming management functions. Recreation staff play an integral part in direct care provision in this setting as well. In the typical age-specific long-term care setting, every member of the facility, from housekeeper, to aid, from maintenance man to administrator, is an integral part of the care process and team (Fabiano, 1989). This is especially important when one considers that the majority of staff come from a variety of backgrounds and disciplines and possess minimal training in this specialty. This is an approach that is not generally encouraged in the acute care or generic setting.

Presently, the majority of age-specific long-term care facilities do not employ social workers. Even though the need and desire may be present to have such a specialist on hand, most generally do not receive the necessary funding to add that position to their staff compliment. Fortunately, this is changing as pressures within the industry to increase funding allow for flexibility to integrate a social worker position within the majority of long-term care facilities.

What is evident to this point in the evolution of the social workers' role within long-term care is that the limits and scope of the role within any one facility depend very much on the initiative and creativity of the individual social worker involved. The challenge for the field of social work is to anticipate the changes before they happen and incorporate new and innovative strategies in response to the increased demands and changes.

V. The Frail Elderly Clientele

The institutional setting in which the older adult is located determines to some extent the problems that they present. In other words, the differences associated with the social, psychological and physical environment of different institutions may result in varied responses in any one client. Therefore, it is important to consider the frail elderly in relation to the types of settings in which they are found.

The elderly admitted as short-term-stay patients (a few days) in the generic settings do not create the same problems as those who become long-stay patients (a period of weeks or months) in an acute care setting. The older adult seldom exhibits one distinct impairment. Rather, he typically demonstrates a variety of disabilities. When placed in a setting that includes younger clients, the differences can cause problems.

The contrasting profiles of the younger versus the older person, their premise for being in generic settings and the impact and prognosis of their diagnosis are contributing factors to difficulties they will inevitably encounter.

For example, a younger person may be admitted to the hospital with a leg fracture suffered in a football game at school. In the bed next to him is an elderly man who fell at home and broke his hip. While the injuries are of the same general nature, the individual needs and responses can be quite diverse. The energy, resilience and recuperative powers of the young man may result in his fracture having little more impact than restricting him to bed. His cognitive and physical energy level is still intact, resulting in his need to be active and occupy his time to relieve the boredom. As a result he does those things he likes to do — play his radio (loudly), watch television, do his homework and visit with his friends [which periodically seem to occur all at the same time!].

Meanwhile, the effect of the fractured hip on his elderly roommate is much more severe. This older gentleman is not so quick to "bounce back" to his normal self. The demands now placed on him both physically and emotionally may be taxing his remaining resources to the limit. In fact, the combination of the injury, its restrictiveness and the effects of the medication given for pain may cause bouts of confusion and disorientation. Any added noise or disturbance in his room represents further stress that he cannot easily deal with at this time. Hence, the conflict. Both patients become increasingly frustrated and agitated with each other. This places demands on staff to resolve the conflicts and smooth over the differences in this imposed relationship.

Furthermore, the pace that staff normally maintain can be constantly challenged by the older client. As a person ages, his functioning levels decrease. Reflexes, muscle strength, co-ordination, cognitive processing, etc., are still intact and working, but are not as fast nor as resilient as when he was younger. This does not create a handicap to any older person in their life course, they simply learn to adapt to the gradual changes as they occur. But when that older person experiences a disability, that limitation now taxes those resources to the limit.

Adding further to such problems may be the approach, perception and focus of the facility and staff toward the long-stay older adult in the general population care centres. In a setting that is focussed on treatment and recovery, and measures its successes by major positive changes in a person's condition, performance or behaviour, working with the long stay older patient may be seen as counterproductive to the organization.

The improvements of the older patient experiencing multiple long-standing problems, associated with a decrease in physical energy, stamina and recuperative power, are often less dramatic than staff are accustomed. When the prognosis shows little gain, those staff who are trained to "cure" are frustrated in what they perceive as the benefits of intense and aggressive efforts.

For facilities and staff who are geared and trained under the medical model of care, the older client can be seen as a source of frustration. Such frustrations are manifested both overtly and subtly. Overtly the facility can point to the back-up of treatment and long waiting lists as evidence of the negative impact older people have on the care system and the reason for the institution's inability to cope. In a way, the older clients are often seen as the source of institutional paralysis.

Negative consequences of staff frustration with the older client can be more subtle and consequently more difficult to identify. Seldom will staff openly express their frustration about the older long term patient. However, it becomes difficult to contain one's frustration over a long period of time. Eventually, staff may not be able to control their feelings and frustrations when performing care with this client. Although it is hoped that the quality of physical care is not jeopardized, the emotional and psychosocial components may be. The older client will often find the staff's time spent with him becomes less and less.

In some settings this can be understandable. Generally, the majority of generic institutions are not environmentally equipped to handle a long-stay patient. The best example is an acute-care hospital. Many medical floors where such a patient will be found do not have lounges, dining areas, etc. The patient is then restricted to his room for extended periods of time because there is really nowhere else he can sit. The general expectation is that the patients will wear hospital gowns rather than being dressed, perpetuating for the older patient the sick role. Staff on such units do not normally consider how a patient must occupy his day. The usual expectation in the generic setting is that patients are too ill to be concerned about fulfilling their time or are well enough to occupy it themselves. The older long-term patient is usually not ill enough that he can be oblivious to the hours passing, nor well enough to be independent in filling those hours. His boredom and isolation can only complicate his frailty, resulting in withdrawal or behaviour outbursts in order to break the pattern and routine of this setting.

The care of older clients in generic institutions will not only continue in the future, but will be accelerated. The implications for such settings are that both the institutional and staff approaches to care for the frail elderly will require significant changes in order to best serve this clientele.

VI. The Age-Specific Institution and The Frail Elderly

One of the most common stereotypes of aging is that all "old people" are alike. In actual fact there are as many differences among the older population as there are between the young and the old (Keith, 1982). This is perhaps easier to appreciate when one thinks in terms of age spans. It is easy to accept that the needs and interests of the 15-year-old are different from that of the 35-year-old. (They don't even know who the musical performers are that each other prefers, let alone like each others music!) On the other hand, there can be an expectation that the person who is 70 years of age has a great deal in common with the person who is 90. Just as there is a 20 year span and differences in interests and needs in the younger age comparison, there are similar differences between these older groupings. They don't all like the same old tune. The difficulty for staff in an institution for older clients is to not only recognize and support these differences, but also be aware that over time the institution must change as the age cohorts change.

One problem that may be perpetuated in an age-specific long-term care facility is that if all clients are older and disabled to some degree, then the range of expectations made of the clientele, by the institution, its staff and the clients themselves can be less. The obvious detriment of such a setting is that there can be this "age-ghettoization" process. There are few, if any, younger people within the facility (other than the caregivers themselves), and the older clients become isolated and surrounded by a diminished level of expectation — a "what else can I expect at my age" response (Fabiano, 1989). This becomes a self-fulfilling prophesy of course — because the client does not expect to be able to do more, it becomes difficult to motivate the client to try harder, to go beyond the current functioning level. And while the personal lifestyles of the younger population can pose frustrations and difficulties for the older client in the institutional setting, the older person can also long for some contact with age groups other than the elderly. It is common in an age specific setting to hear an older client comment about visitors "breathing some life into this place" following a visit by a group of young persons or family members.

Upon entry to the age-specific long-term care facility, the person does become a "resident." The name itself is indicative of the institutional expectation of the person's tenure — this is not for recovery, rehabilitation and return home — this is for recovery and rehabilitation to the point where the person will be able to function at his maximum level given the circumstances he is experiencing. This perception and expectation is reinforced by the operating norms (most people stay long-term, and the staff reinforces the person's settling in and making this home). Residents are encouraged to bring in mementos and some furnishings from home. There are no restrictions on visiting hours, and there are more offerings of seemingly non-therapeutic recreational activities, much like what one would find in the outside community.

The net result of this process has the potential of reinforcing the client's loss of control and choice. Now that the person is in an institutional setting, there generally is little discussion or acceptance of the idea of a return to home. The negative responses (fight or submission) may be heightened in response to this new environment (Fabiano, 1989).

Social workers within the age specific institutions face many problems that are similar to those experienced in generic settings. Both clients (now referred to as residents) and family members are the key target groups for the social worker's efforts. Residents in the long-term care settings exhibit the same responses of resignation, unrealistic anticipation and a realistic acceptance combined with the determination to try to deal with the disability as well as possible. However, there may be differences in the intensity of the response now.

The converse of the resident's acceptance of his or her functioning level provides the social worker with the next challenge. Once the resident has accepted the status of "resident," the problem of resignation and giving up may become more of an issue. The social worker now must work to provide encouragement for the person to continue to try, to be involved in the face of recognizing that things may not get a whole lot better.

Again, the client must come to understand that making the choice to do nothing also has consequences. By doing nothing, there will be change; there will be further deterioration. As bad as things may seem now, the resident must understand that they can get worse if nothing is done and there is withdrawal from the surrounding people and activities of the facility. The social worker provides both individual and group supports for residents in the long-term care environment. While the bulk of such interactions may take place in the early stages following admission, there will also be the need for ongoing support for different residents at different times (Burnside, 1984).

The function of helping residents understand their own responsibilities in their personal care plan is an important element in the process of motivating residents. It is one in which the social worker plays a key role, but not the only role. The social worker must function as a team member, co-ordinating approaches and strategies with all members of the care team. Not only does this have implications for the obvious functioning areas in the facility such as nursing, OT, physiotherapy and recreation, but also the not so obvious areas such as housekeeping and dietary. The social worker must work with all other team members as equal partners in the care process. The dietary aide can either reinforce or undermine the team's efforts simply by casual comments or actions in the course of serving a meal. Similarly, the housekeeping aid can have a dramatic impact on the resident's outlook and approach to life. Most people who work in long-term care generally concede that residents will often disclose more to the housekeeper who comes into their rooms every day than to any other member of the care team. Without encouragement and recognition that they have such valuable insights, the housekeeping staff will often not be aware that they have this exceptional vantage point and will not come forward with their observations. The social worker must not only be open to talking to the housekeepers about what they have seen and heard, but they must also reinforce with them the important role they can serve and encourage them to share this input with others.

Times have changed in long term care. It used to be that the main concern centred around physical issues — programming to prevent bedsores and contractures and dealing with bowels and bladder. The field then progressed to centre attention on social issues such as activation and activities. Now the industry is beginning to focus on the socio-emotional concerns.

Nothing less than 100% of the clientele within long-term care are candidates for depression, one of the predominant disorders of the frail elderly (Butler & Lewis, 1982). Given the variety and severity of losses experienced within a short period of time, from widowhood to a change in lifestyle, to relocation, disability and so on, it is no wonder that these individuals experience what can aptly be termed "compounded grieving" (Fabiano, 1989). The challenges of dealing with the emotional side of these people are only now being recognized in long-term care, and the role of the social worker is crucial to this care process and approach.

PRACTICE ROLES AND RESPONSIBILITIES

The roles and responsibilities of social workers in generic and age-specific institutions are different in the configurations of job responsibilities. However, for the most part, their functions are similar in terms of the specific components that make up the job itself. Therefore, the practice roles and responsibilities are examined here from the broad perspective, rather than from a facility type perspective.

One problem confronting individual social workers is that they face the same moral dilemmas as other health care professionals when confronted by the prospect of working with the elderly in long-term care. For many, the reasons for getting into the field are the same as those that repel them from working with the institutionalized frail elderly.

Individuals are drawn to the social worker field for a variety of reasons, but at the heart of the decision, there is generally a desire to help those who are in need. However, the frail elderly can present too much need. Some care providers find it difficult to deal with people with so many impairments and limitations as those living in long-term care. When confronted with a client whose prognosis presents only short term marginal gains before their condition is further eroded or they are eliminated by death, the care provider's need for personal gratification may take precedence over the desire to assist the client.

The reality is, most professionals believe that working with other populations in the health care sector is seen as more attractive, glamorous and exciting, where the clients have more potential for improvement over a longer period of time. In a society that highly values designer clothes, exotic foreign cars and life in the fast lane, and where people are inundated by a media blitz focussed on drugs, alcohol, sexually transmitted diseases and child abuse, the realities of the needs of the frail elderly are lost. People working in the health care sector, including social workers, are obviously influenced by such societal values and focuses. It is difficult for health care professionals to be motivated by wrinkles, sagging body parts, incontinence, memory loss and the constant presence of death.

The frail elderly represent one of the social worker's greatest challenges. Not only must the social worker help the client overcome her/his response to the various impairments and obstacles, but the social worker must overcome her/his own personal notions and prejudices about the elderly, growing old and the relationship of this to the professional role of the social worker to be effective.

Social workers can perform a variety of functions when serving the older adults in institutional settings. The differences vary depending on both the type of setting and the individual expectations of the specific institutions themselves. In some instances, the social worker is hired to perform typical social work functions, not unlike those that would be performed with a non-age specific group. At other times, the social worker might be hired into an age specific position where social work skills are seen as a benefit, but where there may be an expectation of many other non-social work functions to be performed. In either situation, the social worker is seen as a key player in the provision of care.

The philosophy of age-specific institutions is centred on holistic care that is consistent with the mandate of the social work profession. The skills the social worker brings to the setting are viewed as not only fitting within the philosophical perspective, but are seen as being as important as the provision of physical care for the clients.

The social worker in a non-age-specific institution is usually seen as a member of the larger health care team. In its legitimate form, the social worker has as much input and importance as any other member of that team — be it the physician, nurse, occupational therapist or whomever (Edelson & Lyons, 1985). The reality is that this often falls short in actual practice. The social worker may find that the "hard facts," such as patient temperature, blood pressure and bowel movements carry more weight within the medical model of health care than the less measured and calibrated observances of the social sciences. There are realities about the degree of how holistic the care might be, given such restricted perspectives. The placement of the social work department and personnel within the organization should help to shed some light on the status of the program within the facility. If it is located under the medical umbrella, then there may be a realistic expectation that there will be a dominant role to be played by the medical staff.

The social worker in long-term care takes on a more diverse role than in other settings. The social worker generally has an eclectic approach — counselling residents, family and staff, assessment and placement co-ordination of prospective residents, policy development, leading support groups, educating—almost anything can be expected in this setting. The range of responsibilities and duties of the social worker depend very much on the size and progressiveness of the facility in which that person works and the ability and drive of the individual social worker in each setting. Such a professional may be expected to cover any or all of the following components:

1) Working With The Client
     - direct counselling
     - behaviourial assessment and intervention
     - support group
     - education
     - advocacy
     - resource utilization

2) Working With The Family
     - direct counselling
     - support group

- education
- integration into care

3) Working Within the Organization
   - assessment & placement
   - employee assistance program
   - policy development
   - volunteer co-ordination
   - research
   - co-ordination with psychiatric services
   - staff training
   - community outreach co-ordination

I. Working With The Client

1) Direct Counselling

There are no easy solutions to the problems and dilemmas of those living in long-term care. The social worker is challenged in this setting to broaden her/his expectations beyond the curative role to a qualitative one — qualitative in the sense that the quality of life for the individual is enhanced to the highest possible level, given the losses and impairments that will not go away. There is a major limitation in the social worker fulfilling this role in a long term care setting: limited time. One social worker in a facility of 200 residents cannot invest much time to do one-to-one counselling for all residents and still perform the range and variety of other duties that would be expected. In this environment, it is important that the social worker not concentrate his/her attentions on all residents, but focus on those who the staff cannot handle or who are having the greatest problems.

The social worker takes on a more challenging and creative role in such a setting that can be almost consultative in nature, required to provide the guidance and support for the psychosocial component of care within the entire setting.

Again some social workers in long term care will say that their time is so limited that they cannot counsel any residents. As identified earlier, it is the creativity of the social worker that often dictates job priorities and performance. The effective social worker in such a setting learns to take advantage of and utilize all the available resources. This involves completing the initial and ever important assessment, defining the problems, breaking the ground with specific counselling interventions and then assigning specific staff or volunteers to provide that listening ear (Edelson & Lyons, 1985). The utilization of other residents (Scharlach, 1988) and individual staff (Moss & Pfohl, 1988) as "buddies" for new and troubled residents is proving to have considerable success in the institutional treatment program.

2. Group Support

Group support in long term care is not, as yet, a well developed area (Burnside, 1984). The wide age range, responses and degrees of impairment do not make it easy to have a group of residents interact well in such a setting. The trend has been to move from a restricted group (i.e., only stroke victims or arthritic victims), to general resident support groups (Scharlach, 1988). This allows small groups of residents to discuss and resolve some of the problems of living in a communal setting.

3. Behaviourial Assessment

The skills and insights of the social worker may be most important in getting to the heart of the problem experienced by the resident. It is too easy for untrained staff to see the superficial behaviour of the resident as the problem, rather than identifying the underlying factors that may be causing that behaviour. By not understanding the complexity and interrelationship of this person's circumstances, it is easy for such staff to become critical and impatient with what their client demonstrates, only further compounding the problem (Fabiano, 1987). Providing all staff with a clearer picture and some direction to deal with the problem is probably the most rewarding facet for any social worker's efforts. Tapping the sensitivity and compassion of the staff in long term care, and steering their efforts to a successful conclusion, represents a significant positive role for a social worker in this setting.

4. Resident Advocacy

Our society is inundated with concerns about human rights. Long term care is an industry under that pressure. It is the social worker who is often called upon to become the resident's advocate. The social worker represents the individual resident's wishes and desires on any decisions made by the care team. The social worker's assessment skills and counselling abilities provide the opportunity for the most objective perception, ensuring that the freedoms and rights of the resident are respected.

5. Education

A very limited area of development in resident supports in the long-term care industry is in resident education. It is important that those who are able do understand their disability, circumstances, rights within the facility and how to relate to others living within the same environment with a range of disabilities and limitations. Such perceptions are essential for quality living within such an institutional setting. The social worker, through both individual and group interactions, can be the primary catalyst for such insights.

II. Working With The Family

The other side of the social worker's responsibility within long-term care has to do with the families of the older clients. There exists a strong stereotype that families abandon their older parents in long-term care settings. In fact, many families are very involved with their family members (Butler & Lewis, 1982). The major problems that are encountered by families are the same as the residents' — the sense of helplessness, not knowing how to deal with mom or dad and what their role is in relation to the changing needs of the parent. These feelings of helplessness and undeveloped interactional skills can keep families away over the long term. In many cases, by the time the family member is admitted to long-term care, the family is exhausted.

Typically, the older client will have support from family members, and particularly from daughters. This group has traditionally provided the greatest degree of support for older parents, and the trend continues even as more women enter the work force and share in the provision of the family income. The social worker is confronted by children who are determined to do what is best for their parent and, while well motivated, they are not always well directed.

Family members are often driven by feelings of inadequacy regarding their availability for support for their aging parents. One hears the lament "If only . . ." implying they have been negligent in their support or selfish in their decision to place the parent. With these feelings of inadequacy come feelings of guilt — guilt that they could have or should have done more (Hansen, Patterson & Wilson, 1988). In actual fact, families are left in a "damned if you do and damned if you don't situation." No matter what decision they make, "bad feelings" are associated with it (Fabiano, 1989).

While the family members may have done everything possible, given their time constraints, personal and family commitments, this does not alleviate the immediate feelings of guilt that something more could have been done. The family members' expressions of this guilt may be manifested in less than obvious ways, such as staying away and rarely visiting, or displacing their negative feelings on the caregivers. The care providers can frequently encounter extreme hostility, unrelenting demands and suspiciousness when dealing with family members.

The social worker must be prepared for "real feelings" to be expressed by family members, and these can include not only present circumstances but factors that may stem from long standing-relationship problems with their parent—such as old hurts that have not been resolved or complex family dynamics. Families in long-term care can present the full gambit in terms of family counselling needs. This can include dealing with family issues, relationships, and emotions that have been in place for 50 years or more and are now complicated by current compounded losses and changes within the family structure. Such situations call not only for the social worker to listen carefully to what is being communicated, but also to recognize that such long-standing problems usually cannot be resolved through short-term interventions.

The social worker plays an important role in helping the family members face the realities of their parent's present situation and helping them to establish legitimate expectations for the future evolution of treatment for their aging parent. Ideally, the family members should become an integral part of the care plan process (Hansen, Patterson & Wilson, 1988). If they are involved in the process, they can become important facilitators in the efforts of enhancing their parent's quality of life, rather than becoming deterrents when their dealings with the older client run contrary to the institutional care plan (Shulman & Mandel, 1988).

Family members are usually open to suggestions for helping their parent adjust to her/his situation and progress beyond her/his current functioning level. The social worker can work with the family members through inservice sessions and special family gatherings. Not only do the families gain a better understanding of the social worker's plan, but they can be given specific training and suggestions on how to be more effective visitors. This client group is likely to be dealing with the existing impairments over an extended period of time, and the family will need all the resources it can find to make the visits worthwhile for the client, and enjoyable and meaningful for themselves.

Just as knowledge about options and consequences is crucial for the client, the same holds true for the family. And just as the social worker must leave as much control and choice in the hands of the client as possible, the family too must understand the importance of this approach on their part as well when dealing with the parent.

II. Working Within The Organization

There are a wide range of roles that can be filled by the social worker. They can include any one or combination of the following:

1. Pre-admission Assessment & Placement

Probably the most universal and long standing role of the social worker in long-term care is in the area of assessment and placement. This involves interviewing potential clients for admission, determining whether their admission is appropriate, defining the individual's needs in relationship to the facility and making recommendations to an admission committee. This function involves assessing the potential client at his home or in another health care facility, meeting and interviewing available family members, coordinating the medical assessment and developing the subsequent report and recommendations.

2. Policy Development

In recognition that the social worker in this setting is probably the most knowledgeable person with respect to the psychosocial needs of the client, the social worker is involved in almost all aspects of organizational growth and development that pertain to such concerns (and these concerns impact almost all elements in the care process).

3. Staff Education

Many social workers are required to augment the staff training program by providing regular inservice sessions for staff on aging, emotions and grief, death and dying, behaviourial management, communication skills, etc. Staff within the facility can range from individuals with little or no formal education in the people-caring field to highly skilled health care professionals. Staff training by the social worker must meet the wide range of needs of this diverse staff group.

4. Employee Assistance Programs

Employee assistance programs have not been well developed in many long-term care facilities. It has become the social worker's responsibility in many facilities, especially in the smaller rural settings, to provide staff with assistance with personal problems, from family issues, to drug and alcohol abuse and so on. In many cases this may involve some counselling to determine the problem and then linking that staff member with available community service agencies for follow-up.

5. Volunteer Co-ordination

In some settings the role of overseeing volunteer utilization is assigned to the social worker, either being part of her job directly, or having a full or part time volunteer co-ordinator assigned to her, depending on the size of the facility. The rationale for the social worker to have this under her umbrella, rather than any other department head, has to do with the skills required to direct the volunteer on interacting with the residents and staff, and the importance of linking the volunteer with residents requiring the appropriate support.

6. Community Outreach Co-ordination

Many facilities assign community outreach programs to the social worker's jurisdiction. These programs can range from day centres, respite care and walk-in clinics, to community meals support programs (meals-on-wheels). The attempt is to link the social worker with the community in utilizing the resources available through the facility with contacts made for potential admission. Individuals placed on a waiting list for admission are often those who can best utilize these services on an interim basis. The social worker is often required to maintain that waiting list and ensure it is updated, and it is therefore appropriate for this person to link the services provided by the facility with these individuals while they remain in the community.

7. Co-ordination with Community Services

The social worker is usually the contact person for external non-medical services needed for resident care. This involves psychiatric assessment and consultation with the available psychiatric institution or unit, social service programs such as family counselling to link family and staff, drug and alcohol counselling and treatment centres.

8. Research and Publication

Probably the least developed area for involvement by the social worker (and most other team members as well) in long-term care is in the area of research. More and more facilities are monitoring their progression and results as they develop their strategies in caring for an increasingly complex clientele . This is becoming one of the ways to justify increased funding for new and innovative projects. The skills of the social worker makes this area a necessary component of their role. The result cannot only be recognition for the individual and the facility, but also enhanced service opportunities through increased funding.

POTENTIAL FOR ROLE DEVELOPMENT

The social worker's role and responsibilities within institutional settings seem almost limitless at this point in time. In the generic settings, there will be opportunities to facilitate the organizations' attempts to come to grips with serving an increasingly elderly dominated clientele. In the age-specific settings, there are limited standards or expectations of the social worker role, and there will be tremendous latitude for development of the field in this setting. It will depend primarily on the individual facility, the perception of the need and benefits of such a professional, the philosophy and progressiveness of the facility, the resources and time made available to the individual social worker and the initiative and personal drive of the individual fulfilling the role.

The reality is that the numbers do not match the need. In a relatively new area of specialization such as long-term care, each facility is pressured to evolve in multiple directions at the same time in order to keep up with the increasing demands and expectations placed on it. In the planning of some facilities, the social worker role is seen as a part of that progression. In other facilities it has been a long-established and integrated role, while yet others cannot see the position being of high priority in their immediate growth. The reality is that the changing clientele (changing in terms of needs and numbers) will force the requirement for the increased availability of social workers within such settings.

The future older adults that will be served are the "me" generation, the post war baby boomers. This cohort has been a dominant group throughout their lives in our society and one who has been comfortable and successful in dictating policy directions. There is no doubt that they will probably continue to do so into the future as well. Therefore, there is greater likelihood that services for older adults will increase in magnitude and there will be increased demands for quality services as the baby boomers approach their own old age and see the need for better services. There is also less hesitation on the part of many in this age group to seek out professional help in dealing with emotions and relationship issues as compared to those who are presently over 75 (Lasoski & Thelen, 1987). It will be an expected service by those entering institutional care settings.

As has already been identified, areas such as resident advocacy and community outreach and co-ordination are being recognized as crucial in the health care continuum. These are areas that are ideally suited to the skills of the social worker, and there probably will be opportunities to develop and be involved in such services.

Much of the impetus for the increased utilization of social workers in the age-specific institutions is likely to come from within such organizations in the future. This can only help to reinforce the need for the expansion of services to include social work as a discipline into itself in the future. This self-advocacy on the part of social workers should be facilitated by networking among both practising social workers and non-practising social workers who are functioning in related capacities (Karuza, Calkins, Duffey & Feather, 1988). If social workers recognize the pioneering role that they can assume in the age-specific institutions, the need and value of networking will be obvious, and this will become an increasingly important area of involvement for them in the future.

CONCLUDING REMARKS

Throughout this chapter the focus has been on the current and future role of social workers in institutional settings. At times, the role appears quite established and clear. In other instances it is seen as being buried or almost non-existent — social work practices and skills being implemented through the auspices of other disciplines and functions. Both scenarios are visible in the workplace today. The challenge for social workers of the future is to determine where in this scenario they will be able to function most effectively. Some will personally find the established positions to be what they are seeking and they will benefit most by moving in that direction. Others will be excited by the crusading nature of becoming involved in the less well-defined areas of service and will embark on this more uncertain career path. Either route offers tremendous scope and opportunity for the social workers of the future.

CASE EXAMPLE

Mr. Jones has had a history of relative affluence. He was a bank manager for 42 years until he was forced to retire (with many misgivings) at the age of 65. In retirement he initially had considerable difficulty filling his time and defining his role. He interpreted retirement as "being old." He believed he had little purpose. His pre-retired life was predominantly occupied by his job, and without it he had difficulty defining his personal self-worth and identity.

His relationship with his wife was always strong. In retirement that relationship only intensified. She filled the void, challenging him to become involved, becoming his main companion. For three years she directed him into rewarding activities, with much of their time spent travelling. He was beginning to enjoy his changed status and the freedom it provided him.

At the age of 68 Mr. Jones experienced his first stroke. Although the residual effects of that stroke were minimal, it hit him hard, only further reinforcing his previously held misconceptions of "being old" and his changing role. Again it was his wife who became his main motivational support. It was her encouragement and persistence that drew him away from the abyss of emotional collapse. Two years later he experienced his second stroke. The residual effect this time was much more severe. He lost movement on his right side, as his right arm and leg were completely paralysed.

He was devastated. His time in hospital was a difficult one. His emotional response was expressed in chronic aggressive behaviour. He resisted physiotherapy, activities and almost everything he needed in order to effectively cope and achieve his maximum independent state. The result was that there was little progression beyond being able to transfer himself to a wheelchair. Within a short time, he was ready for discharge. The options given to his family were home or admission to a long-term care facility. His wife decided she wanted to take him home.

Within three months she worked with him to the point that he was able to walk with a quad cane. She had him active to a certain degree. Her constant support became the catalyst to move him through his grieving state to a point where he began to see a light ahead in the tunnel. Within a year of his second stroke he still presented angry outbursts, but maintained a more liveable state. It was at this time that his wife died suddenly.

His inability to care for himself resulted in immediate placement in a long-term care facility. He was allowed only to bring in minimal personal belongings. To him each item he sold or gave away represented a permanent separation from his past— a further loss of his wife and a part of himself.

He now not only had to deal with the loss of his wife, his companion and his mentor, but he also had to forfeit the lifestyle to which he was accustomed. As someone who was used to being in control, he would not accept nor participate willingly now when confronted by directives and routines. The only accommodation available was a semi-private room. He was required to share this room with another man in his 90s who was very frail and noncommunicative due to a recent stroke.

Mr. Jone's daughters were beside themselves as to what to do. Their mother was the dominant figure within their family and the only one who "controlled" Dad. Dad's aggressive response not only made them feel hopeless but frightened them. They had never encountered the full extent of his emotional outbursts before. Mom had always buffered his emotions so they never totally saw this side of him.

Staff in the facility found themselves with an increasingly difficult resident. His aggressive outbursts resulted in an avoidance behaviour on their part. Staff spent only as much time with him as they had to. The more Mr. Jones was left alone, the deeper he sank into his depression and grief.

His involvement within any functions of the facility was almost nonexistent. From admission, he sat himself in a wheelchair and refused to walk or even to stand on his own. He would not transfer from bed to chair and back without assistance. Whenever he did receive help, he was belligerent and vulgar, making accusations that staff moved him the wrong way or were not quick enough to respond. Some nursing staff suggested that he be administered sedation to make him more manageable. There was concern that Mr. Jones' frustration and aggression might be taken out on other residents if they disturbed him.

The social worker became the intermediatory factor within the facility. Her initial assessment of Mr. Jones consisted of reviewing his past history, lifestyle, family dynamics and his response to his two strokes. She started working with him in one-to-one counselling. Initially her attempts to establish any rapport were thwarted. As she got closer to any delicate issues, his aggressive response became more intense. During this initial work-up, she met with the daughters to help them understand their father's behaviour and to assist them in learning how to cope with his outbursts and emotions.

With the background information in hand, the social worker began working on establishing a positive relationship with Mr. Jones. During the same period, contact was made with another long-established resident who had indicated an interest in participating as a "resident buddy." The social worker discussed Mr. Jones with the other resident buddy, and he agreed to start visitations with Mr. Jones in the hope of making him feel more a part of the facility. After a period of four weeks of resident and social worker visitations, Mr. Jones was encouraged to attend a "new resident" support group intended to assist new admissions to understand and deal with the transition to long-term care. At the encouragement of the social worker, he was also assessed by a psychiatrist and placed on an antidepressive agent.

In conjunction with these efforts, the social worker worked with the staff during the care conference to help them understand his behaviour and to develop some techniques to deal with his outbursts. A "staff buddy" system was established, which identified two direct care staff and a volunteer who were willing to work with the social worker in assisting Mr. Jones to work through his grieving.

The result of these efforts was that Mr. Jones' behaviour and emotional state became tolerable for both staff and family. A year after admission, Mr. Jones was walking again with a quad cane. His depressive episodes flared at increasingly fewer intervals. Even though he still had frequent periods of anger, he was able to control his outbursts. His involvement within the activities of the facility was minimal, but he would participate in a few general events. On speaking with him, he would state that he felt he could not enjoy life anymore, but it was tolerable.

Postscript

The focus in long term care is a different one to what most are accustomed to in an acute care setting. The question always arises: What do you do for the person who has virtually lost all of the major components that provide him with the desired level of quality of life?

The client who experiences compounded grieving is one who has gone from one major loss to another without the opportunity to resolve the initial loss. This has a domino effect, where the emotional experience of the first loss only compounds the second, weakening the person's coping skills and support systems (Fabiano, 1989). In such a situation, there is often little opportunity to re-build a person's life. Rather, there is only the potential to patch it together with what is remaining — probably one of the greatest challenges for any in the "people professions."

References

Atchley, R. C. (1980). *The Social Forces In Later Life*. Belmont, California: Wadsworth Publishing Company.

Becker, G. & Kaufman, S. (1988). Old age, rehabilitation and research: A review of the issues. *The Gerontologist, 28*(4).

Bennett, R. (Ed.) (1980). *Aging, Isolation and Resocialization*. Toronto: Van Nostrand Reinhold Company.

Berg, S., Branch, L. G., Doyle, A. E. & Sundstrom, G. (1988). Institutional and home-based long-term care alternatives: The 1965-1985 Swedish experience. *The Gerontologist, 28*(6).

Burnside, I. (1984). *Working With The Elderly*. Monterey, CA: Wadsworth Health Sciences Division.

Butler, R. N. & Lewis, M. I. (1982). *Aging And Mental Health*. Toronto: C.V. Mosby Company .

Edelson, J. S. & Lyons, W. H. (1985). *Institutional Care Of The Mentally Impaired Elderly*. New York: Van Nostrand Reinhold Company.

Fabiano, L. (1987). *Supportive Therapy for The Mentally Impaired Elderly*. Seagrave, Ont.: Education & Consulting Service.

Fabiano, L. (1989). *Working With The Frail Elderly*. Seagrave, Ont.: Education & Consulting Service.

Grossman, H. D. & Weiner, A.S. (1988). Quality of life: The institutional culture defined by administrative and resident values. *Journal of Applied Gerontology, 7*(3).

Hansen, S. S., Patterson, M. A. & Wilson, R. W. (1988). Family involvement on a dementia unit: The resident enrichment and activity program. *The Gerontologist, 28*(4).

Karuza, J., Calkins, E., Duffey, J. & Feather, J. (1988). Networking in aging: A challenge, model and evaluation. *The Gerontologist, 28*(2).

Keith, J. (1982). *Old People As People*. Toronto: Little Brown and Company.

Lasoski, M. C. & Thelen, M. H. (1987). Attitudes of older and middle-aged persons toward mental health intervention. *The Gerontologist, 20*(3).

Marshall, V. W. (Ed.) (1987). *Aging in Canada: Social Perspectives*, (2nd ed.). Markham, Ont.: Fitzhenry and Whiteside.

McPherson, B. (1983). *Aging As A Social Process*. Toronto: Butterworth's.

Moss, M. S. & Pfohl, D. C. (1988). New friendships: staff as visitors of nursing home residents. *The Gerontologist, 28*(2).

Novak, M. (1985). *Successful Aging*. Markham, Ont.: Penguin Books.

Scharlach, A. E. (1988). Peer counselor training for nursing home residents. *The Gerontologist, 28*(6).

Shulman, M. D. and Mandel, E. (1988). Communication training of relatives and friends of institutionalized elderly persons. *The Gerontologist, 28*(6).

Chapter 20

SOCIAL WORK PRACTICE ON A GERIATRIC CONSULTATION TEAM

Bernice Wilson, BSW, EdD

Abstract

This chapter describes the role of a social worker on a multi-disciplinary geriatric consultation team. The objectives and procedures of the team are outlined. The team's philosophy based on a medical model is sometimes incompatible with the theory base of social work practice, especially in the area of helping the family of the elderly hospitalized patient. The conflict of the needs of adult children and their aged parent, when the patient can no longer be cared for at home, is described. A case example to illustrate how this situation creates conflict within the team is provided. The difficulties in collective decision making on a team where members hold different perspectives, value systems, priorities and assumptions about the nature of man is explored. Collaborative practice in an acute care hospital is a challenging environment for social workers.

SOCIAL WORK PRACTICE ON A GERIATRIC CONSULTATION TEAM

Elderly patients in acute care hospitals have special needs because of the complex interaction of their acute illness, concurrent chronic conditions and psychosocial factors. The objectives of the Geriatric Consultation Team are

1) to help patients improve their functional level, regaining as much autonomy and independence as possible by providing comprehensive care in collaboration with the primary care providers;
2) to assist and educate patients and families so that the older person can return to the community, or to a setting where the quality of life can be improved or maintained;
3) to teach the principles of geriatric medicine to health care professionals and students, to improve quality of care and prevent premature institutionalization and
4) to conduct clinical research in health care delivery and impact of the team.

The three main functions of the Geriatric Consultation Team are patient care, education and research.

In most hospitals, regular patient care rounds are held twice weekly, and patients referred for consultation are discussed. There is a sharing of information from each discipline in order to reach an assessment and plan of care for the patient in his family/social context. Goals are set, both short term and long term, and a foll-w up discussion held weekly to monitor, and perhaps change, the plans for intervention. Decisions are made regarding the recommendations to be passed on to house staff. The major role of the team is one of consultation, although some direct practice is undertaken, especially by the physiotherapist, occupational therapist and clinical nurse specialists. Transfers for rehabilitation are considered. Family conferences and meetings with nursing, medical staff, home care, etc., are planned when appropriate.

The teaching of medical, nursing and social work students on a formal and informal basis is considered to be one of the main purposes of the team. Students attend patient care rounds and participate fully in the work of the team. Each discipline brings to the team a different perspective, body of knowledge, value base, skill and experience. There is a sharing of research findings and literature from each discipline. A research committee is helpful to promote relevant projects related to practice and the impact of the team in this setting.

Team members come from the following disciplines: geriatric medicine, psychogeriatrics, clinical nurse specialists in gerontology, physiotherapy, occupational therapy, rehabilitation medicine, public health and social work.

THE CLIENTELE

The patients referred to the team are usually over seventy-five-years of age, most often in their eighties or nineties. Some are alert, intelligent, resourceful, with a sense of humour, while others are depressed, cognitively impaired and disoriented to time and place. Their spouses, if they are alive, are usually younger, but some are fragile and in poor health themselves. The adult children (with whom we work closely) are often in their fifties or sixties. Patients may be located on units throughout the hospital, or they may be assigned to a special geriatric unit (six beds only). Perhaps they came to hospital for hip surgery after a fall, or have suffered a heart attack or stroke. Most often they present a mixed diagnoses at admission, such as weight loss, incontinence, confusion, pneumonia, dehydration, frequent falls or some combination of these medical problems. The medical chart may state a diagnosis of "failure to thrive" or "placement problem." Often this is translated to mean that the person lives alone and is unable to care for himself adequately. Further, there may have been a gradual decline in mental or physical functioning so that the routines of shopping, cooking and self-care are no longer possible. As a result, an elderly spouse, or adult child, may have had to provide almost total nursing care for the patient. These caregivers become exhausted and sometimes bring patients to the emergency department in total desperation.

Family members, friends and neighbours who have supported the patient in the past, eventually become our clients. They need help to continue their caring, and, with support, to help the patient decide on future plans. Often nieces, nephews and grandchildren can become involved in the treatment planning.

Many older people are alone in the world. They may have been "loners" who were always single, or have become widowed or divorced. Perhaps they experienced alienation from their family, or family members moved to distant cities, and now they exchange only letters or phone calls. The social worker carries a major responsibility in planning for future care for these socially isolated people. The social worker must deal with public trustees, community workers, Home Care, public health, etc. The goal is to engage others in forming a support network team to help the older person after s/he leaves the hospital.

Some patients come from situations where they have been housebound, and even bedbound, for weeks or months prior to admission to hospital. For instance, they may have suffered from severe arthritis or a broken hip, and their house was not accessible to the outside without using many steps. In this case, they will have become immobile and they will need weeks of treatment to regain their ability to walk around.

Interviews with the hospitalized elderly are often conducted at the bedside, in a room where other patients can hear, and may even interrupt. This can be uncomfortable not only for the patient but also for the social worker who is accustomed to private interviews in her/his office. The nurse or doctor may arrive in the middle of a meaningful interchange with the patient, or the patient may be removed to take a test. It becomes commonplace after a time to conduct interviews "standing on one foot." As well, many hospitalized older persons have hearing problems. Until a proper hearing aid can be arranged, it may be necessary to talk loudly or place yourself in a position so that the person can lip-read. It is embarrassing at first, especially if you are new to the setting and unsure of your skills. Sometimes language problems arise and an interpreter becomes necessary. This can work well unless the interpreter tries to help the patient give the "right answers." Older patients may respond to a warm smile or holding a person's hand. The human touch often communicates concern when language fails.

I. Social Work Presence on the Geriatric Team

As a social worker on the team, several questions arise. What is the special area of knowledge and skill that social workers bring? What are the relevant social work values and goals related to working on a geriatric team? Finally, how does the social work role come together in practice with older people who have been hospitalized in an active treatment institution?

A major area of social work expertise is in understanding and being able to assess the psychosocial situation of the patient. One of the first considerations as a team member is to deepen and share understanding of the older person or his social situation. As the social worker becomes familiar with the person and her/his family, friends and neighbours, and learns about her/his life, the professional need is to share this with the rest of the team. For example, perhaps there have been conflicts or tensions in the living arrangements and in relationships that have contributed to the breakdown of the patient's health. There may have been a sudden loss of an intimate other who was a major source of support. There is no substitute for a mate of fifty years, no consolation for the loss of an adult child. Loneliness, grief and a sense of isolation may have been overwhelming and may have contributed to this illness.

Social workers know that there is rarely a single event that has disturbed the equilibrium. More often, there are multiple inter-related, physical, cultural and social factors that contribute to a breakdown in healthy social functioning. It is vitally important to interpret the psychosocial context of the illness so that the hospital staff, in an effort to empty beds, will not return the person to the same conditions that helped to make her/him ill. The social work role is to provide this information to the team and to intervene with the patient and the family to build-in adequate supports and services so that the older person might return home if that was appropriate. But, if long term care, or transfer for rehabilitation to another facility, is needed, there needs to be adequate preparation for this change. The older person and the family need enough information, and psychological help, to deal with their fear, or conflict about alternate plans for care. Only then can they make a wise choice, one that they are prepared to live with.

Other considerations are: What is happening to the patient now? Is the patient terrified of their illness, pain and/or the unknown hospital and how they will cope in a large, impersonal institution? Concerns about loss of control over body and destiny abound. The patient needs the intervention of each member of the health care team to accept, respect and share both plans for treatment and expectations of the patient's participation in these plans.

The third and most vital question to ask is: Does the person wish to recover? The social worker needs to observe the patient's willingness, or lack of it, to participate in the treatment process. How is the patient coping with the illness and treatment procedures? Perhaps they want to be left alone or no longer feel important or valuable to anyone. If despair has set in, then perhaps there is one member of the team the patient might be willing to discuss feelings with. Can the team find a way to help the patient shift attitude, regain hope, change perspective? Patients need to feel some sense of autonomy, of control over what's happening, in order to make choices about treatment and plans for the future. If patients no longer perceive themselves as self-determining individuals with some roles intact, some purpose in going on, they may not wish to participate in the medical staff's procedures to cure or make them self-sufficient. As Erikson (1963) stated, "in the last stage of life, the dilemma of ego-integrity versus despair is an ongoing issue." More simply, one cannot make a person healthy who does not choose to go on with her/his life. As a social worker we can bring hope and belief that life is precious and worth living, that s/he is a valuable human being whom we respect and care about. We can participate in a process of "life review" whereby the older person, through reminiscence, may recapture her/his sense of ongoing purpose and identity (Wilson, 1983). But we cannot impose our values on another human being — the choice belongs to each of us as to how we live the rest of our lives. We must choose, sometimes unconsciously, whether to continue to struggle or merely to wait and die with dignity.

PRACTICE ROLES AND RESPONSIBILITIES

I. Organization and Administration

In addition to the administrative tasks of other workers in the social work department in a large hospital, such as keeping statistics, working on standing committees, participating in supervising groups, staff meetings, etc., there are special tasks for a social worker on a geriatric team.

1) Facilitating transfers to a rehabilitation unit, a Home for the Aged or other facility when a bed is available. This task involves preparing the patient, family and staff for the move. Also, the staff at the other facility need to be prepared to visit the patient, and/or have the patient visit the other setting before the transfer so that continuity of care can be maintained.

2) Participation in pre- and post-discharge visits to the older

person is another responsibility for the team social worker. Home visit teams are critical and much planning needs to be done to co-ordinate the services and establish criteria. Who should go on home visits? Should pre-discharge visits be made routinely before the patient's discharge occurs to minimize risk to safety and see that adequate supports are available in the community? How long after discharge should visits be planned to provide adequate follow-up?

3) Team building, communicating and planning. Regular business meetings are important to discuss issues and decisions regarding the way the team functions, how to increase visibility and effectiveness in the hospital. Planning for research projects and new programs, evaluating effectiveness of patient care and collaborative practice are dealt with here. The social worker can play a key role in mediating differences by facilitating regular evaluations of team effectiveness and by helping the team to deal with process when conflicts arise.

II. Education and Research

The education of social work students (BSW or MSW) placed in a hospital for their practicum is a task for the team social workers. It is an excellent learning opportunity for any social work student to participate in an interdisciplinary context and to learn to share their work with other disciplines. The interaction between disciplines can be helpful in establishing professional identity and in understanding and accepting differences in values and perspectives.

As well, research projects are developed by the team that may contribute to understanding the needs of the elderly in hospital and to evaluate the impact of the team on yhe patient's morale, family support, discharge plans, etc. Another task of the social worker is to provide consultation and act as a liaison to other social workers throughout the hospital. Many social workers at Toronto General Hospital are carrying responsibility for service to elderly patients on their units (not all cases are referred for geriatric consultation). It is important for the team social worker to keep the primary care workers informed about the teams' thinking, to involve them in patient care meetings and, when appropriate, to get information from them about their work with the patient to help the team understand the psychosocial factors in the situation.

The team social worker also assists in the planning and implementation of lectures, seminars, journal clubs or educational events for social workers, hospital staff, trainees in medicine and other disciplines.

Sometimes older patients are ignored or patronized in a hospital. Staff may decide that the person is hopeless and will die soon anyway, so "what's the use." This attitude adds to the patient's sense of helplessness and frustration, and may lead to apathy, withdrawal and a defeatist attitude. The patient may then be labelled as unco-operative, non-compliant, "a problem." Even worse than being ignored, or experiencing direct hostility, is being talked down to by the staff. It is difficult enough for the older person to become dependent in self-care, but they are often called "dear," or by their first names, when they have been addressed as Mrs. Smith, for instance, all their adult lives. The patient may be afraid to complain, afraid to ring the bell for fear of repercussions. If s/he wets the bed they may feel mortified at the loss of dignity and control. The social worker can help to alert staff to the patient's needs and feelings, and support the patient in asserting their wants. Some members of the medical and nursing staff become impatient with the slow pace of the older patient. They are frustrated by their inability to provide a "cure" and grow anxious because an acute care bed is being "blocked." The social worker's role is to try to change staff attitudes by example, by discussion, presentations, and by giving medical and nursing staff a chance to express their frustrations and ambivalence regarding working with the aged.

III. Patient Care Services

Assessment: The social worker helps to make the assessment of the social situation prior to the present illness. Such factors as housing, living arrangements, financial status, degree of social isolation and family relationships, are explored.

Counselling: The social worker on the team may engage in direct counselling with patient and family members, or may act as a consultant to other social work staff in the area. Counselling involves dealing with the painful feelings experienced by the patients about the illness, the sense of loss of the previous level of functioning and the fear of possible need for greater care. Planning for future needs, accepting limitations and changes in living arrangements, using community supports or choosing an appropriate institutional setting all need to be dealt with. It is important to help the person and the family prepare for a change of lifestyle when necessary, such as entering an institution. There may be mourning for loss of independence and autonomy. When a patient needs more care, helping family members to take on a new role in planning for and supporting the patient, and accepting changes in their perception of the family member, are important concerns. As well, social workers help to mobilize family involvement with a patient during the illness so that they can cope with the situation after discharge. Family members sometimes disagree with one another about the plans for the patient's care and need help to work through their conflicting feelings and come to some agreement. We help families arrive at decisions they become comfortable with so that they are able to use information, visit facilities and do the necessary work to arrange for the patient's care after discharge.

Family Conferences: The team social worker may facilitate family conferences that include several members of the team. It is then possible for the family to get a well-rounded picture of how the patient is functioning in hospital and how s/he will likely manage after discharge. This is an opportunity for families to question professionals who know their parents or spouse in a different context, to put together a picture of what their parents' needs are likely to be in the future. For example, the occupational therapist will describe how the patient manages in the kitchen, whether they are safe and competent in making a meal, a cup of tea, etc. They can comment on whether the person puts on their clothing backwards or how much help they will need in self-care. The physiotherapist will discuss mobility, how far the person can walk, whether they need a wheelchair, a walker, or some other support. The geriatrician may describe medical problems, whether they can be controlled and what the prognosis may be. From this conference, a tentative plan will evolve for the level of care that will be needed, how well the person might manage at home and what supports are necessary. Perhaps a homemaker and VON three times a week will be enough, or perhaps the person needs to accept the realitiy of moving to a Home for the Aged.

The teamn may return to working further with the patient and meeting the family again with an updated assessment. They may offer to make a pre-discharge visit to the home with the patient to see how well s/he can manage in a familiar environment. In summary, the family conference is an excellent tool to help families and patients (if they are well enough to participate) plan for the future based on clear evidence of the patient's present level of functioning and projected needs. The social worker facilitates this process and follow-up in planning with the family, helping them to deal with communication blocks and relationship problems.

Counselling by social workers in hospital settings is sometimes undervalued by other staff who view social workers as discharge planners or providers of tangible services. Social workers must continue to assert their unique contribution and skill in helping patients deal with the emotional and social impact of illness and hospitalization. A collaborative effort in counselling is desirable but there is often rivalry and overlap between social work, psychiatry, occupational therapy, and nursing. We must learn to be more assertive in claiming our part of the healing process so that patients and their families will be better served.

Social Work With Groups: Social workers also facilitate caregiver groups for spouses and adult children and plan with other team members to develop new groups for patients such as reminiscence, social activation, current events, etc. Patients who are waiting for scarce long term beds in chronic care hospitals become bored, apathetic and hopeless. They need stimulation, companionship and interaction with the community if they are to maintain their present functional level. The social worker can promote new groups to help patients and caregivers cope with the stress of chronic illness.

Co-ordination and Referral to Community Services: Social workers need to assist other staff in preparing the patient for discharge or transfer to another institution, dealing with the fear of getting sick again and the ambivalence about going home, perhaps returning to the same isolation or tension. We try to help the patient make it different by bringing in new supports or using old ones differently. We follow up with the patient, with caregivers, and community agencies to sustain the gains that were made while in hospital.

Other Services: Writing articles for journals, giving presentations for Telemedicine, keeping informed on current literature by reading and attending conferences — all of these are tasks of the social worker on a geriatric team. Writing clinical reports, assessments, summaries and transfer forms for other institutions are also tasks of the social worker. Written reports on the medical chart give information to other professionals in the hospital.

POTENTIAL FOR ROLE DEVELOPMENT

One of the areas in which social work can develop a more meaningful role is in the area of ethics. Biomedical ethics is a growing field of concern for all health care professionals, but social workers have always been deeply involved in ethical issues. As a profession our concern for enhancing the individual's right to make her/his own choices about how to live is of prime importance. We are committed to advocating for the patient's rights. As a social worker on a geriatric team, one is confronted with decisions about the individual's right to be self-determining, to make choices about where to live and about whether to live. This issue is complicated when the patient is not fully competent mentally, when s/he may not be able to make a sound judgment. The patient may be competent in some areas but not able to make informed decisions about others, e.g., finances. Assessing competence is becoming an area in which social workers will be called upon more frequently in the future with the proposed *Substitute Decision Act*. Up to this time, psychiatry has assessed the mental competence in many acute care hospitals.

Further, quality of life decisions, prolonging life versus dying with dignity, are complex issues. For example, the team was recently faced with a decision about whether an eighty-seven-year-old woman who was apathetic, non-communicative, cognitively impaired, refusing to eat should be given a feeding tube to prolong her life. Some team members were quite convinced that the patient was demonstrating her wish to die, that her quality of life was poor and that she had stopped struggling to survive. However, when the team psychiatrist talked with her, in a lucid moment, the patient surprised everyone by being able to express her wish to go on living. She was placed on a feeding tube. Later, we learned that the patient had a gum infection that had caused her withdrawal, depression and refusal to eat. She lived on for several years and enjoyed some quality to her life.

Some elderly people "give up" temporarily, especially if they are in pain or suffering with an infection. Some psychiatric conditions are reversible and attitudes can change with recovery. Patients may be despairing, overwhelmed with losses and fearful of future loss of independence. However, it is possible for patients to become re-engaged in living if given an opportunity to regain some control of their life. We must care enough to challenge them, and offer hope; they may feel a renewed sense of purpose. Sometimes a contact with a child or grandchild can help to turn things around so they can begin to work on their own recovery.

Social workers need to lead the way in involving families of older patients, encouraging their involvement on whatever level they can sustain. Family members are valuable allies to the medical team and also advocates for the patient.

Social work assessments need to be sharp and our interventions skillful if we wish to have an effective voice in ethical decision making. Now that medical technology can keep people alive longer, families and patients need help to decide whether a "do not resuscitate" order should be signed. Feeding tubes, dialysis and transplants are some ways physicians can help patients go on living, but what about the quality of that life? What is unacceptable to one person may be tolerable to another. Patients and families need help to make these difficult decisions, and all members of the team have a contribution to make. Only the patient can know if s/he is willing to take the risk when there is uncertainty about the outcome of a medical procedure, whether to go on or to die with dignity. When the patient is impaired cognitively we must rely of the family members to know their wishes. If there is no family what can we do? Perhaps a good friend or neighbour can be helpful in knowing what the person would have wanted.

Sometimes team members disagree on the ethical stance the team should take. Physicians may not understand the patient's resistance to a medical procedure or the family's resistance to taking the patient home again. Self-awareness is sometimes lacking, and a doctor may disagree when her/his judgment is questioned. Social workers can bring a different perspective in these situations, appreciating the physician's reactions and helping her/him to deal with them, but interpreting the client's fear and the need for time to work through their ambivalence. The social worker's value of advocating for the patient's right to autonomy may be viewed negatively by other members of the team. Physicians have been educated to take charge, use persuasion, educate and impose decisions. Social workers value consensus and negotiation, providing alternatives. These differences can lead to difficulties and strains in inter-disciplinary teamwork. It is through articulating the differences in values and learning to respect one another's perspective that some resolution may come about.

When the social worker cannot agree with the team's decision after all attempts to reach a consensus have been made, it may be necessary to withdraw from active involvement with a particular patient situation (Abramson, 1984). Abramson recommends guidelines to help teams deal with collective responsibility. She recommends that teams learn a common moral language, developing shared meanings for concepts like "autonomy" or "quality of life." She suggests also that team members learn to be articulate about their feelings and thoughts on moral issues, allowing for healthy disagreement rather than suppressing conflicts between team members. Group members should spend time clarifying and prioritizing group values and professional principles. Developing a procedure for analyzing complex ethical issues is suggested and a mechanism for dealing with an individual member's dissent. I believe that the social worker could take leadership in this area to help the team become more effective in collaborative practice.

A trend in geriatric care for the 1990s appears to be increased home visiting. A team of geriatric experts will visit older patients in their homes, offering a combination of preventive and treatment interventions. These programs are designed to help people remain in their own familiar environments, prevent the over-use of expensive hospital beds and return them quickly to their homes if a hospital procedure were deemed necessary. Social workers who are skilled in planning support services and co-ordinating a care plan will be able to make a big contribution in this area. There is always an issue of setting priorities, assessing the urgency of referrals and helping patients and families wait for service when waiting lists grow. Social workers have much experience in dealing with the latter kinds of issues. Family systems need to be understood in order to recognize the stress on caregivers and the resentment of the "cared for" spouse who has become partially or wholly dependent. Family and couple counselling needs to be one of the services offered by a home visit team.

Social workers in health care settings may find that they are faced with value clashes in many areas but particularly in working with families. Some disciplines in an acute care hospital view the family members in a negative way. According to Rosenthal (1989) families are often scapegoated by staff. They are blamed for not taking the patient home or for being too protective and interfering with nursing care. Sometimes health care workers feel a commitment to the patient only and do not see the patient as part of a family. If the needs of the spouse or adult children seem to conflict with the patient's needs, they may take sides, not perceiving the family as an interactive system. For example, if the family is not able to cope with the patient's care at home, the physician will be quite ready to impose a plan of care on the family that they do not agree with and cannot sustain. The patient is often returned to the hospital within a short time because the plan falls apart and the whole process may be repeated. There are many sources of strain between social workers and physicians and, as Mizrahi and Abramson (1985) point out, they are the result of countervailing perspectives that are rooted in the professional training of both disciplines and are reinforced in practice settings. If we can understand and accept these differences we will not take them as personal failures and will learn to have more realistic expectations of collaborative models.

CONCLUDING REMARKS

In summary, social work roles and functions on a multi-disciplinary geriatric team demand the following skills and knowledge:

1) generic social work skills dealing with individuals, couples and families and small groups;
2) a knowledge of systems theory, small group theory and intergenerational theory;
3) ability to form links with the community;
4) knowledge of legislation and policies affecting services to the aged and
5) knowledge of gerontology and research methodology.

We need to learn new skills in working in a collaborative way, holding to our own values, disagreeing openly yet respecting other team members' ethical stances come from their training and philosophy. This requires continuous learning and stretching of ourselves, emotionally and intellectually, to find a way of sharing responsibility for patient care. We need to accept and value the unique contribution of each team member. Patients and their families will benefit from this collaborative effort. Each discipline must give up some degree of autonomy and self-determination in order to gain our common purpose of competence in patient care.

Social workers in medical settings often find themselves in situations where they feel powerless. The physician is the leader of the team and makes the final decisions. The medical establishment sets the norms, builds the structure and disapproves of the deviant. It is easy for a social worker to withdraw into a defensive, self-protective shell, guarding comments, fearing to write on the medical chart, taking the "safe position" in a controversial situation. The biomedical model permeates the thinking and behaviour of most physicians, nurses and other health care professionals (Weick, 1986). There are clinical nurse specialists and other health care professionals who, because of a different kind of education, question the disease orientation, the authoritarian, hierarchical structure, challenge labels (such as "unco-operative" patient) and value the patient's perception of the situation. Since medical research is based on a positivistic philosophy of science, where cause-and-effect thinking, quantitative measurement and outcomes are valued, it is to be expected that they are suspicious of the social work emphasis on process, non-judgmental attitudes, offering alternatives, multiple causation and descriptive data. They are committed to the patient, but do not view the patient as part of an interactive family system. The social worker's body of knowledge and skills are often undervalued (Mizrahi & Abramson, 1985). The relationship and conflicts between team members is a topic that is beyond the scope of this paper. It has been addressed however by several writers: (Germain, 1984; Lowe & Herranen, 1978; Mizrahi & Abramson, 1985). It is important to recognize that there will always be potential for overlap in roles and functions between various team members and thus, conflict. It has been suggested that by anticipating problems and planning joint solutions, many conflicts can be avoided or minimized. It is in the interest of patient well-being and team effectiveness that conflicts be resolved as quickly as possible.

If social workers are to survive and help humanize the medical setting, we must build alliances with other health professionals. We need to find support from social work colleagues. It is in the interest of patients and their families, the consumers of health care, and also our own interests (if we live long enough) that we continue to individualize patients, offer alternatives, challenge labels and stereotypes and respect each person's right to decide about her/his life. We must learn to negotiate differences and perspectives when possible and to accept that some differences are not negotiable. Respect for one another as caring professionals with a common purpose of wanting to promote healing is a crucial ingredient in successful collaboration.

CASE EXAMPLE

Mrs B. is an eighty-year-old Latvian woman who lived with her 45-year-old daughter Mary in a two-storey house before coming to hospital. Mary, an only child, did not get along well with her mother. Their conflict started during her teens when she saw her mother as hostile, stubborn and demanding. She moved out of the family home, married at an early age and lived in a different city. She only came home for Christmas and Easter. Unfortunately, Mary's husband died at age 35 and shortly thereafter, Mary learned that her father, whom she adored, was terminally ill. She returned to her parents' home to take care of her father until his death. Her mother became ill shortly after her husband died, then suffered a stroke, becoming incontinent, cognitively impaired, immobile and needing constant care. Mrs B. had always been a demanding woman, but now with Mary at her beck and call, no amount of time spent with her was enough. Mary cared for her mother for eight years, managing the house and renting out rooms to support the family. She had also the responsibility of a schizophrenic son who sometimes went off his medication and acted irrationally. This time when mother was hospitalized, Mary decided she could no longer care for her at home. She had a new relationship with a man she wished to marry, and she was "sick to death of coping with mother's constant demands." She told the geriatric team in a family conference that she was not willing to take her mother home again. She visited her mother daily and was willing to continue being responsible for her finances, etc., but she wanted her mother to live in a nursing home. The relationship between these women was a stormy one, as nursing reported after the daily visits. The team physician was disappointed and he voiced his disapproval that after all our attempts to rehabilitate Mrs B., her daughter was no longer willing to have her mother at home. He wanted the social worker to persuade the daughter to change her mind, to take her home temporarily, to wait for placement. Mother was slightly more continent, could feed herself a little and could ambulate to the bathroom and back. The daughter was firm, and the social worker supported her right to decide what care she could sustain as an only daughter.

The team members were split on this issue. We had worked hard to rehabilitate Mrs B. and, therefore, "the daughter should keep her word" (she had initially said if mother were continent and mobile she could come home). I felt this was a difficult decision for the daughter to make, that she had a great deal of guilt and anger, that she needed support to get on with her life. Ideally, mother and daughter would decide together what plan would meet both their needs. But the mother was too impaired cognitively to be involved in the decision making. Mrs B. indicated that she wished to be at home, but if her daughter resumed care against her better judgment, I assessed that she would be resentful and might be neglectful or even abusive to her mother. Her behaviour was angry in relation to her mother, accusing her of stubbornness when she was simply forgetful. I felt that Mary had the right to begin a new life without the burden of her mother's care. Caring for her son was a heavy enough load for a second marriage. I predicted that Mrs B. would probably adjust to an institutional setting, if it were carefully chosen and she was prepared by advance visits. She would not be alone as much as she had been at home and might enjoy the companionship of the other residents. I stated my disagreement about any attempts to pressure the daughter or make her feel guilty.

These kinds of decisions can become divisive for a team. Geriatricians value getting older people back to the community and are opposed to institutional care unless absolutely necessary. They are committed to what they believe is the best interest of the patient, and they often see institutions as all bad and home as always preferable. Social workers also prefer to help older people remain in the community, but we are concerned with all members of the family and see the older person as part of an interactive system. Caregivers need advocates in a hospital setting, as they are often blamed for not taking the patient home (Rosenthal, 1989). Sometimes there is a conflict of needs. What is best for the patient may not be what is best for their spouse or child. An institution that provides a good quality of care may increase life satisfaction by providing higher levels of social interaction for an elderly person who is physically disabled (Myles, 1980).

References

Abramson, M. (1984). Collective responsibility in interdisciplinary collaboration: An ethical perspective for social workers. *Social Work in Health Care, 10*(1).

Erikson, E. (1963). *Childhood and Society* (2nd ed.). New York: Norton.

Germaine, C. (1984). *Social Work Practice in Health Care: An Ecological Perspective.* New York, NY: Free Press.

Kirkland, J., Maser, J. & Redman, P. (1985-1986). Geriatrics Service Proposal. Unpublished manuscript.

Lowe, J. I. & Herranen, M. (1978). Conflict in teamwork: Understanding roles and relationships. *Social Work in Health Care, 3*(3).

Mizrahi, T. & Abramson, J. (1985). Sources of strain between physicians and social workers: Implications for social workers in health care settings. *Social Work in Health Care, 10*(3), 33-51.

Myles, J. F. (1980). Institutionalizing the elderly: A critical assessment of the sociology of total institutions (pp. 257-268). In V. Marshall (Ed.), *Aging in Canada: Social Perspectives.* Toronto, Ont.: Fitzhenry and Whiteside.

Rosenthal, C. J. (1988). Families of elderly patients in acute and long term care settings. Paper presented at meeting of Scarborough General Hospital on Alternative Solutions for the Aged Population. Scarborough, Ontario, Sept. 15-16.

Schwenger, C. W. & Gross, M. J. (1980). Institutional care and institutionalization of the elderly in Canada (pp. 248-256). In V. Marshall (Ed.), *Aging in Canada: Social Perspectives.* Toronto, Ont.: Fitzhenry and Whiteside.

Weick, A. (1986). The philosophical context of a health model of social work. *Social Casework: The Journal of Contemporary Social Work, 67,* 551-559.

Wilson, B. (1983). Major issues of older adults confronting institutional living: What to keep and what to give away. Unpublished doctoral thesis. Ontario Institute for Studies in Education.

Chapter 21

SOCIAL WORK PRACTICE IN GERIATRIC ASSESSMENT UNITS

Patricia A. Mackenzie, MSW

Abstract

The gradual deterioration of function with increasing age is so widely perceived and so expected that all difficulty experienced by an elderly person tends to be attributed to age. Geriatric Assessment Units are built upon the premise that it is disease not senescence that leads to disability in the elderly. GAU programs provide an environment where it becomes routine for an older person with problems of mobility, mental change or functional disturbance to be assessed for disease, and for remedial action to be taken. Composed of both social and medical and functional investigations, geriatric assessment can address the complexities that accompany many acute and chronic conditions of old age. It is within this investigative environment that social work finds a natural home and the opportunities for creative and challenging practice.

SOCIAL WORK PRACTICE IN GERIATRIC ASSESSMENT UNITS

From the widowed world traveller in Nova Scotia to the 80-year-old marathon runner in Calgary and the "Raging Grannies" of the West Coast, the older population in Canada uses imagination, energy and creativity to use retirement and aging as an opportunity to accept new challenges and master new skills. These individuals engage in such activities with a zest and passion for life that was beyond their grasp when saddled with ties to jobs, families and the other trappings of the "productive years." There are presently more than 3 million Canadians over the age of 65 and there is every indication that this number will increase in the ensuing years. Projections by Health and Welfare Canada (1986) estimate that by the year 2021, Canadians in the 65-plus age group will make up one-fifth of the total population (1988). Skelton (1986) predicts that the 65 and older age group will enlarge more rapidly than any other segment of the population and those in their 9th decade will increase by more than 200% in the next two decades.

Despite the "joie de vivre" and independence of the majority of aging Canadians, society as a whole tends to hold fast to negative stereotypes of the older population and to equate "old" with "debilitated." Social workers often join other helping professionals, economists, statisticians and politicians in alarmist reactions over the doom and gloom predictions of the "greying of our society." As a result, we tend not to see the old realistically. Part of the problem might be that the word "old" conjures up images of brittle bones, wrinkled skin, fragile health and forgetfulness, all of which serve to obscure the strengths and abilities of the majority of aging Canadians. Seniors', advocacy groups have begun to challenge societal perceptions and acceptance of the equation that relates chronological age with infirmity and dependence. These new cohorts of the aging population are beginning to question the ministrations of helping professionals and social scientists and suggest that society must recognize and appreciate the political and economic power of a large segment of this group (see Hooyman et al., 1988).

Although the trend is reversing, academics continue to obtain considerable professional mileage from the study of the aged as if this group were comprised of some strange new species of being. Recent research on the biological, health and social correlates of aging as described by Cox (1988) indicates that the lives of older persons are not nearly as foreboding or as unhappy as the literature may have led the public to believe. As a society, we need to redefine our perceptions of exactly what the ageing of our country is all about. Indeed, McDaniels (1988) points out:

> the aging of Canada is not new and alarmism about aging fails to recognize some very important points. Societal aging is the unexpected consequence of successful planned parenthood. The average age of the population has increased because of declining numbers of babies and young children. What is new will be the aging trend in the Twenty-First Century as the baby boom generation swells the ranks of the elderly.

Neugarten (1974) has distinguished the young-old from the old-old and fortunately gerontologists, social scientists, helping professionals and economists have begun to listen and recognize that chronological years alone do not an "old" person make!

It remains, however, that we cannot make broad assumptions about the elderly as being a completely homogeneous group. Each person's lifetime experiences are widely dissimilar and responses to these experiences result in important variations in personality. Consequently, aging enhances our individuality. It is this uniqueness that adds an attractive and challenging dimension to working with elderly people.

Perhaps another reason for our inability to see the elderly in a more positive and differentiated light is that the media and other interested groups limit their focus on that part of the experience of aging that results in the fiscal responsibility of providing increasingly scarce resources for this segment of the population. The sheer business of living weakens the body. As people begin to age and fail to recover quickly from the insults of illness or injury, they often present for care and treatment in a health care facility. It is this entrance into the service delivery system that requires expenditure of public funds and this financial burden seems to be the issue that causes great distress for policy-makers, economists, politicians and health/social service agency personnel. As a society, we worry about the raging geriatric tide that supposedly threatens to bankrupt the health care system. Hertzman (1985) questions this fear and suggests that an economic redistribution of health and social resources would help to better prepare the state for the interventions required in the coming years.

Caring professionals often neglect to give credit for the benefits this group has conferred upon society and need to adopt a critical review, not only of some of the negative stereotypes of ageing, but also of the pessimistic predictions regarding the costs of caring for an elderly population. Negative stereotyping of the elderly must be eliminated and education and experience can serve as effective means to that end. Gaitz (1974) points out the necessity for relieving ourselves of repressive attitudes toward the aged when he states:

> If one mistakenly assumes that psychiatric disorders of the aged are beyond treatment, then neglect of elderly persons with remediable conditions may occur. If one assumes that an elderly person is only waiting for death to relieve him, his family and society of a burden, a practitioner may become the instrument of implementing the unwitting inadequate treatment plans of a society unwilling to invest the time, energy and money to obtain the best resources available to all citizens.

THE CLIENTELE

It has been pointed out in the previous comments that old age is not a monolithic, static condition that guarantees dependency. However, while it is true that the majority of persons over the age of 65 enjoy reasonably good health and independent function, what of the elderly who do suffer a health crisis that is sufficiently complex or severe to compromise both their physical and psychosocial functioning?

One of the great economic and social frailties of the present health care system is a failure to respond in such a way as to provide services tailored to meet the specific needs of the elderly. Rathbone-McCuan (1977) has suggested that our society has been ineffective in generating strategies for providing preventive or restorative health care to the elderly. When an older person is thought to be coping poorly, there is a tendency to focus on appropriate facility-based care rather than on creative alternatives and helping strategies. As Watson states (1984), "too often, the individual is made to fit the system, rather than the system being adapted or modified to meet the needs of the person." It is, there-fore, essential that, before any action is taken, every frail elderly person has a proper assessment and review of potential alternate resources and ways of coping.

I. Assessment

This assessment process is described by Rubenstein (1982) as one that "can lead to the discovery of new important and treatable problems, simplification of overly complex drug regimes, arrange-ments for needed rehabilitation and development or remediation of a supportive physical and social living environment to enhance patient functioning." The goal of any assessment procedure is to maximize the abilities and minimize the dysfunction that might result from an insult to an elderly person's vitality.

Therefore, when health crises strike, it is important that the elderly person has available to her/him a continuum of care that includes programs designed to treat the treatable, reverse the reversible and maintain a state of physical, functional and psycho-social well-being. Novak (1988) suggests this continuum should range from programs that have maximal institutional support, such as hospitals and long-term care facilities, to those with little such support as exemplified by adult day programs, senior's cen-tres, etc.

This goal of maintaining, enhancing and restoring both the physical and psycho-social vitality of the elderly receives little real criticism from any sector. The challenge, however, involves the actual development of creative and broad-based care delivery sys-tems that can provide the care continuum required. An inherent difficulty in this task is described by Skelton (1986) when he cautions that:

> The present strain the elderly impose on the health and welfare services will not be relieved simply by the provision of more beds. Too frequently the problem is addressed by hasty and thoughtless provision of larger and more expensive long-term care institutions, or by suggestions that favour rationing health and welfare services to the elderly. Better basic planning and the development of integrated and comprehensive geriatric services offer the only viable long-term solutions.

II. Geriatric Assessment Units

One of the components of this integrated and comprehensive geriatric service delivery system involves formal Geriatric Assessment Programs, and, before one can successfully examine the clientele, it is necessary to describe the parameters of these particular practice settings.

Geriatrics is that branch of gerontology that studies pathology, treatment and prevention of disease amongst the elderly. Specialized geriatric assessment units (GAUs) have been established in major urban centres across Canada, patterning trends established in the UK, the USA and Europe. These programs have developed in response to the growing recognition of the many unmet needs of the frail elderly and are motivated by the conviction that GAUs can have major beneficial impacts on the health and well-being of elderly patients. GAU programs trace their origins to Great Britain and were pioneered by the work of several people including Dr. Marjory Warren and Sir Ferguson Anderson. Geared to specific local needs and available resources, these programs vary in many of their structural and functional components including: how the program is financed, institutional affiliation, which types of patients are accepted, staffing composition, etc.

Rubenstein (1987) defined geriatric assessment as a " multi-dimensional and interdisciplinary diagnostic process designed to quantify an elderly individual's medical, psychosocial, and functional capabilities and problems with the intention of arriving at a comprehensive plan for intervention and follow-up." Kane reviews the growing body of literature that outlines the different types and purposes of GAU programs and also describes the positive health care outcomes of GAU intervention (1987). Wooldridge et al., (1987) point out the need for more cautious and inclusive program evaluations when measuring program effectiveness, arguing that,

> Successful treatment of severe cardiac congestive failure in an 85 year old woman which leads to successful discharge home may lead to frustration for all if the presence or absence of family or other caregiving support, the possibility of drug compliance, or the suitability of the patient's housing are not taken into account.

This example demonstrates the social parameters that must be taken into account when dealing with the frail elderly and lends credibility to the increasing involvement of social workers in GAU programs.

Elderly patients typically present with complex and interrelated medical and psychosocial problems that often do not fit into a limited biomedical model of care. The focus therefore, needs to be expanded beyond the description of the impact of physical disease to encompass the effect of functional, psychosocial and financial problems on the health and happiness of elderly persons and their subsequent ability to remain independent. The interrelationship between the biological and behavioural aspects of human existence, important for all ages, is no less important for the elderly. Medalie (1986) expanded the traditional approach of assessing the elderly, which generally focusses on the biological changes of the aging process, to include a review of the multiple interrelating factors associated with the patient, her/his intimate associates, cultural sub-groups and society.

Rubenstein (1981) identifies the three major services of geriatric assessment units as assessment, interventions, and/or placement of the frail elderly patient (1981). Studies reported by Flathman and Larsen (1976) have noted that patients involved in such programs improved their physical, mental and social well-being. It is well known that elderly patients have more varied problems and health care needs than younger patients, although Barer et al., (1986) suggest that the reason for the increased utilization of health care resources by the elderly has less to do with the intensity or frequency of disease and more to do with the way the health care system responds. Schumann (1984) also identified the challenge of designing new interventions to meet these needs.

In order to address the multiple problems of the frail elderly, most geriatric assessment units are designed to provide intensive, comprehensive assessment and therapeutic planning by an array of health care professionals. This expanded system of care reflects a broader concept of health and illness than is included in the strictly biomedical model. Central to GAU program philosophy is the belief that careful assessment of frail elderly patients can often reveal remediable conditions, and help to better match services with needs. The GAU social worker, therefore, finds it possible to follow the principal social work objective described by Rosenfeld (1983), "the aim of social work is to match resources with needs and increase the goodness of fit between them by harnessing potential provider systems to perform this function." It is within the GAU environment, then, that social work can find a natural home as this setting offers the opportunity to participate in a system of care that is congruent with the commitment of the profession to person-in-environment interactions. The subsequent intervention strategies (possible in a social model of health care delivery) involve efforts to keep people in their own homes when appropriate.

Since no single professional group is capable of meeting all of the elderly patient's needs, teamwork is essential. Interdisciplinary GAU teams typically consist of geriatricians, other medical consultants, nurses, social workers, occupational therapists, physiotherapists, speech therapists, dietitians and psychologists. Each team member is responsible for patient assessments in her/his field of expertise. Usually the entire team monitors patient progress and continually plans and re-evaluates therapeutic goals for individual patients. Social work is comfortable with Brill's (1976) definition of the team approach to patient care which suggests that:

> There needs to be a mix of professions each of whom possess particular expertise; each of whom is responsible for making individual decisions; who together hold a common purpose; who meet formally and informally to communicate, to collaborate, and to consolidate knowledge from which plans are made, actions determined and future decisions influenced.

PRACTICE ROLES AND RESPONSIBILITIES

As Westberg (1986) points out, shifts in the age of a client group do not require the abandonment of all generic or specialized social work skills but do require that those skills be tailored to a new client group whose needs and resources may have special features. This is most certainly the case for the social worker employed in a GAU. For example, it is essential that the social worker acquire a familiarity with medical terminology, enabling her/him to understand the common physical ailments and medical interventions performed with this population.

While it is true that social work alone cannot begin to harness all the resources needed by the frail elderly GAU patient, it remains that the principle feature of social work practice in this setting requires the worker to meet the objectives of social work practice outlined by other authors. The required "tailoring of skills" can be demonstrated by taking the liberty of inserting the appropriate adjectives into Hepworth and Larsen's (1986) stated *Objectives for Social Work Practice*. This process helps to lend additional relevance to this practice setting allowing one to re-write that GAU social workers:

1. Help (frail elderly people) enlarge their competence and increase their problem-solving and coping abilities;
2. Help the (elderly patient) obtain resources;
3. Make health care and other social service organizations responsive to (frail elderly people);
4. Facilitate interactions between (older individuals) and others in their environments;
5. Influence interactions between organizations and institutions which serve (elderly people) and
6. Influence social and environmental policy to respond to the health and social needs of the (older person).

Social work practice in GAU's can be described by using the concepts of primary, secondary and tertiary intervention as outlined by Beaver (1985). A discussion of the application of these concepts to GAU social work practice follows.

I. Intervention

Primary intervention suggests that it is best to try and identify problems *before* full manifestation occurs and to design strategies to either eliminate or minimize the potential harmful effects. Primary intervention, therefore, leads the GAU social worker into a role of both consultant- educator and advocate. As such, energy is focussed on a review of the conditions necessary for healthy and satisfactory life-styles of all citizens including the elderly person. The social worker is also responsible for identifying harmful influences and scarcity of resources in the physical and social environment that may have deleterious effects on the clientele served.

This practice role is easily adhered to in GAU settings as the social worker strives to provide early education of patients/families about the resources available to enhance coping. In the combined consultant-educator role, the GAU social worker is called upon to interpret agency/hospital rules and regulations and to teach or transmit information about a host of services to patients, families and other caregivers.

The social worker in a GAU must also act as consultant/collaborator with other health care professionals, both within and without the GAU, to design effective care plans for individual patients and thereby ensure quality service to the clientele. Virtually all types of GAU programs have some interrelationship with community services. As Williams (1987) points out, "It is obvious that, if the geriatric assessment is to contribute to the further care of the patient, its results and recommendations must reach the appropriate community services." Maintaining this community communication network is often the responsibility of the GAU social worker.

GAU social workers in the advocate role are usually "client-focussed." Not only does the advocacy role of social work direct the worker to help patients cut through bureaucratic red tape and other systems related problems, but it has expanded to encompass a conscious movement on the part of the worker to address inequities in social and health policy decisions that adversely impact upon clients. For GAU social workers then, advocacy is an inherent feature of practice as efforts are made to challenge, among other things, agist discrimination, limited or rationed health and social services and the assumption that to be old is to be sick and that sickness is to be expected and is beyond treatment.

The main emphasis in secondary intervention is on early diagnosis and treatment and it is at this level that the bulk of direct practice responsibilities are found. The GAU practice setting offers opportunity to participate in strategies that are designed to improve and enhance the older person's well-being. In order to bring about a resolution of the patient's problems, or to prevent exacerbation of same, intervention is offered in the form of standard clinical casework. The goal of such intervention includes patient recovery and restoration of the previous level of social functioning. This involves the social worker and patient in problem assessment and problem-solving exercises, all of which are designed to enhance coping abilities.

As social workers assess the presenting problems of geriatric patients, it is helpful to reflect on a modified version of the psychosocial systems perspective as outlined by Beaver et al., (1985). This approach offers a set of generic guidelines for the following: engaging the client; conducting the assessment; formulating the intervention pla; and finally, evaluating outcomes. These concepts can be easily transcribed to GAU social work practice and offer a broad overview of the total physical-psychological-social function-ing of the patient. Another assessment tool that the reader may find helpful and that can be readily adapted to GAU social work practice is the 4 Rs of Medical- Social Diagnosis as described by Doremus (1976).

Yet another way to assess areas of the patient's life that may have been affected by current difficulties involves a review of sev-eral key "arenas" or "spheres of influence" that describe aspects of healthy, productive human functioning. These have been described by Gilmore (1973) as vitality, community, identity, accountability, activity and frivolity. An adaptation of these ideas provides a conceptual framework for understanding the depth and breadth required for a complete gerontological social work assessment. It is reasonable, for instance, to suggest that any depletion of the patient's "vitality" will have an impact upon how capable s/he is of continuing her/his level of involvement in her/his social world or "community." As well, a limitation in the "activity" of the patient may change that for which the individual patient is "accountable," i.e., that which gives her/him "identity" and a sense of "frivolity," (defined as accomplishment/ purpose in life). This situation may hasten feelings of loss of self-worth, self-doubt and depression. The following case example illustrates the interconnectedness of the "spheres of influence" concepts.

Mrs. B. was referred to the GAU for consultation after a recent mild CVA and subsequent problems with erratic blood pressure. The GP and visiting Home care nurse were concerned about Mrs. B.'s apparent total disregard for her medication regime/diet. She was described by the family physician as mentally intact but depressed. While talking with Mrs. B. during the home visit, the social worker discovered that her husband had died just one month previous. Her only child, a daughter in Toronto, had made a quick trip to Victoria after her father's death and found her mother "incapacitated with grief." The daughter made all the arrangements for her father's funeral, saw to the details of the estate and, just before returning to Toronto, convinced Mrs. B. to put the large home she and Mr. B. built 15 years ago up for sale. Arrangements were also made by the daughter for Mrs. B. to visit a new "senior's condominium" complex and put a deposit on the purchase of a suite. She also contacted the lawyer to draw up "power of attorney" forms for her mother to execute in her daughter's favour. Mrs. B. mentioned to the daughter just after the funeral that she was feeling apprehensive about learning to manage the family finances as that was "always your father's responsibility." With that information, the daughter contacted an accountant and made arrangements for all cheques and other finances to be managed by his firm with "consultation" from Mrs. B.

The tragedy in this case study involves the well-intentioned but misdirected effort of a concerned daughter to make major decisions on mother's behalf and "in her best interests," which had serious negative impacts on her mother's feelings of self-worth, control and competence. By making the assumption that mother was either not capable of or interested in learning how to manage money and other business dealings, the daughter did her mother a great disservice.

By applying the "spheres of influence" concepts, the social worker recognized that Mrs. B. had a recent insult to her physical vitality, (mild stroke with complications), which compromised her ability to cope with some of the social problems of a recently bereaved widow. The resources in the environmental system, i.e., the daughter, failed to recognize the importance for Mrs. B. of maintaining a sense of identity, accountability, community, activity and frivolity. Time, and a system of instruction and support, were required to help her learn or re-learn to perform the "activities" that enabled her to continue to function in the mainstream of life, meeting the usual opportunities for success or failure present for all.

Fortunately, Mrs. B. recovered well from her bereavement and stroke episode and, through counselling by the social worker and other members of the GAU team, recognized that many of the arrangements made by her daughter were unnecessary. A team meeting with the daughter on her next visit West helped to clarify and allay some of her very real fears, ("mother is all alone and I'm so far away"), and when she was able to understand that her mother was in fact capable of continuing to make decisions and call for help from various sectors when required, the situation for both mother and daughter was much more relaxed.

Social workers must expand their perception of the nature of the patient's clinical condition to include a view of the person as being in transaction with their environment. It is this ability to bring an ecological perspective to GAU settings which provides social work with an important and distinct role in these particular practice settings.

IV. A GAU Example

It was the author's experience and good fortune to be employed as a social worker in a Geriatric Assessment Unit in Victoria B.C. This GAU operates adjacent to both an Acute Care Hospital and a Long-Term Care facility. Funding for the Unit is from the Continuing Care branch of the Ministry of Health. Wooldridge et al., (1987) list the main purposes of the program as :

1) to diagnose and treat those elderly who were failing at home for uncertain cause;
2) to diagnose and treat those elderly at home or in long-term care facilities who manifested behaviourial problems, based on the well-recognized premise that much disturbed behaviour has a basis in physical disease and later
3) to admit from the acute hospital, including the emergency department, those elderly presenting with multiple diagnoses who had been admitted for an acute illness. This latter group of patients was accepted in recognition of the fact that elderly patients frequently remain in hospital longer than is optimal and develop conditions that make their discharge difficult.

Most referrals are telephoned into the Unit Medical Director and an initial screening process occurs to determine which particular "area" of the GAU service would best meet the needs of the patient in question. This GAU offers service to patients in 3 main areas: a 50 space geriatric day hospital, a 28-bed inpatient unit and an outpatient/domiciliary visit service. Social work service is available to patients in all three service areas via a "blanket referral" system. It is important to note that this particular GAU functions as a "whole" with interrelated components. This structure was developed with the conviction that only with a broad range of flexible services, available at the moment of referral, can the patient be helped to reach her/his best level rapidly and cost effectively. Patients are often admitted to one particular branch of the program and later transferred for treatment to other branches as their care needs change.

In this particular program, the medical director conducts a preliminary review of the patient's condition to assess the acuity/urgency of the referral. On occasion, requests are made by the referring agent to admit patients to the inpatient unit when it is clear that their needs are chronic in nature and would best be met by either expanded home supports or admission to some form of long-term care facility. Continued vigilance has to be maintained to ensure that only those patients with some remedial condition are admitted to the inpatient unit. An active community education program by the GAU staff aids in the clarification of objectives and purposes of the GAU for physicians and other community caregivers; i.e, the assessment and treatment of episodes of recent and reversible illness.

MacKenzie (1982) confirms that all provinces and territories in Canada now have some type of Home Care Nursing and community support service. British Columbia began a comprehensive Long-Term Care program in 1978, which has expanded to co-ordinate both home help/nursing service and the waiting list for all government funded long-term care facilities in the province. Before any individual can be placed in a government funded LTC facility, s/he must have her/his physical and psycho-social care needs reviewed by a staff member from the local LTC office. Needless to say, many patients referred to the GAU require either a complete re-direction to the local LTC office for service and direction or a consultation by the GAU social work staff and LTC about the types of community or facility supports that can be offered to the patient while s/he is rehabilitated or treated through the efforts of the GAU program. This liaison work between the GAU and the local Long-Term Care office is a principal and vital role of the GAU social worker.

Although there may be variations in the practice styles, modalities and procedures to be found in GAU social work departments, most casework intervention in these settings begins with a review of what is known about a patient. Since most GAU's operate on a referral basis, information is provided to the Unit by the attending physician or other referring agent. Equipped with this knowledge, members of the GAU team are invited by the Unit director to become involved with the process of helping the patient regain, or compensate for, what was lost.

Considerable emphasis is placed on maintaining the elderly person in her/his home environment. To this end, the majority of the patients seen in this GAU service become patients in the Day Hospital branch of this GAU service. As reported by Wooldridge et al. (1987), the majority of patients referred to this program, (95 percent), are usually seen at home by the social worker. The remainder comprise a patient group whose physical needs are sufficiently acute to require an urgent house call by the geriatrician, usually followed by a direct admission of the patient to the Geriatric inpatient ward or transfer to the Acute Care hospital.

V. Social Work Assessment

For the majority of the patients referred, the social work assessment process begins with the practitioner visiting the patient in her/his own environment. This makes it possible to truly, " begin where the client is." A relationship is established with the patient on the patient's home turf and is facilitated by the social work practitioner demonstrating an interest and desire to understand the nature of the patient's present difficulties, and her/his interests, goals and strengths. All of this is done in the reflective light of the patient's personal, family and community support systems.

VI. Home Visits

Mary Richmond (1917) summed up this aspect of practice well when she observed that, we make home visits not to, "find our clients out but rather to find out how to help them better."Home visits afford the opportunity for the GAU social worker to perform three very important but often overlooked duties. The first involves preparing patients for GAU intervention by outlining the nature and the types of services offered. It is a sad fact, that many elderly patients are referred for various health treatments/interventions, but are seldom prepared for the rigours of these encounters. Not surprisingly, these processes are met with anxiety and reluctance by many individuals. Just as is the case for the younger patient, an elderly patient also needs to know what the helping process will contain, what will be required of her/him, and receive answers to more practical questions such as cost, transportation, etc. Provision of clear and concise information about the complexities of the process will assist in reducing anxiety and potential feelings of powerlessness.

A second essential duty of the social worker conducting the home visit is the review of the patient's presenting problem. Although the social worker has had some idea of the reasons for the GAU referral, often this information has come via the attending GP and/or family and other caregivers. Although this information is valuable, it requires supplementation by the patient. There are instances, of course, where the very nature of the patient's difficulties may preclude her/him from having the ability to communicate problems accurately—i.e., speech difficulty, cognitive failure or denial/resistance—but it remains that engaging the patient in a discourse about her/his perceptions of the problem(s), thereby coming to an understanding of what the problems *mean* to the patient, is an essential element of good social work practice!

The third duty involves an analysis of the personal and environmental resources available to the patient. The availability of intrapersonal, interpersonal, and environmental resources is a significant part of any social work assessment. It is important to try and obtain a perception of the personal coping strategies of each individual patient, including a review of personal strengths such as the motivation for getting well.

The role that formal and informal caregivers play in the ability of the older patient to mobilize the appropriate resources to regain their independence is also extremely important and must be included in the social work assessment. Considerable literature is available outlining some of the special roles and characteristics of formal and informal caregivers of elderly patients (see Chappell et al., 1988; Snider, 1981; Fengler & Goodrich, 1979).

VII. Assessment Stages

In the beginning stages of geriatric assessment, the social worker may find it helpful to reflect on the eclectic theoretical orientation of crisis intervention as described by Golan (1986). Patients who are seen for geriatric assessment are usually responding to the impact of internal stressors such as injury or illness and/or the external stressors of recent intra- or interpersonal losses. This can create disruptions in the person's equilibrium or homeostatic balance and often thrusts the patient into a state of crisis. The significance of these events for social work practice is that when problems occur and the physical and psycho-social resources of this clientele cannot return them to a state of equilibrium, functioning may become more impaired. Such setbacks result in the elderly person developing feelings of loss of control or purpose which may lead to depression, increased dependenc, lack of motivation for getting better, and may be followed by the need for institutional care.

After the home visit, the social work case notes are shared with the medical director and other members of the interdisciplinary team as all prepare to admit the patient to the program. As one can see, the information collected by the social worker during this pre-admission home visit provides a solid baseline from which to begin to plan therapeutic interventions with the individual patient. An example of GAU social work intervention is out-lined in the case study presentation at the end of the chapter.

Upon admission of a patient, the social worker continues to maintain contact with both the patient and her/his caregiving con-stellation by providing the social casework services identified earlier i.e., patient and/or family counselling, liaison and referral to community resources, participation in case conferences with other members of the GAU team, etc.

Interventions at the tertiary level stress prevention or delaying the possible consequences of illness or other dysfunctional pro-cesses which may already be occurring. Aging is often accompa-nied by decline, and threats to vitality have consequences that impact negatively on all aspects of an elderly person's personal and social world. The preventive efforts of the GAU team encour-age early diagnosis and, hopefully, treatment that will remedy some of the acute problems and chronic conditions of age. This can lead to renewed interests, new hope and a re-vitalized lifestyle for the elderly patient. Typical preventive intervention strategies offered to patients in GAUs are expanded beyond the treatment of the presenting problem to include suggestions for improved diet, home renovations leading to increased safety, access to expanded home or community supports such as Adult Day Care and Medical Alert Systems, programs to improve medication compli-ance, individual and family counselling, etc.

The very essence of a discussion about prevention needs to go beyond superficial strategies however. For preventive or restora-tive efforts to be successful, it is necessary to know the "root cause" of certain functional or social problems. This requires a dili-gent examination of many factors. As Hepworth and Larsen (1986) point out, "direct social workers should not limit them-selves to remedial activities but should also seek to discover envi-ronmental and other causes of problems and sponsor or support efforts aimed at enhancing the environments of people." For example, the difficulty of getting patients and their families to admit that they have some unresolved interpersonal problems, and the belief that these can be resolved with professional guid-ance and support, presents an interesting, exhilarating, but occa-sionally frustrating challenge for social work practitioners and other team members. As well, depression is too frequent a diag-nosis in the elderly and requires careful assessment and creative treatment approaches. The availability of psychological and geri-atric psychiatry services to patients of GAUs is extremely important but often not available, although research findings document that elderly couples and family units frequently need and can benefit from individual, marital, sex and family therapy (see Sander, 1976; Toseland, 1977; Butler, 1975). Social work needs to advocate for the expansion of these and other services and make continued efforts to influence social policy decisions that affect this group.

POTENTIAL FOR ROLE DEVELOPMENT

As the provision of health care moves into the community and away from the constraints of institutional medical care, the role of the social worker may become less tied to institutional demands, thereby freeing the profession to respond to the broad range of social factors that shape the health of individuals, families and communities. Social work must be prepared to assume this responsibility as both direct practitioners and as health and social service policy planners/ analysts.

At the same time, however, caution must be used not to embrace the concept of "community care" so tightly as to restrict access to the diagnostic and treatment services that will continue to be offered in institutional settings. Rather than designing the service delivery system based on concerns over cost or program ideology and then trying to "fit" the target population into the system, social work, and other service providers, need to ensure that all health agencies continue to identify and respond to the needs of the population to be served. Opportunities for creative and rewarding social work involvement with the frail elderly population should exist in every component of the health care continuum; from the Acute Care Hospital to early Rehabilitation and Convalescent Care Centres such as Geriatric Inpatient Units, to ambulatory care programs such as Geriatric Day Hospitals, to community support programs i.e., Adult Day Cares, Home Help agencies, Senior's Centres etc. and to Long-Term Care Facilities. These practice opportunities have become more available within the last decade and will grow as the country continues to respond creatively to the challenge of caring for our aging citizens. Social workers need to educate themselves to the particular needs of the frail elderly and focus on ways to empower this population to use its strengths and resources in mastering the difficulties associated with illness and disability.

The ideal service delivery system of the future will acknowledge that the accumulated impairments and chronic conditions of the older patient should be seen comprehensively and attention must be given to the structure or "flavour" of the helping agency or institution. Hospitals take great pride in becoming "Centres of Excellence" for Neonatology, Pediatrics, Cardiology, etc. Social workers should encourage hospitals and health care centres to recognize the need to elevate the care of the elderly person to the level where we can also identify this population as deserving care from such "Centres of Excellence," which would guarantee a program of care offered to every elderly patient rather than labelling this entire population of health care consumers as "bed blockers"!

As the health care system becomes more responsive to the needs of the elderly patient, a focus on more comprehensive models of health care will help to redefine and refocus energies and resources away from institutional, disease-related concepts of health and illness to more community-based services that stress the social and health promotion models of health care service. Social work has much to contribute to this movement and can be on the leading edge of program and policy initiatives which, will help to make health care organizations more responsive to the people. All health care professionals should be delighted with the recent statement by the new federal minister of Health, Perrin Beatty (1989), when he suggests that strategies need to be developed that "promote the independence and quality of life for seniors' as this is what they are entitled to as citizens." Representatives of government need to be reminded of the promises in this statement and since such strategies do not come cheaply, nor from mere rhetoric, be persuaded to support new and creative strategies for caring for society as we all age, releasing the resources needed to enhance the existing programs of care.

The relatively recent development of geriatric assessment programs in this country makes it difficult to cite examples of research about the efficacy and health/social benefits to patients reviewed. Follow-up studies would provide much information relevant to social work practice with this population and would also provide support and direction to those individuals currently involved with the design and operation of GAUs. Obviously, a tremendous practice opportunity exists for social work research and publication in this "new" field.

CONCLUDING REMARKS

As life is a progression of events that requires individuals to make transitions, there is no better way to perceive old age than to think about continuing change. GAU social workers as "agents of change" find the frail elderly struggling to adapt rapidly to change with diminished personal and environmental resources. The recognition of multiple disabilities, particularly psycho-social disability, is of particular interest to social work in this practice setting. The social work practitioner in these programs has much to offer as efforts are made to understand the interrelationship of all factors that lead to dysfunctional change and then to design interventions to return the elderly patient to good health and as much independent function as is possible or desired.

Since reversible health problems and individual problems in social functioning may incorrectly be attributed to the infirmities of age, continued efforts must be made by social workers to ensure that stereotypical perceptions of elderly persons do not distort assessments, limit goals, nor restrict interventions. Unless such efforts are made, the elderly of today, and we as the elders of tomorrow, will have to endure the final years of life with services that are designed to provide less than adequate support and opportunities to compensate for human frailties.

CASE EXAMPLE

GERIATRIC ASSESSMENT UNIT— SOCIAL WORK REPORT
PRE-ADMISSION VISIT—MR. JOE BLOGGS

Mr. Bloggs is an 83-year-old gentleman who was visited today in his home on Main Street where he lives with his well and active 81-year-old wife. He has been referred to the GAU by his attending physician at the urging of his son, George. George lives in Calgary but manages to visit his parents every 3-4 months. On a visit last weekend, he was alarmed to note a rapid deterioration in his father's physical and mental functioning. He is concerned that his mother is becoming exhausted with caring for Mr. Bloggs and " wants something done."

MENTAL FUNCTION AND MOOD

Mr. Bloggs appeared listless and depressed during the home visit. Efforts to engage him in conversation were difficult and most questions were answered by his wife before he had opportunity to respond. A gentle direction was given to Mrs. Bloggs to allow Mr. Bloggs to respond in order to allow an assessment of how well he was processing information. On further questioning, Mr. Bloggs appeared oriented to person and place but disoriented to time, but his poor response may be related more to his feelings of poor physical health than a dementing process.

AMBULATION

Mrs. Bloggs reports that her husband has been having difficulty walking lately and has had many falls. He gets up often at night to use the bathroom and frequently stumbles enroute. His most recent fall was four days ago when he suffered a severe "bump" on the head from the edge of the bathtub. She feels his condition has become worse since then.

MEDICAL BACKGROUND

Appendectomy – 1923
Prostatectomy – 1987
Hiatal Hernia
Borderline Diabetes
Hypertension
Recent Falls

MEDICATIONS

Tagamet 300 mg. tid
Dalmane 30 mg. @ hs
Diabeta 0.5 mg. OD
Moduret 25 mg. bid

SOCIAL HISTORY

Mr. Bloggs is a retired accountant who moved to Victoria from Calgary with his wife 11 years ago. He is described by his family as a shy and quiet gentleman who kept to himself and had few interests outside the home, save his woodworking hobby. Even though Mr. Bloggs has a fully equipped workshop in the basement of their home, it seems he lost interest in this pastime some 6-7 months ago. He takes great pride in his business competence but had his ego sorely bruised last spring when he made a number of errors in preparing the tax returns of several friends from their bridge club. Mrs. Bloggs reports that he has appeared depressed and withdrawn since that time and rarely responds positively to social invitations with the individuals he feels he "wronged."

PATIENT/FAMILY PERCEPTION OF THE PRESENTING PROBLEM

Mrs. Bloggs appears to be very perplexed by her husbands behaviour and confided that she really does believe that he has the beginnings of "senility." She states that she is desperate for some assistance or will have to make arrangements to place her husband in a long-term care facility.

SOCIAL WORK IMPRESSION AND PLAN

It appears this gentleman was having some problems with depression over the past several months but was otherwise functioning relatively well. His behaviour has changed significantly in the past week. His wife is his primary caregiver and is quickly becoming exhausted. The nature of the Geriatric Assessment Program was explained to both Mr. and Mrs. Bloggs and after some gentle persuasion and coaxing by his wife, Mr. Bloggs agreed and arrangements were made for him to be seen in the Geriatric Day Hospital in two days time.

SOCIAL WORK CASE NOTES – MR. JOE BLOGGS

Mr. Bloggs was seen in the Geriatric Day Hospital in December, 1988. The Geriatrician noted a number of neurological deficits during his physical examination and arranged for an immediate CT Scan after learning of Mr. Bloggs recent fall and head injury. The CT Scan showed a subdural hemotoma. Mr. Bloggs was admitted to the geriatric in-patient unit for further observation and transferred the next day to the acute-care hospital for surgery to release the intracranial pressure from the hematoma. He returned to the geriatric inpatient unit after a 6 day stay on the acute care ward for further investigation of some other physical problems (borderline diabetes, urinary tract infection) and where his medication regime was restructured (including an anti-depressant) and a physiotherapy program begun to restrengthen him. Both Mr. and Mrs. Bloggs were seen by the nutritionist for counselling for his diabetic condition.The social worker arranged to have the local long-term care office send homemaker help once per week to help Mrs. Bloggs with the heavy cleaning. Both Mr. and Mrs. Bloggs rejected the idea of any home help coming to assist in the personal care needs of Mr. Bloggs such as assistance with bathing. The occupational therapist arranged to visit the Bloggs at home to install railings around the bathtub and a raised toilet seat. Mr. Bloggs responded well to the music program while on the inpatient ward and was encouraged by the OT to return to his long neglected hobby of restoring musical instruments. The staff reported at case conference that he was thinking more clearly although his mood remained somewhat depressed. Mr. Bloggs remained on the inpatient ward for three weeks and was then discharged home to the care of his wife with the understanding that he would continue his rehabilitation by attending the geriatric day hospital program of the GAU three days each week. His attendance at the GDH program was somewhat sporadic as he often would find excuses not to be ready when the GDH bus came to call for him. The social worker made subsequent house calls to follow-up on the concerns of the Geriatrician and other members of the team that Mr. Bloggs continued to be depressed and unmotivated.

With some reluctance Mr. Bloggs began to discuss his feelings of apprehension, despair and " uselessness." He stated that he felt "ridiculous" having to depend on his wife for assistance with his personal care as he had been rarely ill and needy of this type of care before. He was very fearful that he might become ill again and that caring for him would be "too much" for his wife. A subsequent exploration of the sense of failure he experienced when making errors on the tax forms for his friends was structured around helping him to modify his negative self-thoughts and subsequent sense of embarrassment and frustration. Further sessions with both the social worker and the visiting psychiatrist allowed Mr. Bloggs to ventilate some of these feelings and come to some resolution over disappointments he had experienced both in the past and recently. Mr. Bloggs also responded well in group settings with the social worker and other patients of the GAU. He admitted coming to the realization that many other older people like himself struggled with similar feelings of depression over the dependency sometimes associated with ill health. Mrs. Bloggs was seen both separately and conjointly with her husband as the team attempted to help her understand her husband's care needs and to recognize her need for support in dealing with the situation. Mrs. Bloggs was initially very resistive of the idea of accepting home help as she was very proud of her own homemaking abilities. After some discussion with Mr. Bloggs, the son and the GAU team, Mrs. Bloggs recognized that relinquishing some of the more mundane and exhausting household duties would free her time and energies to allow more opportunities for Mr. and Mrs. Bloggs to become re-involved in a social world they had neglected for some time. The Bloggs were referred to a local senior's activity centre and encouraged to participate in the organization as one way of re-developing a sense of activity, community and frivolity. Mr. Bloggs was encouraged to re-define his sense of identity, which to this point had always told him that he " must be in control at all times." Mrs. Bloggs and the son, George, had a tendency to mistakenly assume that Mr. Bloggs would not recover from his recent illness and were about to make arrangements with the bank and the accountant to "take over" their financial affairs. Fortunately, staff were able to convince Mrs. Bloggs and the son that this potential insult to Mr. Blogg's sense of accountability and identity was not necessary as his vitality returned. Mr. Bloggs was discharged from the Geriatric Day Hospital Program of the GAU after an 8 week stay.

DISCHARGE NOTE — Six Month follow-up

The Bloggs were contacted by the social worker for follow-up information. Mr. Bloggs recovered well from his numerous physical problems, although he continues to struggle with feelings of depression. He is seen monthly by his family physician for re-evaluation of his anti-depressant medication. Mrs. Bloggs reports that they have taken a number of short day trips with a group from the senior's centre and hope to participate in a six-day tour of the Southern United States next month. Mrs. Bloggs cancelled the homemaker help as she found she had " plenty of free time" since Mr. Bloggs had returned to his wood-working hobby.

References

Barer, M. L., Evans, R. B., Hertman, C. & Lomas, J. (1986). Toward efficient aging: Rhetoric and evidence. Paper presented at the Third Canadian Conference on Health Economics, Winnipeg, Manitoba.

Beatty, P. (1989). Notes from an Address to the Canadian Club. Ottawa, Ontario.

Beaver, M. L. & Miller, D. (1985). *Clinical Social Work Practice with the Elderly*. Illinois: The Dorsey Press.

Brill, N. I. (1986). *Team Work: Working Together in the Human Services*. Philadelphia, PA: W.B. Saunders Co.

Butler, R. (1975). *Why Survive? Being Old in America*. New York: Harper and Row.

Calkins, E., Davis, P. & Ford, A. *The Practice of Geriatrics*. Philadelphia, PA: W.B. Saunders Co.

Chappell, N. L., Strain, L. & Blandford, A. (1986). *Aging and Health Care*. Toronto, Ontario : Holt Rhinehart and Winston of Canada Ltd.

Cox, H. G. (1988). *Later Life — The Realities of Aging* (2nd edition). Englewood Cliffs, New Jersey: Prentice Hall.

Doremus, B. (1976). The four R's of medical social diagnosis. *Health and Social Work, 1*(4).

Fengler A. P. & Goodrich, N. (1979). Wives of elderly disabled men: The hidden patients. *Gerontologist, 19*, pp. 175-183.

Flathman, D. P. & Larsen, D. E. An evaluation of three geriatric day hospitals in Alberta. Calgary, Alberta. Unpublished report, Division of Community Health Services, Faculty of Medicine, University of Calgary.

Gaitz, C. M. (1974). Barriers to the delivery of psychiatric services to the elderly. *Gerontologist, 14*, pp. 210-214.

Germain, C. B. (1973). An ecological perspective in casework practice. *Social Casework, 54*, pp. 323-330.

Gilmore, S. K. (1973). *Counsellor- in- Training*. Englewood Cliffs, New Jersey: Prentice Hall.

Golan, N. (1986). Crisis theory. In F. J. Turner (Ed.), *Social Work Treatment: Interlocking Theoretical Approaches* (3rd edition). New York: The Free Press.

Health and Welfare Canada (1988). Health Promotion Directorate, Health Service and Promotion Branch, 27(2).

Hertzman, C. & Hayes, M. (1985). Will the elderly really bankrupt us with increased health care costs? *Canadian Journal of Public Health, 76*, pp. 373-377.

Hepworth, D. H. & Larsen, J. A. (1986). *Direct Social Work Practice: Theory and Skills* (2nd edition). Chicago, Illinois: The Dorsey Press.

Hooyman, N. R. & Kiyak, A. (1988). The importance of social supports: Family, friends and neighbours. In *Social Gerontology — A Multi-disciplinary Perspective*. Needham Heights, Massachesetts: Allyn and Bacon.

Kane, R. (1987). Contrasting models: Reflections on the pattern of geriatric evaluation unit care. In L. Z. Rubenstein, L. J. Campbell & R. L. Kane (Eds.), *Clinics in Geriatric Medicine*. Philadelphia, PA: W.B. Saunders Co.

MacKenzie, J. A. (1982). Aging in Canadian society. *Issues in Canadian Social Policy: A Reader, II*, Canadian Council on Social Development.

McDaniels, S. A. (1988). Prospects for an aging Canada: Gloom or hope? *Transition*, pp. 9-11.

Medalie, J. H. (1986). An approach to common problems in the elderly. In E. Calkins & A. Ford (Eds.), *The Practice of Geriatrics*. Philadelphia, PA.: W.B. Saunders Co.

Neugarten, B. (1974). Age groups in American society and the rise of the young-old. In *Political Consequences of Aging*. The Annals of the American Academy of Political and Social Science, *415* pp. 187-198.

Novak, M. (1988). *Aging and Society*. Scarborough, Ontario: Nelson Canada.

Rathbone-McCuan, E. & Levenson, J. (1977). Geriatric day care: A community approach to geriatric health care. *Journal of Gerontological Nursing, 3*(4), pp. 43-46.

Richmond, Mary (1917). Social Diagnosis. New York: Russel Sage Foundation.

Rosenfeld, J. (1983). The domain and expertise of social work: A conceptualization. *Social Work, 28*, pp. 186-191.

Rubenstein, L. Z., Abrass, I. & Kane, R. L. (1981). Improved care for patients on a new geriatric evaluation unit. *Journal of the American Geriatrics Society, 29*, pp. 531- 536.

Rubenstein, L. Z., Rhee, L. & Kane, R. L. The role of geriatric assessment units in caring for the elderly: An analytic review. *Journal of Gerontology, 37*, pp. 513- 521.

Rubenstein, L. Z. (1987). Geriatric assessment: An overview of its impacts. In L. Z. Rubenstein, L. J. Campbell & R. L. Kane (Eds.), *Clinics in Geriatric Medicine*. Philadelphia, PA: W.B. Saunders Co.

Sander, F. (1976). Aspects of sexual counselling with the aged. *Social Casework, 58*, pp. 504-510.

Skelton, D. (1986). The future of geriatric medicine in Canada. *Gerontion,* pp. 19-23.

Schumann, J. Z. (1984). Maintaining ability in the elderly. *Canadian Family Physician, 30,* pp. 607-610.

Snider, E. L. (1981). The role of kin in meeting health care needs of the elderly. *Canadian Journal of Sociology, 6,* pp. 325-336.

Toseland, R. (1977). A problem-solving group workshop for older persons. *Social Work, 22,* pp. 325-326.

Watson, M. (1984). Alternatives to institutionalizing the elderly. *Canadian Family Physician, 30,* pp. 655-660.

Westburg, S. (1986). An aging population: Implications for social workers in acute hospitals. *The Social Worker — Journal of the Canadian Association of Social Workers,* pp. 107- 109.

Williams, T. F. (1987). Integration of geriatric assessment into the community. In L. Z. Rubenstein, L. J. Campbell & R. L. Kane (Eds.), *Clinics in Geriatric Medicine.* Philadelphia, PA: W.B. Saunders Co.

Wooldridge, D. B., Parker, G. & MacKenzie, P. (1987). An acute inpatient geriatric assessment and treatment unit. In L. Z. Rubenstein, L. J. Campbell & R. L. Kane (Eds.), *Clinics in Geriatric Medicine.* Philadelphia, PA: W.B. Saunders Co.

Chapter 22

Social Work Practice in Hospice Care

Nina Millett Fish, RN, BS, MSW

Abstract

Hospice is a relatively new component of the health care system, having its beginnings in London in the early 1960s. Its phenomenal growth in the United States since the early 1970s emphasizes its value in today's society. Differing from traditional health care, its focus is on palliative (comfort) rather than curative care for terminally ill persons and their families. Symptom management for the patient is the first priority, and emotional and spiritual support is provided for both patient and family. From the beginning, social workers have played integral roles in the development of hospice, both in management and in direct service to clients, helping to meet non-medical needs of patients and their families.

Social Work Practice in Hospice Care

In medieval times, hospices were way stations for sick and dying travellers on pilgrimages to and from the Holy Land. They were places where special care was given until travellers either died or were able to continue their journey. The modern hospice movement began in the early 1960s when Dame Cicely Saunders, a British nurse, medical social worker and physician, distressed by unmet needs of dying persons she saw in London hospitals, founded St. Christopher's Hospice in 1967. Her primary goal was to manage physical symptoms of persons in the final stage of a terminal illness and to provide emotional and spiritual support for both patient and family, ultimately enhancing the quality of remaining life for all concerned.

Saunders' concept of care soon spread to the United States, with the formation of a model hospice program based on St. Christopher's, in New Haven, Connecticut. The movement flourished, and now there are over 2000 such programs representing every state in America.

Hospice programs have specific characteristics resulting in care that differs from traditional health care. Their characteristics include:

1. physician-directed care;
2. co-ordinated home and in-patient care under a central hospice management;
3. management of symptoms (physical, emotional and spiritual);
4. provision of care by an interdisciplinary team, including (at least) a physician, nurses, social workers, clergy and volunteers;
5. patient and family together are the unit of care;
6. use of volunteers as an integral part of the team;
7. 24-hour availability of care and services and
8. bereavement follow-up for family members.

Hospice is "care" rather than "cure" oriented. This means that despite the best efforts of medical care, the disease has progressed to the stage where further aggressive, curative treatment is considered inappropriate, and the patient's physical, emotional and spiritual comfort becomes the focus of care. Defined as palliative care, the prescribed treatment is designed to relieve pain and other distressing symptoms of the illness, in addition to being attentive to the needs of family members.

THE CLIENTELE

Hospice patients are persons experiencing the end stages of a progressive terminal illness (usually estimated at six months or less life expectancy) and their families. Most suffer from cancer, but those with other illnesses such as end stage heart, liver or kidney diseases, ALS (Lou Gehrig's disease), multiple sclerosis and AIDS are also appropriate for hospice care. Whatever the diagnosis, the focus is always on symptom management for the patient and on emotional and spiritual support for both patient and family.

In the United States, most hospice care is provided in the home by family members, with availability of in-patient care coordinated and managed by the hospice team, if needed. In the home, hospice staff and volunteers are available to assess, assist, monitor and support both patient and family as they care for the patient. The staff also functions as liaison to or advocate for the patient with the physician, the health care system and community agencies. In-patient care may take place in an acute-care hospital, extended-care facility or free-standing hospice, depending on organization of individual programs. Usually, in-patient care is provided on a specially designed and organized hospital unit, staffed for specific needs of hospice patients and families. Customary institutional rules such as visiting hours are relaxed, allowing family, including children, to remain with the patient 24 hours a day if desired. Family members are encouraged to participate in the patient's care.

Hospice patients are diverse, coming from all income levels, ages, ethnic and racial backgrounds. Unless children are excluded by individual program admission criteria, ages may range from one to 101. Their commonality is a terminal illness, usually accompanied by symptoms that are needing to be managed, and their families are experiencing emotional and spiritual turmoil as well. Frequently, after having fought the disease for months or years, their physical, emotional, spiritual and financial resources are exhausted.

As a group, their physical symptoms are similar, usually including pain (the most frightening and often the easiest to manage), extreme weakness, nausea and vomiting, loss of appetite, constipation, edema and weight loss. However, since physical comfort is the first priority, similarity of symptoms in no way diminishes the importance of their management. Without physical comfort there is no quality of life, and psychosocial and spiritual needs cannot be dealt with. Reflecting this concept, Sylvia Lack (1977, p. 162), an early hospice physician, said, "there is far too much talk...in this country about psychological and emotional problems, and far too little about making the patient comfortable.... Counseling a dying person who is lying in a wet bed is ineffective."

Psychosocially, emotionally and spiritually, each patient/family is unique. They are products of their culture, values, racial and ethnic origins, spiritual beliefs, developmental age, families of origin, socio-economic status and numerous other factors. Their family skeletons may include drug and alcohol abuse, poverty, spouse or child abuse, incest and mental illness, to name only a few. Not uncommonly there has been a divorce and remarriage, so "family" expands to include all the step-relatives as well, and all the additional problems that may accompany these situations. In some instances, patients are referred for care in the midst of a bitter divorce and/or custody battle. For example, one woman who had lived in one state moved to another while terminally ill. She was virtually penniless because in the midst of her bitter divorce, her estranged husband, a friend of the judge, refused to send any support. He also encouraged the judge not to proceed with a court hearing, waiting instead for the patient to die. In the meantime, she was cared for by a daughter who was herself in the midst of a divorce and custody battle.

A diagnosis of terminal illness never occurs in a vacuum. According to Dobkin and Morrow (1986), the experience of cancer fundamentally disrupts a patient and her/his lifestyle. Future plans are halted, roles are reversed, financial savings are depleted, and life becomes suddenly unpredictable. In discussing a diagnosis of terminal illness from a "task-interrupted dimension," Pollin (1984, p. 28), states that "normal living is replaced by conditional living — the realization that one cannot go on with one's life as planned." Certainty becomes uncertainty, and patients encounter intense fears, anxieties and frustrations that are unexpected and unfamiliar.

Regardless of other problems, a common theme of hospice patients and families is coping with losses of all kinds. The patient grieves for past, present and future losses. Rando (1984, p. 227) lists numerous potential losses common among terminally ill persons: control; independence; productivity; security; physical, psychological and cognitive abilities; predictability and consistency; future existence, experiences, dreams and hopes; pleasure; ability to complete plans and projects; significant others; familiar environment and possessions; aspects of the self and identity; and meaning. Families grieve for similar losses, and both grieve for the family unit as it has been, for it is irretrievably changed and will never again be the same. According to Pollin (1984, p. 28) the impending death of a loved one awakens their own fears about loss and separation. "Life becomes an awesome mingling of hope and despair, courage and fear, humour and anger, and constant uncertainty."

It is in these areas of psychosocial and emotional problems that social workers can have an impact on the lives of patients and families. Assessing for strengths and weaknesses, coping strategies and defences, communication patterns, availability of social support beyond the nuclear and extended families, the need for legal or financial assistance and interpreting these issues to other team members helps the entire team to better understand the overall situation and to plan care within the appropriate framework.

PRACTICE ROLES AND RESPONSIBILITIES

The majority of social work time is spent in direct service to patients and families. There is valid potential for involvement beyond direct service in areas such as education, management, policy development, research, planning, consultation and collaboration (Millett, 1983), and these will be discussed further in another section. Given realities of staffing, funding and reimbursement, however, most time and effort of staff social workers is directed toward patient/family concerns.

An initial psychosocial assessment is completed for each patient/family admitted to the hospice program. A thorough assessment serves as a vehicle for follow-up care and interventions and helps team members understand the uniqueness of each family system beyond symptoms experienced by the patient. A framework for a comprehensive assessment discussed by Lusk (1983), and adapted by the author, includes a social and developmental history, assessment of the family system and physical and environmental resources.

Included in the social and developmental history are cultural, educational and psychological issues prior to the illness, focussing especially on coping skills associated with loss. Loss of control, independence, self-esteem and body image, financial security, relationships with family and friends and other losses mentioned previously are all faced along the way to the ultimate loss of life itself. Purtilo (1976) suggests that each "little death" is a reminder of the ultimate loss of life itself. It is crucial to understand how the patient/family has dealt with previous losses, since it is likely that current losses will be handled in a similar manner.

Assessment of the family system includes both nuclear and extended families and also the social support network; its size, capabilities, structure, stability and ethnicity, the roles various members play, its strengths and vulnerabilities. It also includes assessing for mental status, mood and affect, appropriateness of behaviour, patient and family's reaction to the illness, defence mechanisms and coping strategies, the relationship between the patient, caregiver and other family members, altered communication patterns, how family roles have been affected by the illness and how these roles and responsibilities have been reallocated and accepted by others.

Assessing for physical and environmental resources refers to such things as adequacy of the home environment, health and capability of the caregiver to provide necessary care, financial status, health insurance and need for referral to community agencies for equipment or other services. Medical bills may be overwhelming and insurance forms are complex, and sometimes beyond the capability of the patient or caregiver to complete while all energies are focussed on caring for the patient. Ensuring that patients and families are receiving services to which they are entitled, i.e., equipment loaned by the American Cancer Society rather than paying rental costs, is part of the social worker's responsibility, as is helping with wills and trusts, if requested by the family. Practical issues after the patient's death, including helping to file insurance claims, obtaining information on death benefits and similar assistance can be helpful to the survivors.

Several years ago, Koenig (1968) conducted a study that examined non-medical needs of 60 persons suffering from terminal cancer. The study reported over 700 instances of problems the group found moderately or severely difficult to manage. Included were financial problems (71 separate problems were reported), illness and symptom problems such as fear and anxiety about the course of the disease; i.e., fear of pain, loss of energy, physical limitations, changes in body image and fear of painful medical tests. Additional problems identified were changes in communication patterns with family and friends, sexual concerns and feelings of worthlessness due to inability to function in familiar roles. Patients were also concerned about the effects on family and friends of their mood changes, anxiety, depression and hostility. Koenig concluded that unless these non-medical needs were addressed, patients would not receive the full benefits of medical or palliative care.

In providing direct services, social workers will utilize their skills in crisis intervention (sudden, unexpected patient or family problems), short term casework (to help make decisions about specific problems), longer term therapy (especially during difficult bereavement) and collaboration and/or consultation (with other team members or professional colleagues) (Millett, 1983). Pilsecker (1979) provides a helpful summary of four social work tasks in working with terminally ill patients and families:

1. helping patients and families to get in touch with their feelings and understand their behaviourial options;
2. assisting patients and families to develop or maintain meaningful communication;
3. assisting patients and families to locate and utilize other community resources as needed and
4. helping health professionals involved with the patient/family to get in touch with and acknowledge their own feelings, and to understand and respect patient/family needs and to meet them in a sensitive manner.

In accomplishing these tasks, the social worker may find her/himself functioning in a variety of roles, as discussed by Foeckler and Mills (1980), including

1. enabler/extender — to help patient/family talk about death and dying, as appropriate, to reach out and assist others involved to talk to each other about the approaching separation, in addition tos letting them know that negative feelings such as anger, irritability and depression are also acceptable and valid;
2. comforter - listening to the patient/family and sharing their pain, joy and sorrow;
3. interpreter — utilizing knowledge of human behaviour to interpret feelings and behaviours, and to understand and work through difficult situations;
4. advocate — protection and defence of the patient/family when appropriate, i.e., helping them navigate the health care or welfare system;
5. mobilizer — searching for additional internal resources within the extended family and support system;

6. team member — working as a member of a team rather than independently;
7. consultant - discussing with a member of another discipline the most effective way they might help in a particular situation; and,
8. teacher — with patient/family, other team members, the community and students.

In reference to functioning as a team member, it is essential to recognize that with such close teamwork, role overlap or blurring is inevitable. Rather than well-defined roles such as in traditional health settings, all team members perform, from time to time, tasks other than those traditionally allocated to them. For example, a nurse may counsel about a psychosocial issue, a social worker may perform a basic physical task or pray with a patient if asked. For an effective, smooth-functioning team, it is essential that team members accept that role blurring is inevitable. To provide quality hospice care, the combined resources and skills of all disciplines are necessary (Millett, 1983).

Families vary greatly in their need for social work intervention. Some may need assistance primarily with concrete services, others may need help with specific issues or problems, yet others may need counseling to help resolve long-standing issues. Whatever the need, there are ample opportunities for utilization of a challenging blend of social work skills.

POTENTIAL FOR ROLE DEVELOPMENT

The social work role in hospice is varied and challenging and has potential for expansion beyond provision of direct service into management, planning, policy development, education, research and involvement in legislative issues.

The social work perspective easily lends itself to management of aspects of a program such as volunteer or bereavement co-ordinator, or as executive director of an entire program. Management requires a variety of skills familiar to social workers, including organizational behaviour, communication, negotiation, policy development, planning, leadership, stress management and collaboration with other organizations/agencies and community work.

Education is a continuing process for self, colleagues, patients/families, community and students. Issues of separation and loss are universal, and with the social workers knowledge of coping and defence mechanisms, family dynamics, developmental life span issues and concerns and the grieving process, s/he is a valuable resource to provide education at many levels. There is ample opportunity for staff education within agencies and institutions throughout the community. Churches, service organizations, schools, hospitals, nursing homes, colleges and universities are all examples of areas needing education about loss and separation. Serving as a practicum advisor for students working with individuals and groups, to learn about issues of loss and separation s/he will deal with throughout her/his career, is a challenging social work function.

Research on management of physical symptoms has come a long way in the past decade, but there are other less well researched areas in which social workers may become involved. Effective ways to help children and adolescents cope with loss and grief is such an area, as is the role of humour as a coping mechanism, both for staff and patients/families. The effect of terminal illness on families, spiritual needs of patients/families and clergy involvement are little researched areas, as is the relationship between physical pain and emotions such as fear, anxiety and depression.

Legislation to date has dealt successfully with reimbursement and licensing issues, with hospice now reimbursable by Medicare, Medicaid (in some states) and numerous private carriers. Many states have licensing laws, also. Other legislative concerns affect hospice patients/families directly or indirectly, such as the need for affordable respite care and financing home care for persons without caregivers. The advent of AIDS and the overwhelming needs of these patients and their families, and the many ethical issues associated with this disease, are potential areas for legislative involvement.

CONCLUDING REMARKS

The birth and rapid growth of the hospice movement emphasizes its value as an important part of the overall health care system. For those persons for whom life-prolonging treatments are no longer appropriate, it offers a human and humane alternative to the cold technology of many medical centres.

Hospice is not a panacea. It cannot meet all needs of each patient/family it serves, nor can it often change family problems and dysfunctions of long-standing duration. What it *can* do is manage symptoms, provide support, help families mobilize resources, supplementing when needed, to ensure quality palliative care for the patient during her/his final weeks or months.

From the beginning, social workers have been an integral part of the hospice movement, helping to insure its focus on the value of human life, dignity and worth of each individual. In return, hospice practice offers social workers challenging career opportunities, utilizing a broad range of roles and responsibilities. Both can only benefit from continued association and involvement.

CASE EXAMPLE

This case study is presented because it represents the team nature of hospice work, rather than focussing on a single discipline.

Rosa was an 87-year-old white female Christian Scientist referred to hospice after being brought by her family to the hospital emergency room (ER) on a sweltering, humid summer evening, suffering from heat exhaustion. While in the ER, she was found to have a large fungating, infected, foul smelling, protruding lesion on her right breast, about the size of a large grapefruit. Admitted to the hospital overnight, Rosa quickly became alert and refused any type of treatment or diagnostic procedures, because they would conflict with her religious beliefs. Because of this refusal, and because of her expressed desire, she was to be discharged the next day, after being seen by someone from hospice.

Rosa was a spry, thin, angry, stoic, very private person who did not want to be in the hospital. She was difficult to communicate with, and a poor historian. She agreed to allow hospice to be involved with her care at home, providing we did not require her to take any medicine or treatments that were contrary to her reli-

413

gious beliefs. We assured her we would defer to her wishes in any such matters.

A widow, Rosa lived alone in a small, cluttered, dilapidated, unairconditioned house, and her limited income came from Social Security, supplemented by food stamps. Her family consisted of the following: Ruth, a divorced, marginally functioning, diagnosed schizophrenic daughter; Kathy, a granddaughter who worked full time and was struggling to hold together a shaky second marriage; and two great grandchildren (Kathy's), aged 19 (from her first marriage) and 3 (from her current marriage). Kathy and Rosa were very close, Kathy having been raised by Rosa because of Ruth's mental illness. Although Rosa had suffered from this condition for approximately three to five years, no one in the family had been aware of it. Eventually Rosa described it to Kathy as "a pimple that wouldn't go away, and just kept getting worse." There was some social support, mainly from church friends, but they were unable to provide care for Rosa. They visited when they could. Clearly, the burden of responsibility and decision making would be on Kathy.

Determined to return home, a shaky plan was devised for Rosa's care. Ruth was very dependent on her mother and routinely spent much of each day with her. At this point, she totally denied her mother's condition, which was her usual coping mechanism with stress or loss. Ruth agreed to spend each day with her mother, and Kathy spent some time each evening, but Rosa was alone at night. The financial resources of the whole family did not allow for hiring help in the home. Hospice nurses visited each day to change the dressing on the lesion and to monitor for further infection. Volunteers were utilized for a few hours each day, although this was a difficult assignment for them since Rosa remained essentially non-communicative and angry, even though she had agreed to allow the volunteers to come. Her great-grandchildren were her favourite topics of conversation, and about the only thing she would talk about. Application was made to the local Department of Aging for additional daytime care, but by the time the bureaucratic wheels turned and help was approved, Rosa was back in the hospital.

Rosa's condition actually improved briefly, the infection decreased and, with use of dietary supplements, she became stronger. However, problems with reimbursement soon developed. Operating under Medicare's Home Health guidelines, Medicare questioned the need for daily RN visits since no treatments were being given. We attempted to teach Kathy to change Rosa's dressing, but it was embarrassing for Rosa and, due to the nature of the lesion, too difficult for Kathy. A volunteer RN agreed to see Rosa twice a week to change the dressing, so the hospice RN decreased her visits accordingly, satisfying Medicare briefly.

After a few weeks, Rosa's condition began to deteriorate. One evening she fell, was again brought to the hospital ER and was admitted to the hospice unit. She continued to refuse any treatment and stoically denied any pain.

Within a few days, Rosa stopped eating and drinking and quickly became comatose, with death appearing imminent. Kathy was very distraught. While fully aware of Rosa's condition, she had a great deal of difficulty "letting Grandma starve to death," a common issue for families of hospice patients. After several lengthy discussions with Kathy, during which she agonized over her own feelings and Rosa's religious beliefs, she made the decision to request intravenous fluids for Rosa. Although contrary to the hospice team's wishes, we supported Kathy in this decision. Rosa responded somewhat, but remained semi-comatose. Because she was restless at times, Kathy was afraid Rosa was in pain, so she made another difficult decision and asked the physician to order some mild pain medications.

After about two weeks, the hospital's Utilization Review Department, which reviews all Medicare patients for appropriateness of in-patient care according to Medicare guidelines, could no longer "look the other way." The social worker began talking to Kathy about extended care. The only Christian Science nursing home in the area refused to take Rosa because she was receiving medical care. Others refused to accept her because of her fungating lesion. Eventually, an administrative decision was made by the President of the Medical Centre that Rosa could remain in the hospital and the hospital would absorb the cost.[1]

Rosa lived another two weeks. Hospice team members read to her from the Christian Science Handbook and the Bible and played tapes of hymns. The hospice chaplain visited and prayed with her. She visibly relaxed during these times. Meanwhile, Kathy became more comfortable with her decisions, and was able to "let go" when Rosa died. Kathy supported her mother as much as possible. Ruth had visited her mother only once in the hospital, but was unable to handle the stress.

After Rosa's death, Kathy was an active participant in the

bereavement program as she grieved painfully for Rosa. Although she received little support from her husband through all of this, the marriage seemed still intact. Between meetings of the bereavement program, Kathy called the hospice staff frequently just to talk and express her grief. Eventually, she came to terms with her loss and no longer felt the need to remain involved in the bereavement program.

As stated previously, Kathy bore the responsibility and the burden for decision making. Hospice staff spent almost as much time with Kathy as with Rosa. She was forced to come to grips with Rosa's illness and impending death in a very short period of time. Kathy's marriage was shaky, she had no contact with her father and, due to her mother's illness, she was more like a parent than a child to her. Rosa was her primary family.

Rosa's death was pain-free and comfortable, but not the way she would have chosen. Kathy was our "patient" almost as much as Rosa. She was deeply grateful for our help and support and expressed it over and over again. We were her main source of support from the beginning. While caring for Rosa (and Kathy), we dealt with issues of denial, mental illness, dysfunctional family, religious beliefs, ethical issues surrounding those beliefs, inadequate housing and caregiving support, Rosa's anger and reimbursement problems. All of these are common issues faced by many families when there is a terminal illness.

This case was selected for discussion because it is representative of the complexities and ethical issues involved with patients and families when a member is dying, and also the need for all disciplines to work together as a team.

References

Dobkin, P. & Morrow, G. (1986). Biopsychosocial assessment of cancer patients: Methods and suggestions. *The Hospice Journal, 2,* 37-57.

Foeckler, M. & Mills, T. (1980). Preparing social work students for thanatological roles. In B. Orcutt et al. (eds.) *Social Work and Thanatology* (74-78). New York: Arno Co.

Koenig, R. (1968). Fatal illness: A study of social service needs. *Social Work, 13,* 85-90.

Lack, S. (1977). The hospice concept — the adult with advanced cancer. In *Proceedings of the American Cancer Society Second National Conference on Human Values and Cancer* (160-166). Chicago: American Cancer Society.

Lusk, M. (1983). The psychosocial evaluation of the hospice patient. *Health and Social Work, 8,* 210-218.

Millett, N. (1983). Hospice: A new horizon for social work. In C. Corr and D. Corr, (eds.), *Hospice Care: Principles and Practice* (135-147). New York: Springer Publishing Company.

Pilsecker, C. (1979). Terminal cancer: A challenge for social work. *Social Work in Health Care, 4,* 367-379.

Pollin, I. (1984). The talk-interrupted dimension: Understanding the emotional components of a traumatic medical diagnosis. *The American Journal of Hospice Care, 1,* 28-31.

Purtilo, R. (1976). Similarities in patient response to chronic and terminal illness. *Physical Therapy, 56,* 279-284.

Rando, T. (1984). *Grief, Dying and Death.* Champaign, Il.:Research Press Co.

Endnote

1 Hospice care in the U.S. is reimbursable by one of two mechanisms, either through Medicare's Home Health guidelines or through Hospice Medicare certification. Prior to passage of Hospice Medicare certification in 1983, the majority of programs operated under Home Health guidelines, and many still do. At the time of this case, the program was functioning in this manner. Since many hospice patients do not fit increasingly stringent Home Health criteria, reimbursement problems such as these described do occur. Initially a controversial piece of legislation, the Hospice Medicare benefit is now becoming more readily accepted, and increasing numbers of programs are electing to participate in it. Such reimbursement problems would not have occurred under the Hospice Medicare benefit.

Chapter 23

SOCIAL WORK PRACTICE
IN PALLIATIVE CARE

Margaret R. Rodway, PhD
Judith Blythe, MSW

Abstract

Palliative care is a unique and growing part of the Canadian health care delivery system. In a 1988 survey conducted by the authors it was identified that half the palliative care facilities in Canada do not employ social workers. However, in identifying the patient's problems and service goals of palliative care the authors clearly describe the natural roles that are classically associated with social work and that are critical to providing supportive and caring counselling to this particular patient population. Characteristics important for social workers in palliative care, together with issues concerning working with relatives in bereavement and the problems that arise in working on a multi-disciplined team, are reported on and analysed in terms of the present and future functioning of social workers in palliative care units.

SOCIAL WORK PRACTICE IN PALLIATIVE CARE

"Terminally ill patients are living persons in the process of dying who may require palliative care to sustain both their physical and emotional integrity" (Allison, Gripton & Rodway, 1983, p. 29). In Canada, "palliative" is the commonly used term for hospice care and it reflects the hospital bias of terminal care in this country. Palliative care implies alleviation of distressing or painful symptoms associated with patients' physical deterioration and infirmity and combines empathic care with professional understanding directed towards the physical, emotional and spiritual needs of both patient and family (Saunders, 1978; Simpson, 1979).

There is considerable debate regarding whether palliative care is a discipline or speciality and both affirmative and negative arguments have been put forward. While recognition of it as a discipline would be "the quickest route to acceptance of palliative care as a unique and respected component of the health care delivery system" (Scott, 1988, p. 11), perhaps it can never be confined within such boundaries because it is as broad and diffuse as the individual needs of each patient. Presently, the literature supports the idea that palliative care is best delivered by a number of health care providers representing several professions. While there are many advantages to a team approach to palliative care, the lack of a clearly delineated model of palliative care may well be the result of its interdisciplinary nature (Brockopp, 1987).

While care of the sick and dying in shelters has been documented since the fourth century, the contemporary hospice movement began with St. Christopher's House in Britain and was partially built on a voluntary tradition. While hospice care in Britain and the United States has been in the direction of autonomous free-standing hospices, Canadian pioneers have committed it to the university teaching hospital (Scott, 1981). In 1975, a palliative care service was opened at the Royal Victoria Hospital in Montreal, Quebec. It was the first comprehensive hospital-based hospice service in the world (Manning, 1984).

In Canada, there are now a wide variety of programs referred to as hospice or palliative care services. These are based primarily in existing hospitals. However, palliative care concepts may be operationalized through free-standing hospices as previously mentioned, designated beds in hospital patient care areas, palliative care units in chronic-care or long-term facilities, roving pallia-tive-care teams or finally community-based programs. Ley (1985), commenting on palliative care in Canada observes that while its initial and major thrust has been institutional, community pro-grams are being developed in response to perceived community need. The majority of new programs have a community oriented component. She suggests that in the future, institutional programs will remain cancer related while programs caring for other patients will be more community oriented. Ley also observes that although palliative-care programs have increased greatly in the past decade, they only serve a small fraction of the people who die. For example, only 10% of patients dying with cancer are in palliative-care programs.

In a survey of Canadian hospitals in 1983 (Palliative Care Foundation), it was determined that there were sixty-two hospice programs in existence. It should be noted, however, that the sur-vey did not include community-based programs.

In a 1988 Canadian survey conducted by the authors, letters were sent to 347 palliative-care programs listed in the 1987 Palliative Care Directory. A 35.3% response rate was received. It should be noted that the responses were descriptive in nature and the findings should be interpreted with caution. Only the facilities that employed social workers in palliative care were considered. However, it is interesting to consider that fully half the functioning palliative-care programs had no social workers attached to them. This is similar to Alperin's (1985) survey finding, which indicated that in a study of 463 hospices in the United States, only 48% included social workers in their programs. While many of these programs admire the value of social work involvement, they choose either not to fund this involvement or offer no comment as to why they are not used. This is particularly significant when one considers that one of the basic tenets of palliative care is the psy-chosocial care of the patient.

THE CLIENTELE

Patients in these settings ranged in age from infants to 100 years of age. The majority of patients, however, tended to be more elderly, averaging about 60 years of age. In those settings in which AIDS patients were served, the average age tended to be around 35 years.

The majority of palliative-care clients have cancer. However, many respondents reported that they also have small numbers of patients with cardiac, respiratory, neurological, trauma, post surgical and chronic pain problems. Palliative care patients are represented in all ethnic, racial and marital status groups. They are male or female, from either rural or urban settings and from a wide variety of educational, employment and socioeconomic backgrounds.

I. Settings

Responses were received from a variety of health care settings. Palliative-care social workers practised in acute-care hospitals with and without specialized units. They were employed by long-term, chronic- or convalescent-care facilities including pediatric-care settings.

Some of the facilities had a home-care component while other settings were exclusively home care. Some respondents were involved with volunteer agencies, that is to say they co-ordinated a group of volunteers who performed direct service to patients. Other agencies offered no direct service to patients but served as a co-ordinating body for other community services.

II. Presenting Problems

Most of the settings reported that the primary presenting problems for palliative patients were pain and symptom-control problems. Beyond that, however, the presenting problems were by and large psychosocial, systems related or instrumental. These could apply equally to both patients and family members.

More specifically, psychosocial problems were identified as those involving depression, denial, anger, fear, anxiety, sadness, blame and issues of loss. System problems included the lack of co-ordination of the treatment approach, dissatisfaction with care, lack of social support, placement issues and the need for education or information. Practical or instrumental concerns involved aspects such as finances, arrangements for wills and funerals and nursing care.

All these problems affect the quality of life of the dying patient. Social work that is based on a philosophy of caring and concern for others and on a person-in-environment perspective can serve as a vital dimension in meeting many of these patient needs.

PRACTICE ROLES AND RESPONSIBILITIES

"The provision of palliative care to the terminally ill is a natural extension of social work, which has traditionally provided supportive services in times of crisis" (Allison, Gripton & Rodway, 1983, p. 31). There are a number of essential goals for social workers in palliative care. The overriding focus is on involvement and sharing with patients so that their lives can be affirmed and they can live more fully until death occurs (Allen, 1980). Weisman (1972) identifies "safe conduct" as an essential goal. This refers to the pledge given to those patients who are ultimately obliged to surrender their autonomy and yield control to someone else.

The unique roles and functions of palliative social work have been addressed by a number of authors (Alperin, 1985; Bolling, 1980; Stark & Johnson, 1983; Rusnack, Shaefer & Moxely, 1988). The following social work roles have been identified as essential to work with patients, their families and staff and service networks: advocate, counsellor, educator, enabler, facilitator, innovator, mediator, maintainer, organizer, participant and sustainer. Advocacy is highlighted for work with patients, particularly when they are unable to act on their own behalf and when their needs must be interpreted to family members and staff members.

Social workers in the various settings surveyed by the authors reflected a broad spectrum of tasks, functions and duties similar in scope to those identified in Alperin's study (1985). This range also reflected Dush's (1988) two general types of functions: those directed toward general support and those with a specific objective.

Based on the presenting problems of the clientele, social workers reported that pain and symptom management was the most important first step in treating palliative patients. The contributions of Saunders (1978) and others in the management of severe pain have made it possible to address the psychosocial aspects of palliative care. Very few respondents addressed the role that social workers could play in providing adjunct therapies for pain and symptom management. Relaxation, hypnosis and meditation

424

are but a few of the many interventions that can assist patients to gain some control over their situation and to participate in their own pain management.

The provision of psychosocial counselling to patients during the dying process and families through the grief process was ranked second in terms of importance. Vachon (1988) in a study of hospice patients and families found that one-quarter to one-half of them wanted or needed help in dealing with their situation. Many, however, such as the aged or poor, would not ask for the needed help. Vachon (1988) asserted that counselling should be immediate, action oriented and have limited goals.

Assessment is the first phase in palliative counselling. Dush (1988) asserts that assessment should take a broad view of the patient and family and should include: screening for psychopathology, risk assessment, identification of specific symptoms or concerns that would benefit from intervention, indications for preventive interventions and identification of coping skills and resources. Treatment plans can then be developed from the assessment that can help the patient sustain present coping abilities or develop new strategies to cope with stress. The treatment plan often should include developing problem-solving techniques, establishing a clear communication network with the family and health professionals and increasing staff awareness of psychosocial needs of the individual (Sakadakis, Bonar & MacLean, 1987). Generally, intervention is seen as being supportive and client- and family-centred with the focus on coping with the present situation. The resolution of specific problems and the provision of appropriate resources are also primary aspects of intervention. Some of the particular interventions that have been described for palliative care include

a) facilitating the expression of strong feelings, such as anger and depression (Manning, 1984; Pilsecker (1979);
b) validating the patients' strengths;
c) promoting the patients' optional coping and well being (Dush, 1988) and
d) encouraging the patients to focus on presenting problems and helping them formulate specific plans of action (Sakadakis, Bonar & MacLean, 1987).

The importance of the therapeutic relationship cannot be over-emphasized. Qualities of acceptance, concern and understanding recognition of abilities and availability are essential to this relationship.

While psychosocial counselling is one of the primary services provided in most palliative care services, respondents in the authors' study indicated, however, that the value of psychosocial intervention was not fully understood or appreciated.

Similarly, much was said about the need for bereavement service to survivors. However, rarely was it stated that grief counselling was provided on a consistent, well-organized basis. Rather, it seemed as if it was provided only in the most critical cases.

In terms of other practice functions and responsibilities, some respondents stressed that one of the most important functions for social workers was the co-ordination of available services. Patients facing death can be overwhelmed by the health care system. Health care personnel tend to deal only with their own areas of expertise. Each patient could use someone to lead him or her through the difficult maze of the health care system. Social workers could fulfill that function very well indeed. Their advocacy role could facilitate the successful negotiation of some of the hazards.

Referral services to other institution or community services, discharge planning and practical or instrumental support were provided. Resource information and a wide range of educational programs were organized and presented by social workers.

Teamwork was often mentioned in the authors' study as an important part of the social worker's duties. They not only worked as part of a team but provided co-ordination of the team, staff support and education, orientation of new team members and liaison between the team and allied health services or patients and families. The importance of this function has been stressed by Stark & Johnson (1983) and Lusk (1983).

Administration is part of the responsibilities of few social workers in palliative care. Those who indicated that they had administrative duties referred to consulting on policy and procedures, planning and program development, committee work within and outside their facilities and, for some, accounting for monies.

Some workers supervised social work students in practicum placements. A few were involved in research projects. One person described the worker's role as "an observer of ethical attitudes"—an important area in palliative care.

Most social workers were involved to a greater or lesser extent in education. Some provided education to the staff members in the facility. Others had a major focus on education, providing short presentations and extensive workshops in their settings and in the community to a broad range of audiences.

Finally, an important function of some social workers was patient room decoration. Palliative care settings should be as home-like as possible. The sensitivity and caring of this profession can be a valuable asset when deciding how best to make the patients and families feel comfortable and at home.

POTENTIAL FOR ROLE DEVELOPMENT

Silverstone (1984) has noted that social work's involvement in palliative care has been a significant step forward for the profession with a number of social workers taking leadership positions in a new movement to help the dying. He also observed that social workers more generally have not "flocked eagerly into practice with either the dying or the elderly. In fact, they have tended to demonstrate an aversion to these client groups although often confronted with the dying in their practice" (page 3).

It appears then that there is great potential for the services of social work professionals to those in palliative care. While, as a profession, it has more generally focussed its efforts on those client groups who are seen as more amenable to change, the deep sense of satisfaction and meaning experienced by those social workers working in palliative care attests to the challenging opportunity available for more of the profession.

What are the some of the essential characteristics of social workers who experience such job satisfaction in their work with the dying? They need to be sensitive, flexible, knowledgeable of others and themselves in terms of needs and feelings, able to skillfully apply professional methods and techniques and have the capacity to individualize their work (Bolling, 1980). They must be able to collaborate with other professionals and facilitate team efforts (Stark & Johnson, 1983). Finally they must have the ability to openly communicate and appropriately share information about the patient among patient, family and staff (Parry, 1987).

A team approach to palliative care has a tendency to blur distinctions between the types of care offered by different health professionals. Davis (1983) in a study of hospices in Illinois found

427

that both social workers and nurses claimed as their area of expertise the meeting of psychosocial needs of patients and families. Because social work has a long term involvement and training in psychosocial aspects of care, this is a crucial area in palliative care that should be identified and most appropriately met by our profession. Hence, this is an area with a potential for considerable development.

Another area where social work role development could occur is that of providing health care professionals and volunteers with emotional support. Because professionals' involvement in palliative care involves the use of self in their relationships with patients, professionals are sometimes subjected to inordinate stresses. These would include repeatedly experienced feelings of sadness, loss and helplessness. Social workers are by virtue of their professional training and experience specifically qualified to offer the necessary support and assistance to help combat the stresses.

While the results of the authors' survey suggested that the majority of social workers in palliative care are not visionaries, they do see a need for increasing their services in palliative care. Most settings could use more staff for assessment and counselling. Many social workers would like the time to do individual and group bereavement follow-up. Earlier involvement, increased opportunity to provide education, networking and more time for staff support have all been identified as areas that required further development. Some social workers stated that they would like to develop management responsibilities and skills. One worker indicated that preventive work with healthy families was a goal worth pursuing and one respondent saw social workers as team leaders due to their abilities in communication and group process.

CONCLUDING REMARKS

Social work practice in palliative care has been described through an examination of the clientele served, the roles, functions and interventions of the social worker and the potential for role development. While a broad range of interventive functions and activities have been detailed, these are based primarily on practice, wisdom and experience. Increased research is seen as essential in helping to define which of the specific interventions involved in palliative care are most helpful for which patients under which circumstances. Models of assessing risk need to be developed and tested, as do interventions to meet specific needs of patients and their families.

Teamwork between other health care professionals and volunteers and among the patient, the family and the community is viewed as essential. The potential for conflict and lessened collaboration between team members always exists in such interdisciplinary functioning, particularly when there is a blurring between professional knowledge and roles. "Each member of the health care team has his or her own special knowledge base, value system and methods of communication. A lack of firm control or understanding of professional function adds to ambiguity and role strain" (Mallick, 1979, p. 127).

Palliative care may be seen as a philosophical approach to health care wherein its basic concepts were developed as a response to inadequacies of the health care system. The philosophy of social work practice thrusts many social workers directly into involvement with dying patients and their families. The profession can make a tremendous contribution to an area of practice often characterized by medical technology, cash containment and non-humanistic values.

The "essential" nature of social work practice has been identified as the dual emphasis on the individual and his environment (Rodway, 1986). This dual perspective could shed more light on the process of palliative care: its social and cultural dimensions, adaptations required by others and the interaction of patients, families, professionals and the larger systems within which they function.

CASE EXAMPLE

Prior to discussing an actual case example we would like to present some information on the organizational setting for palliative care and a model for practice.

I. A Model for Practice:

As is the case in many settings in Canada, palliative care in Alberta relies on discretionary funding to provide a variety of services to dying patients. Palliative-care services in Bethany Care

Centre were established in 1984 through a grant from a private foundation. These grant monies were distributed on a short-term basis to a number of health care facilities in the city. When those funds were depleted, all but one institution chose to maintain the service using discretionary funds. The grant provided funding for a part-time or full-time (depending on the population of the institution) palliative care co-ordinator. Initially, all the co-ordinators were nurses. In 1986, when the Bethany Care Centre committed itself to providing funding to maintain the position, those involved made a conscious decision to give the program a decidedly psychosocial concentration along with the necessary medical focus. They chose to hire a social worker with an MSW for the position. She then became the only co-ordinator within Calgary who was not a nurse. As a result, the program in this centre functioned quite differently from the other institutions.

Pain and symptom control are not the primary concern of social workers. It would have been presumptuous for the co-ordinator to have became involved in that area. That left her with the psychosocial concerns, which were her area of expertise and thus were her focus in working with the dying elderly, and with the co-ordination of a variety of disciplines who had expertise in the medical areas.

Being a 544 bed long term care facility, it was clear that the one person in Bethany assigned specifically to palliative care could not effectively deal directly with patients, particularly considering the fact that over 100 patients a year die within the facility. Decisions had to be made. Choices needed to be taken. Quickly, the co-ordinator made the decision to concentrate on: a) developing a strong Palliative Care Committee that was responsible for policy and planning for the program; b) concentrating on administration with a view to developing a proposal for a palliative care unit and c) recruiting and nurturing a solid core of mature volunteers who would provide support and caring to help ease the loneliness many of the dying patients experienced. Some members of the Palliative Care Committee are part of a treatment team that is formed (under the leadership of the co-ordinator) whenever specific problems warrant attention.

The training social workers receive in communication, in ethics, in allowing self-determination in others and in providing support prepare them well for leadership tasks. At this point in the program, the Palliative Care Committee is functioning extremely well. It is a strong, cohesive body that has developed a solid base of philosophy, goals, objectives and roles of team members, all of which is contained in a program policy manual. A proposal has been sent to the provincial government requesting funding for a palliative care unit in the facility. There is an excellent core of volunteers who are readily available and are widely respected in the institution. They too form a strong, cohesive group who, although the numbers keep building, admit new members while still maintaining group strength.

The program at this point has its own unique strength. Much of the literature points out that the primary need is for pain and symptom control. Consequently, it tends to be medical staff that develop programs. There is often a tendency for a medical model to trivialize the psychosocial component of palliative care. At the Bethany Care Centre it was decided to lend this aspect of care the consideration it deserves. The committee has designated the Palliative Care Co-ordinator's role to remain as an MSW position. This has interesting ramifications for responsibilities of administrative staff on the unit being proposed (see Appendix A).

The committee is in the process of developing a structural model in which the MSW Co-ordinator's position remains strong in order to preserve the psychosocial functioning of the unit. This would see the Palliative Care Co-ordinator and the Nursing Unit Supervisor as sharing many responsibilities while maintaining their own areas of expertise.

It is an exciting model in that it focusses more on the psychosocial needs of the patients than most programs do. Often the medical personnel (and particularly nurses) comment that they have too little time to spend talking with patients and providing psychosocial, as opposed to strictly medical, care. The intention of this model with its emphasis on that aspect of caring for patients is to stress that need and provide enough volunteer support so that all staff will have more time to devote to caring holistically for patients.

II. THE CASE:

Peggy (not her name) is a 78-year-old resident of the Bethany Care Centre who was diagnosed approximately 35 years ago with rheumatoid arthritis. She also suffers from hypertension and a diverticular disease. Her primary medical problem, however, is the arthritis, which causes constant pain along with severe eye problems (corneal degeneration due to rheumatoid disease). She has lived in Bethany since 1983.

Peggy was born in London, England, the daughter of a physician. She attributes much of her independence and success in life to her father who was extremely supportive of her. As well, she attended a number of boarding schools during the First World War, which she believes taught her survival skills for life. She came to Canada where she completed normal school in 1932. During her career, she has tutored Chinese immigrants, supervised a dorm in a community college and taught at a Hebrew school. She married in 1933 and had five children, all of whom provide good support to her.

A review of her charts indicated that she was an intelligent, highly motivated, alert woman who, despite her disability, possessed a positive attitude toward life. She had been described as independent, pleasant, a good problem solver and a woman with the capacity for turning adversity to advantage. She was the Chairman of the Residents' Council in the Bethany Care Centre and participated in programs within and outside the facility. Her method of transportation was an electric wheelchair, which she handled skillfully.

In April of 1988, Peggy developed a very painful, swollen right elbow. She was transferred by ambulance to an acute-care hospital where she was given intravenous antibiotics and a significant increase in her cortisone therapy. After eighteen days, she returned to Bethany, but to a different location and a higher level of care (auxiliary hospital as opposed to nursing home).

Peggy was first seen by the Palliative Care Co-ordinator (PCC) in August of 1988 following that admission. She complained of frightening nightmares and hallucinations about her hospital stay. Peggy was convinced that she had been locked away in a basement. She also harboured bad memories of a doctor who had cared for her. Initially, in order to help her by reality testing, it was decided that she would return to the acute care setting accompanied by the PCC. However, after several sessions, Peggy decided she was resolving some of her delusions and did not need to return to that setting. Her family physician was beginning to reduce her level of steroids.

In September, Peggy began to have serious difficulty with her eyes. At this point in time, she was still very alert, cheerful and independent, although, due to her hallucinations and her reduced vision, she was now using a manual wheelchair, which limited her movement within the building. She was again admitted to a different acute-care hospital where she received eye surgery under a general anaesthetic. After thirty-one days, she was returned to auxiliary care. She had deteriorated considerably and it was believed that she indeed might not recover.

The pain in Peggy's eyes was acute and her vision was extremely poor. She was suffering as usual from her arthritic pain and from the after-effects of the general anaesthetic. Her steroids were still at a fairly high level. All this contributed to a considerably reduced quality of life, which left Peggy feeling extremely depressed and helpless. She approached both her family physician and the PCC with a request that they help her to end her life.

At this point, the PCC began to see Peggy on an almost daily basis. As well, she co-ordinated a team meeting at which the physician, nurse, pharmacist and rehabilitation therapist were represented. Peggy's request to end her life was considered very seriously. All members felt that in all conscience, they could not support that. It was left then to see how they could contribute to improving the quality of her life.

The following interventions occurred:
1. Peggy continued to be seen frequently by the PCC for therapy.
2. The family physician reduced her steroids to the point where she received none at all. Her pain was controlled with Tylenol administered on a regular basis.
3. The PCC accompanied her to the opthalmologist who prescribed medications that caused significant improvement to her eyes.
4. Rehabilitation services were increased. Peggy was seen by physiotherapy, occupational therapy and/or recreation therapy on an almost twice daily basis.
5. Peggy's room location was changed to a much lighter room and with an alert roomate with whom she had much in common.
6. The PCC requested that staff validate Peggy's successes and assume that she was going to improve to her normal condition.
7. The palliative care volunteers were recruited to provide added social and emotional support.

By March of 1989, this combination of interventions had clearly produced positive results. Peggy was no longer suicidal. She was feeling infinitely better, both physically and emotionally. Her humour had returned and she was able to look back objectively at this experience and reframe it to her current advantage.

The importance of this case study lies in the significant contribution of the PCC. While there were some pain, symptom and medication problems, they were handled quickly and efficiently by the physician and nursing staff. What remained were psycho-social problems that required time and the therapeutic and co-ordination skills that are best met by social workers. The current medical and nursing curricula are providing today, more than ever before, more psycho-social awareness. This training still cannot provide the depth of understanding of human behaviours and needs required in palliative care. Professional social work training, however, results in clinicians who have the necessary knowledge and skills. In short, social work in palliative care is important and vital. It should not be allowed to be trivialized.

APPENDIX A

PALLIATIVE CARE CO-ORDINATOR RESPONSIBILITY

Program Administration

- Palliative Care Committee organization
- policy and procedures
* - evaluation of services
* - budgets
* - evaluation of cost-effectiveness
* - hiring and termination of psycho-social staff (in conjunction with appropriate Department Heads)
- fund raising
- public speaking
- organizing special case conferences

Support and Education

- group building/term building
* - staff support - individual and groups
- staff education
- consultant to disciplines indicated on organizational chart
- research
- attendance at conferences, other programs
- supervision of MSW student

Networking

- public relations re program
- collaboration with departments indicated on chart
* - networking with other Calgary palliative-care programs
- networking with U. of C. students
- consultant to prospective providers of service (e.g., adjunct therapies)

Direct Patient Care

- advocacy for patients and families
- counselling with problem families
- clinical work as required
- consultant to Volunteer Co-ordinator on unit
- community visiting where appropriate

Note: * In collaboration with the Nursing Unit Supervision

References

Allen, C. (1980). *Royal Victoria Hospital Manual on Palliative Care.* p. 233.

Allison, H., Gripton J. & Rodway, M. (1983). Social work services as a component of palliative care with terminal cancer patients. *Social Work in Health Care,* 8(4), 29-44.

Alperin, D.E. (1985). Hospice social work: Support for generalist training. *Social Work in Health Care,* 10(3), 119-123.

Blythe, J. & Rodway, M. (1988). A survey of palliative care programs in Canada. Unpublished manuscript.

Bolling, G.V. (1980). The social work role in caring for the dying patient and family. In B.A. Orcutt, E.R. Prichard, J. Collard, E.F. Cooper, A.H. Kutscher & J.B. Seeland, (Eds.), *Social Work & Thanatology.* New York: Arno Press.

Brockopp, D. (1987). Essential concepts in the education of health professionals. *Journal of Palliative Care,* 2(2) 18-23.

Davis, M.A. (1983). Social services in hospices. Unpublished doctoral dissertation: University of Illinois at Chicago.

Dush, D.M. (1988). Psychological research in hospice care: Toward specificity of therapeutic mechanisms. *The Hospice Journal,* 4(2), 9-36.

Ley, D.L. (1985). Palliative care in Canada: The first decade and beyond. *Journal of Palliative Care,* 1, 32-35.

Lusk, M.W. (1983). The psychosocial evolution of the hospice patient. *Health and Social Work,* 8(3), 210-218.

Mallick, M. (1979). The impact of severe illness on the individual and family: An overview. *Social Work in Health Care,* 5(2), 117-129.

Manning, M. (1984). *The Hospice Alternative: Living with Dying.* London: Souvenir Press.

Palliative Care Foundation (1983). *The Canadian Palliative Care Directory.* Toronto: The Palliative Care Foundation.

Palliative Care Foundation (1987). *The Canadian Palliative Care Directory.* Toronto: The Palliative Care Foundation.

Parry, J. K. (1987). The significance of open communication in working with terminally ill clients. *The Hospice Journal,* 3(4) 33-49.

Pilsecker, C. (1979). Terminal cancer: A challenge for social work. *Social Work in Health Care,* 4, 371-375.

Rodway, M. R. (1986). Systems theory. In F. Turner, (Ed.), *Social Work Treatment Interlocking Theoretical Approaches.* New York: The Fress Press.

Rusnack, B., Schaefer, S.M. & Moxley, D. (1988). Safe passage: Social work roles and functions in hospice care. *Social Work in Health Care*, 13(3), 3-19.

Sakadakis, V., Bonar, R. & MacLean, M. (1987). The role of the social worker in terminal care with institutionalized elderly people. *Journal of Palliative Care*, 3(2), 19-250.

Saunders, C. M. (1978). *The Management of Terminal Illness*. London: Arnald.

Scott, D. H. (1988). Is palliative care a discipline? *Journal of Palliative Care*, 4(1 & 2), 10-12.

Silverstone, B. (1984). Social work practice with the dying: Where are we and where are we going? In L.H. Susycki, M. Abrainson, E. Prichard, A.H. Kutscher & D. Fisher (Eds.), *Social Work in Terminal Care*. New York: Prager Press.

Simpson, M. A. (1979). *The Facts of Death*. Englewood Cliffs, New Jersey: Prentice Hall.

Stark, D. E. & Johnson, E. M. (1983). Implications of hospice concepts for social work practice with oncology patients and their families in an acute care teaching hospital. *Social Work in Health Care*, 9(1), 63-70.

Vachon, M. L. S. (1988). Counselling and psychotherapy in palliative/ hospice care: A review. *Palliative Medicine*, 2(1), 36-50.

Weisman, A. D. (1972). Psychosocial considerations in terminal care. In B. Schoenberg, A.C. Carr, D. Peretz & A.H. Kutscher (Eds.), *Psychosocial Aspects of Terminal Care*. New York: Columbia University Press.

Chapter 24

SOCIAL WORK PRACTICE WITH ORGAN TRANSPLANT PATIENTS

M. Jane Bright, MSW

Abstract

Organ transplant, as discussed in this chapter, pertains to a major organ without which the patient will die, specifically lung, liver and heart. Characteristics of and issues for patients and their families anticipating transplant are discussed. In addition, the role of a social worker, as a member of a transplant team throughout the process, including assessment for transplant and maintenance of the patient and family pre, peri and post transplant, is discussed with particular attention to individual and group interventions. Some ethical and staff issues are addressed, concluded by a typical case example.

SOCIAL WORK PRACTICE WITH ORGAN TRANSPLANT PATIENTS*

THE CLIENTELE

I. Settings and Conditions

A transplant patient is normally admitted to hospital for a one to two week assessment to determine if s/he is a suitable candidate for transplant. In addition to various medical tests, a psychosocial assessment should be conducted with the patient and her/his family. If the patient is well enough, all the interviewing should be conducted in the social worker's office allowing for total concentration and confidentiality. Otherwise, the patient interview will have to occur at the bedside with the possibility of distractions from others. Ideally, it is helpful to see the patient and family together and then see each separately. When together, the relationship may be more accurately assessed whereas, separately, each may feel freer to divulge information and feelings that s/he is not able, for one reason or another, to share with the other being present.

Once a patient is accepted into the transplant program, s/he is required, if not already residing in the vicinity of the hospital, to move within "beeper" range of the hospital. During the waiting period for the transplant, s/he will attend outpatient appointments, clinics and, possibly, physiotherapy. It is very helpful if a regular support group can be offered, preferably facilitated by a social worker, maybe in conjunction with another team member. Not infrequently, the patient requires hospitalization during her/his wait, with regard to complications related to illness.

After transplant, the patient is transferred to the Intensive Care Unit until stabilized enough to return to the ward. Social work contact is usually with the family in the waiting area or office during the ICU stay. If the patient is awake and aware enough, a few words of encouragement from the social worker or a positive acknowledgement from the doorway will usually suf-

---

*Organ in this chapter means a major organ without which a patient will die, specifically lung, liver or heart.

fice. It is stressful enough for the patient to cope with the tubes, intravenous lines, medical and nursing staff and their families, etc. and more important to offer support to the family so that they can then cope better with stress they feel while visiting the patient. Once the patient is out of the ICU, interviewing is usually in the patient's room, hallway, lounge or office.

After discharge, the patient usually remains in the vicinity of the hospital for three months, followed frequently and regularly by the team, after which s/he returns home, coming back to the hospital at specified intervals determined partly by the medical condition and partly by distance. The social worker remains in contact as needed by the patient and his family throughout this phase.

II. Descriptive Features of Clients

The patient requiring transplant is experiencing a terminal illness for which medical intervention is no longer beneficial. Thus, s/he is faced directly with mortality and with the possibility of impending death. When transplant is presented, s/he sees a faint light at the end of the tunnel. It may carry great risk but it is the only option other than death. When s/he arrives for assessment, the patient is usually very anxious, fearing that s/he may not be accepted into the program. Once in the program, there is no guarantee that a compatible donor will be found before the patient becomes too ill or dies. Thus, s/he oscillates between hope and fear of death. Although the risks of transplant may be considerable, the patient often hears little of what the doctor says as it is the only chance for life and s/he desperately wants it at any cost.

The upper age limit of patients depends on the organ being transplanted and the criteria of the particular transplant program. Further, patients may live within the range of the hospital or may need to relocate from elsewhere. Most have been unable to work and finances may be tight if the patient has been a major financial contributor to the family. Occasionally, a patient is receiving social assistance. As well, some are able to manage the living costs; others may have family and friends who have raised funds for them or may be sponsored by a service organization.

Patients are usually required to have a support person with them, which can be a problem for those from far away. As well, they may have young children or a spouse who is the wage earner or they may be single or divorced. In these cases, a friend, another family member or a team of persons may provide their support.

Waiting for transplant may be long and stressful (Levinson & Olbrisch, 1987). Lung transplant patients, for example, may wait a year or longer for transplant. All the while, the patient's condition continues to deteriorate, often requiring periodic hospitalization. It is very important for the patient to believe that s/he will survive long enough for a transplant. Patients are much more able to accept death after transplant as they feel that they at least had their opportunity, even if it was unsuccessful.

The patients awaiting transplant become a close group; out-of-town people look to each other as their "family away from home." They are with others who are experiencing similar illnesses, feelings and challenges. This creates a very meaningful experience for them. They gain important mutual support from each other, but also keenly feel each others "highs" and "lows." If a patient dies, they feel for the family and fear for themselves. At times, they may be reluctant again to get close to anyone in case they lose another friend.

The patient is often concerned about his status on the "list" of patients awaiting transplant although, in fact, few are in competition for organs as they vary in size, blood type, etc. When a patient is transplanted, the others are very pleased for them but naturally wish it could have been them. Not infrequently, a patient may be brought into hospital for transplant only to have to return home as the donor deteriorated. This seems to result in a mixture of feelings for the patient specifically, disappointment over a lost opportunity, but encouragement that there was a donor and the physicians selected her/him.

Often, immediately prior to the transplant, the patient's feelings about the donor rise to the surface. For example, he is happy for himself, but very sad for the donor and his family, sometimes feeling guilty that someone has to die in order for him to live. Almost invariably, once well, the transplant recipient writes a letter of condolence and thanks to the donor family. As the law requires that no information may be given to the recipient that could identify the donor, this letter is transmitted through the organ procurement program and forwarded to the donor family.

443

PRACTICE ROLES AND RESPONSIBILITIES

I. Team Members

The social worker is a member of the transplant team that may include medical and surgical physicians, a program co-ordinator, a clinical nursing teacher, nurses, physiotherapists and a nutritionist. A psychiatrist and psychologist may also be members of or consultants to this team. It is very important that the team establish clear lines of communication so that each is cognizant of a patient's status, thus ensuring a high quality of service to the patient and his family. In addition to informal communication, there should also be regular and frequent team meetings. The social worker should share appropriate information about each patient's social or emotional status and glean information from other team members that may impact on the patient's coping ability.

II. Psychosocial Assessment

The social worker conducts a psychosocial assessment with each candidate as part of the team's overall assessment of eligibility for transplant. The patient should be viewed in the context of his illness and feelings about transplant, his family, his community, etc. The goal of a social work assessment is to evaluate the persons emotional status and support system with a view to predicting his ability to cope with the transplant program and its subsequent lifetime regimentation (Christopherson, 1987). Also, it is important for the social worker to identify any areas with which s/he may require assistance throughout the process. For example, one young patient, accompanied by her husband, was being assessed for liver transplant. She was from an Indian reserve three hundred miles away. They were homesick and unhappy with the arrangements they had made for the care of their children, placing added strain on their usually strong relationship. It was clear to the social worker that these areas would need to be addressed in order for the couple to be able to sustain the process of transplant.

The patient must not only wait for, undergo and recuperate from the transplant, but also be prepared for compliance with medical expectations, adopting a lifestyle conducive to continuing health, taking and adjusting medications to prevent rejection, and participating in medical follow-up at regular intervals (Mai, McKenzie & Kostuk, 1986).

A general outline of the areas covered in the assessment is as follows:

(i) **History of Illness** — the progress of the patient's illness from its initial stages and diagnosis to the present, level of functioning, feelings about illness.

(ii) **Transplant** — how the patient heard about the program, the process of coming to assessment, feelings about transplant — with both patient and family.

(iii) **Family, friends, community** — identifying the immediate and extended family, individual roles, how the illness affected the family, who the patient sees as a major support person (s).

(iv) **Education and work history** — level of education, job(s) held, duration and stability, does s/he plan to return to her/his last job, will he require a career change. (The expectation of the team is that the person return to being a contributing member of society.)

(v) **Financial situation** — assess the patient's financial status — independent, disability pension, social assistance, etc., plans for relocation if necessary, medical insurance if from out of country.

(vi) **Substance abuse** — assess the history of smoking, alcohol or drug abuse, or of eating disorder, e.g., does patient still have this problem, has he sought help, if so, when?

(vii) **Coping Mechanisms** — assess how the patient coped with previous hospitalization, stressful situation, what defences does patient use, are they adaptive, maladaptive, etc.

III. Pre-Transplant Phase

Once the patient is accepted into the transplant program, the social worker may need to provide some concrete assistance regarding housing, transportation for hospital appointments or co-ordinating social assistance from other cities, provinces or countries. It is important that the social worker, alone or in collaboration with the psychiatrist and/or psychologist, be available for emotional support to the patient and the family as s/he waits for transplant. This may be accomplished through individual, couple or family interviews. It is also important for the social worker to maintain contact informally with patients and offer support to people when they come in for hospital appointments in order to assess how they are coping and offer assistance if necessary.

The social worker often, alone or with a team member, facilitates a support group for patients and their support people. Such a group should be held regularly and frequently. It is unique, as it is mainly for the patient awaiting transplant and his support person, but can also be open for recently transplanted patients, those returning for follow-up and other friends and family who visit on occasion. The agenda should, for the most part, be decided by the group. They may wish to discuss current progress informally, or request that a team member provide information on the program, etc. Facilitating a transplant group is challenging, as the members are in such a tenuous situation that they are very sensitive to staff sounding negative or unrealistically positive; they keenly feel the imposing potential of death, but find it hard to talk about. Also, transplant patients are given considerably more attention than other surgical patients. That, together with the closeness they feel as a group, sometimes leads to their feeling that they should be privy to information, usually confidential, about other patients. It is important that the social worker be especially aware of these issues and handle them carefully and sensitively, respecting their need for reassurance, but also protecting the confidentiality of the patient and family.

IV. Peri and Post Transplant Phase

When the patient is admitted and waiting to go for the scheduled transplant, the social worker should try to spend time with the patient and the family. This is a busy time as many staff are involved in preparing the patient for surgery, specifically, the nurse, anaesthetist, surgeon and x-ray technician. It is also important that the patient have some time alone with his loved ones to allow themselves to say things they want to say before transplant. However, also at this time, the patient usually expresses feelings not only of pleasure for the opportunity of transplant and fear of the risks, but also appreciation of sadness for the donor's family. There is often some guilt expressed by the patient that his life has to be born out of another's tragedy. The patient is also usually grateful for the opportunity to express this to the social worker. The patient seems to need to confirm that s/he has had no part in the donor's death. Once the patient has gone to the operating room, the family may wish to ventilate some of their feelings as they begin their long wait. For instance, transplant may take from 5 to 12 hours, depending on the organ being transplanted, barring any complications that would extend that time indefinitely.

After transplant, the patient will be in the Intensive Care Unit. This can be a very critical period as the patient may be very unstable medically. It is also a time when the social worker can offer the family emotional support, allowing them to ventilate their worries and fears. Occasionally, they may need help with any guilt they may feel if the patient is faring badly and they are concerned about their role in encouraging the patient to have a transplant. It is also important for the social worker to ensure that the attending physicians are communicating with the family and advocate on their behalf, if necessary. Most families find it much easier to cope with most situations if the physician is honest and straightforward with them. As the patient improves and progresses, the social worker should continue to remain in frequent contact with patient and family, taking into consideration their need for support and the availability of other support people to them.

Occasionally, the immunosuppressive drugs may cause irritability, paranoia and depression along with the other natural reactions after surgery. It will be important for the social worker to recommend a psychiatric consultation to the attending physician as medication may be needed and/or need to be altered.

It is not uncommon for the patient to survive several medical crises and, ultimately, die. It is vital for the social worker to be in close contact with the family throughout this time to help them with their pain and grieving. While they are always consoled by the fact that their patient received the transplant for which they so desperately wished, they may be very upset that the patient endured pain and suffering without a positive outcome. They also mourn the loss of a loved one who endured such hardships so bravely with the illness, their wait, often a long one, for transplant, etc.

V. Discharge

Once the patient is feeling better, s/he may start anticipating discharge with both excitement and fear. The family may be quite apprehensive about the patient being well enough for them to manage at home. It is common for both patient and family to fear separation from the doctors, nurses, etc. The social worker should be actively helping them with these natural feelings of ambivalence. Sometimes, it is helpful for the patient to go home for a few hours or overnight before discharge in order to help all concerned develop some confidence.

After discharge, it may be important for the family to see the social worker throughout the readjustment period at home when the patient comes in the hospital for appointments. The patient may require admission periodically through episodes of rejection or other complications which may be quite frightening. The social worker should follow the patients closely at these times.

POTENTIAL FOR ROLE DEVELOPMENT

As transplant programs grow and develop, it is important for social work to continue to be an integral part of the team. Physicians realize, very early into a program, the need for the patient to be able to cope with the emotional stresses if the transplant is to be successful. It is vital that the social worker and physician(s) establish working relationships based on mutual respect and trust, characterized by frequent and clear communication, especially *ad hoc*.

Unfortunately, there is a shortage of donors largely due, it is thought, to hospital staff not asking families if they would like the opportunity for something positive to come out of their tragedy. It is not an easy task to approach a grieving family about donating their loved one's organs. Also it requires more concentrated work for the physician and staff to maintain a donor until transplant. Many families have indicated that they would have wanted their loved one to be a donor but no one asked them and they did not think of it in their sorrow. There is a role for the intensive care social worker working with these families to help them consider organ donation. In one well-known transplant centre, the ICU social worker has developed this role extremely effectively. She initiates, where appropriate, the subject of donation with the family and is a key person in linking the physicians and staff with the family while remaining with them throughout the entire process. It is not appropriate for the transplant recipient social worker to act in this role as it is a conflict of interest.

CONCLUDING REMARKS

Transplantation is a relatively new option for patients with end stage disease. It is a very challenging and exciting area for social work, involving assessment, crisis intervention and counselling opportunities. The social worker can bring continuity and humanity into this area of high technology.

However, it is still a very controversial procedure as it is costly to the health care system and stressful for staff. Other specialties are not pleased when their surgeries are postponed or cancelled because of a transplant. Ethically, staff may be very opposed to time, energy, and money being spent on a patient who may have abused themselves through smoking, alcohol, etc., especially if s/he is not compliant and may not survive. Post transplant patients require a great deal of care and are very stressful for and demanding of time from nursing and other medical staff (Mishel & Murdaugh, 1987). The social worker who is constantly working with the feelings of the patient and families in crises, where death happens frequently, can become very stressed and needs to find ways of relieving it through mutual collaboration with other team members, ventilating to supervisors, etc.

However, it is truly amazing and gratifying for staff to see a patient be transformed from one who is so close to death to one who is able to regain much of their functioning and return to her/his family and community. It makes all the stress and heartache from the crises worthwhile.

CASE EXAMPLE

Mr. N is a 45-year-old man from western Canada who had been working as a salesperson in a small company owned by a friend. Three years ago, an inherent lung condition began to develop and progress quickly, with the result that he had frequent hospitalizations with pneumonia. Eventually he had to stop working. Finally, his physician indicated that his condition could no longer respond to current medical interventions, that he might have less than two years to live and suggested he consider lung transplantation. He was stunned and found it impossible to believe that this could really be happening to him and that his condition was that bad. Once he got over the initial shock and talked it over with his wife and family, he decided that, considering his only other option was death, he would come for assessment for transplant. By the time they arrived, he and his wife had, despite being very anxious, decided that they really wanted the transplant. Mr. N found the tests quite arduous and was concerned about his performance; was he going to be accepted, what about the question one physician had about his heart function, etc. He and his wife participated actively in the psychosocial interview with the social worker. Mr. N's wife had been working at home to support the two of them; they have no children. Their medical costs were covered but they had insufficient savings to relocate, so their friends and family had held a large fund raiser for them. This was very generous but, knowing the potential wait for transplant, the couple would have to manage their funds carefully. The social worker deemed he would be a good candidate for transplant, was well motivated and well supported and had handled previous crises in his life appropriately.

Mr. N was accepted into the transplant program. He and his wife had met some of the other waiting candidates during the assessment and had heard there was an apartment available, which they rented. They came to a weekly support group co-facilitated by the social worker and psychologist where they felt very comfortable; other group members were experiencing very similar medical, emotional and social challenges as themselves.

Mr. N contracted an infection requiring hospitalization and was terrified he would not make it to transplant. However, he recuperated and was able to leave the hospital. He and his wife had become close friends with another couple; the husband had been waiting a long time for transplant. This person was called one night to come in for transplant. The Ns came down to sit with his wife, feeling very pleased that he was to have the opportunity for his transplant. The operation was successful, the patient was recuperating well, when he contracted an infection and, eventually, died. Mr. N was devastated; he had lost a friend. For a time, he appeared quite withdrawn, then indicated he was finding it hard to get close to another patient in case that person died as well. He began to have anxiety attacks requiring some therapy and medication with a psychiatrist. His wife, who was not only serving as his support person, but trying to keep all the business, insurance, etc. in place was really feeling a lot of pressure. She, too, was grieving the loss of their friend who had died and his wife, who had returned home. She was relieved to be able to talk with the social worker as she felt she could not burden her husband who already had more on his plate than he could handle. After a nine month wait, Mr. N was called in for his transplant. He progressed well but soon after coming out of the ICU began feeling very depressed again requiring psychiatric and social work intervention for himself and his wife. After six weeks, he was able to leave hospital and return to his apartment six weeks before going home. He has returned once for follow-up and is starting to think about returning to work.

References

Allender, J., Slusslak, C., Kasuiak, A. and Copeland, J. (1983). Stages of psychological adjustment associated with heart transplantation. *Heart Transplantation, 2,* 228-231.

Bright, M.J., Craven, J.L., Kelly, P.J. and Tweedell, D.E. (1988). Management of psychosocial stress occurring in lung transplant applicants and candidates. (submitted for publication).

Christopherson, L.K. (1976). Cardiac transplant: preparation for dying or for living. *Health and Social Work, 1*(1), 59-71.

Christopherson, L.K. (1987). Cardiac transplantation, a psychological perspective. *Circulation, 75*(1), 52-62.

Christopherson, L.K. & Lunde, D.T. (1971). Selection of cardiac transplant recipients and their subsequent psychosocial adjustment. *Seminars in Psychiatry, 3*(1), 36-45.

Craven, J.L. (1989). Cyclosporin associated organic mental syndromes in liver transplant recipients. (Submitted for publication).

Levenson, J. L. & Olbrisch, M.E. (1987). Shortage of donor organs and long waits. *Psychosomatics, 28*(8), 399-403.

Mai, F., McKenzie, N. & Kostuk, W. (1986). Psychiatric aspects of heart transplantation; pre-operative evaluation and postoperative sequelae. *British Medical Journal, 292,* 347-355.

Maier, F. A second chance at life. *Newsweek.* (Sept. 12, 1988), 52-63.

Mishel, M. H. & Murdaugh, C.L. (1987). Family adjustment to heart transplantation: redesigning the dream. *Nursing Research, 36*(6), 332- 337.

Suszycki, L. H. (1988). Psychosocial aspects of heart transplantation. *Social Work, 33,* 205-209.

Suszycki, L.H. (1986). Social work groups on a heart transplant program. *Heart Transplantation, 5,* 166-170.

Sangster, S. (1987). I had North America's first double-lung transplant. *Chatelaine,* Sept., 46-95.

Chapter 25

SOCIAL WORK PRACTICE WITH CHRONIC PAIN MANAGEMENT

Mario Spiler, MSW, CSW

Abstract

Chronic pain is a complex problem for the individual, the family and the health care system. Three million Canadians suffer chronic pain, costing the health care system billions of dollars. The Chronic Pain Program at St. Joseph's Health Centre, London, Ontario, Canada, is, as described, a unique program that addresses this issue. The role of the social worker as an interdisciplinary team member is detailed, demonstrating current and potential contributions to the program with a case example. The value of the social work psychosocial family-centred approach in the area of chronic pain is highlighted.

SOCIAL WORK PRACTICE WITH CHRONIC PAIN MANAGEMENT

The debilitating effects of chronic pain impose severe and progressive limitations on an individual's ability to cope. The psychosocial impact, generated by suffering and subsequent increased disability, has made chronic pain a major health problem. About 15 years ago it was estimated that the cost of chronic pain in the United States was over $10 billion annually (Bonika, 1973). Today, the cost is estimated to be as high as $90 billion (Philips, 1988). In Canada, about 3 million individuals are reported to be suffering from chronic pain (Corey and Solomon, 1988; Hibler, 1988).

According to Dr. Corey (1988), a first step in controlling pain is acquiring an understanding of it. This advice is as applicable to service providers as it is to individuals with chronic pain. A definition that offers some insight is that pain is an "unpleasant experience we primarily associate with tissue damage or describe in terms of tissue damage or both" (Merskey and Spear, 1967). A wide variety of explanations for the existence of pain have been offered as well. Regardless of how pain is defined or what explanation is offered for its existence, the fact is that "pain is when it hurts" (Hibler, 1988).

One vital distinction regarding pain is whether it is "acute" or "chronic." "Acute pain" is usually when pain begins, and refers to either its intensity or short duration. The reason for the pain is clear. For example, the pain experienced immediately after an injury, like a fall or cut, is acute pain. "Chronic pain" refers to pain that persists long after the tissue or other damage has healed, and/or original painful event has ended. It can end up being entirely out of proportion to the original injurious event. It is the experience of chronic pain that can lead the individual to experience anxiety and avoid activities which may contribute to improved functioning and recovery (Corey, 1988).

Chronic pain is a complex problem due to its effect on every facet of the person's life. The contribution of the family to perpetuating chronic pain, aand to influencing treatment outcomes, is well documented. As well, differences in pain behaviour and responses between cultural groups have been noted. Therefore, one can easily understand Roy's (1986) contention that "for any kind of comprehensive approach to the treatment of chronic pain, social work has to be an integral component of an interdisciplinary team" (p.

35). Social work has made valuable contributions to the understanding and treatment of chronic pain, and has also assisted patients and their families network more appropriately with their communities.

THE CLIENTELE

The Chronic Pain Management Program, part of a 30-bed General Rehabilitation Unit, is located at St. Mary's Chronic Hospital, a facility of St. Joseph's Health Centre, London, Ontario. The Rehabilitation Unit offers comprehensive treatment using an interdisciplinary team approach for each disability group. Other disabilities treated in this Unit include strokes, amputations and other orthopaedic problems.

The Chronic Pain Team consists of a physiatrist (rehabilitation specialist), a nurse manager, a nurse, a psychologist, a social worker, a physiotherapist, an occupational therapist, a pastoral care worker and a recreational therapist. Since its inception in January, 1985, the Program's evolution has evidenced changes affecting the number of inpatients served at one time, the criteria for and the length of admission and team-membership size. Currently the Program provides service to four inpatients at one time who are admitted for a six-week period. However, there are times when patients require a shorter stay and can be discharged after only three weeks.

The objectives of the Program are to determine the contributing factors influencing the chronic pain disability, provide treatment utilizing an interdisciplinary team approach and provide recommendations for care to the patient, the family and the local health care community. The Chronic Pain Team aims to educate the patient and the family in adopting useful management strategies to cope with the chronic pain, to increase the patient's activity level and general physical fitness, to eliminate dependence on narcotic medication and to reduce the inappropriate use of the health care system.

Patients come to the Program through referrals from their family physician or a medical specialist. Final acceptance into the Program continues to be determined by the directing physiatrist. Admission of the patient is based on the degree to which individuals are disabled by their chronic pain and the extent to which the health care system is being unproductively utilized. The patients are selected from a lengthy waiting list. If patients are able to obtain significant relief from their chronic pain as a result of a single procedure or approach, then they are inappropriate for this Program. The approach taken by this Program is multi-modal in accordance with the team's perception that chronic pain is a complex, multi-faceted phenomenon.

Between 1985 and 1988, there were approximately 158 admissions to the Program, with an equal distribution of male and female patients. A total of 83 of these patients were from the local area, and the remainder came from surrounding counties and other areas. The age distribution of these patients showed that 75% fell between the ages of 26 and 55.

The presenting problems evident in patients diagnosed with chronic pain disability include intractable, non-malignant pain in such areas as the back, neck, arms, knees and legs. The pain is usually brought on by a physical injury that is work related, a motor-vehicle accident or a disease like bone degeneration of the spine. The current pain is usually out of proportion to the original injury. In addition, patients may also present with such problems as depression, narcotic and/or other addictions, social isolation, relationship difficulties, financial limitations and obesity and/or physical unfitness. Patients that enter the program typically request that their pain be taken away in order that they can "get on with life." However, their presenting lifestyle is indicative of being totally consumed and subservient to their pain. Having lived with pain for a significant length of time, and having it play such an overriding part in all aspects of their lives, their pain has become part of their very identity.

PRACTICE ROLES AND RESPONSIBILITIES

The role of the social worker is one of an active team member, whose family-focussed approach (Harthan & Laird, 1983) assists the pain team in its unified efforts in assessment and diagnosis, development and implementation of the rehabilitation plan and evaluation of the program's effectiveness. The areas in which the social worker makes unique contributions are

i)   information/education;
ii) assessment;

iii) therapy and
iv) discharge planning.

As part of the orientation program at admission, each patient is provided with a predetermined schedule of interviews and activities. This provides some structure while safeguarding against becoming overwhelmed by the reality of the admission, the setting and the numerous staff involved in the program. The schedule is organized to reflect an optimum balance between treatment, meals and free time. The patient is encouraged to go home on weekends, except for the first weekend following admission.

During the first week, the social worker sees patients regarding their understanding of why they have been referred to the pain program and why they have been admitted at this time. Some patients respond to their family doctor's suggestions, and agree to enter the program simply because the "doctor said so." Other patients' motivation to enter the program is based on their never-ending quest for a "cure." Still others recognize their inability to continue coping effectively and request assistance in attaining some measure of control over their chronic pain.

The social worker adds to the overall orientation given to the patient and the family on the nature and function of the Chronic Pain Management Program. They receive additional information from the social worker on the rationale for the interdisciplinary team approach. A brief description of the multidisciplinary team composition is also provided in order to further emphasize the multi-modal approach used in the program. Clear and careful emphasis is placed on the **management** of the chronic pain rather than its elimination. However, this directive is balanced by indicating to the patient and the family that there is a real possibility the patient will acquire a greater tolerance for the pain and therefore experience it with less intensity. What the patient stands to gain is a reduction in or elimination of their dependency on narcotic medication, an increase in activity level and overall physical fitness and a renewed interest in other aspects of her/his life previously neglected, avoided or denied.

The initial information-orientation session with which the social worker provides the patient and the family serves four functions:

1) it provides an overall perspective to the admission process and hospital stay;
2) it assists the whole family in dealing with anxieties they may experience;

3) it provides them with a more detailed explanation about the social worker's role in regards to the admission process and
4) it initiates the learning in the family about the nature of pain, its chronicity, its psychosocial manifestations and their ability as a family to gain control over it.

During the first week of the Program, the social worker begins to assess the psychosocial dynamics of the patient and the family. Although the patient may be interviewed alone initially, the family's involvement is emphasized throughout as being crucial in order that the social worker can assess and intervene appropriately. The social work assessment involves gathering information mainly under the general heading of "Demographic Data," "Relevant Social Information," "Current Situation/Functioning" and (Plan and Recommendations."

Gathering relevant psychosocial information initially involves obtaining a chronology of family life events and paying close attention to those events that have been perceived as stressful by individual family members or by the family as a whole. The social worker obtains family observations of their functioning and coping prior to and following the onset of the patient's pain. Areas explored by the social worker include the behaviourial responses of individual family members, how they have contributed to the maintenance of the patient's pain behaviour and how attempts to cope or change have been rendered ineffective or self-defeating. A written psychosocial assessment is made available to the team by the social worker within the first two weeks. This is useful as a point of departure for the pain team to focus on relevant issues and areas in need of further exploration. The assessment process continues through the hospitalization and complements the counselling function.

The provision of social work counselling to the patient and the family focusses on the main issues collectively identified by the Team. Short-term family therapy is provided in order to encourage ways to evolve from their present situation to a more desired one. One of the beliefs that makes treatment a challenge, is that the chronic pain is closely tied up in the individual's identity and self-worth. Therefore any alteration of the pain experience must be balanced with incorporating other methods of attaining self-esteem. The therapeutic aim of the social worker, given the program's time frame, is to create a beginning appreciation for the family regarding how their situation, which they claim is beyond their control, is, to a large extent, of their own making and therefore within their control.

Interdisciplinary team rounds take place on a weekly basis. Team members have the opportunity to exchange information, document progress made by patients and focus on current issues. Along with the other team members, the social worker is currently making attempts at quantifying patients' weekly progress. Following the team rounds, each patient is seen by the whole team and provided with feedback on identified issues. Recommendations for a treatment plan to be implemented by the following week are also agreed upon.

The social worker schedules a family conference for each patient during the latter part of the six-week hospitalization. The family conference provides an opportunity for the patient and her/his family to obtain a verbal report from each team member on the progress they have made. Recommendations regarding a family approach to the management of the chronic pain are offered. The family is encouraged to ask questions, express concerns and contribute, along with the team, to the development of a workable plan of action to be implemented following the patient's discharge. The family and the team agree on a team member who is then designated as the follow-up person either to provide additional treatment on an outpatient basis or remain a "contact" for the family in the future.

The social work role as discharge planner involves networking with the patient's home community. This involves ensuring that the patient and family receive information and have access to community resources such as welfare assistance, vocational rehabilitation, public health, etc. As part of the overall plan to assist the patient and the family to manage more appropriately, representatives from appropriate community resources may be invited to the conferences in order to assist with the development, implementation and follow-up of the patient's discharge plans. Prior to discharge, the social worker also ensures that a follow-up medical appointment is scheduled with the pyschiatrist approximately six weeks following the discharge date. The social worker also ensures that community agencies to be involved are ready to begin their involvement with the patient and family.

A recent addition to the social worker's responsibilities includes a research component. This involves administering a questionnaire to each patient and other family members in order to elicit their individual perception of how their family is presently functioning and would like to function in the future. The questionnaire is then administered again three and six months following the patient's discharge. Presently, the information obtained from the initial questionnaire response is used both for diagnostic and educational purposes.

POTENTIAL FOR ROLE DEVELOPMENT

The social work role has potential for development in two main areas: prior to the patient's admission and post-discharge. With additional time allocated in these two areas, coupled with the contribution made during the patient's hospital stay, more comprehensive social work involvement in the areas of assessment, treatment, community networking and research could be achieved.

With pre-admission involvement, a social work assessment would be carried out earlier and would provide psychosocial information to assist in determining who would have the greatest need for the program and who would benefit the most from it. At this stage, the information obtained from the assessment would contribute to the efficiency of the program's in-patient information gathering process. For those individuals considered inappropriate for the program, the social worker would function as an information and referral source and a link with appropriate community agencies available.

The preventative function performed by the social worker would more effectively assist those individuals who may more appropriately utilize assistance from the program on an out-patient basis. However, it needs to be acknowledged that knowing how to access resources may not be sufficient if the necessary community agencies are not available for the chronic pain population. The social worker could be instrumental in assisting with the establishment of community-based self-help groups for chronic pain sufferers and their families.

Pre-admission social work involvement would further enhance the current social work role in the program during the hospitalization phase. The social worker would be able to devote more time to providing casework intervention since the assessment would have been completed prior to admission. The social worker would also be able to exercise a higher degree of efficiency by instituting pre-admission discharge planning, ensuring earlier mobilization of community resources.

In the post-discharge phase, the social worker would continue to function as the link between the patient and family and the community, in order that the management of chronic pain and the effectiveness of the program are monitored through proper follow-up procedures. The social work research potential at this phase of involvement would help in evaluating the program's effectiveness and in identifying the need for additional follow-up interventions.

CONCLUDING REMARKS

The multi-dimensional nature of chronic pain requires a multi-disciplinary approach to its management. The area of chronic pain offers exciting challenges and opportunities for social workers. It is a relatively new speciality as marked by a small but growing number of publications.

As an interdisciplinary team member, the social worker in the chronic pain program reflects the family-centred approach in the psychosocial assessment, and also in the development and implementation of the treatment and discharge plans. Another challenge is to remain consistent with the objectives of the entire team. Collaboration, negotiation and communication are essential elements in an efficient, effective, and enthusiastic approach to the treatment of chronic pain.

CASE EXAMPLE

Mrs. J. is a 36-year-old woman from a small town sixty miles from London. She has been married for sixteen years and has two sons, ages nine and thirteen. She was referred to the program by her family physician due to complaints of low back pain. She was admitted with a diagnosis of chronic pain disability with dependency on narcotic medication. She reported sustaining a gymnastics injury to her lower back in her high school years, which resulted in a short-lived disability. In her early twenties, during labour with her first son, she experienced a "popping sensation" in her lower back while receiving an epidural needle. The resulting pain lasted about two months. About a year later, Mrs. J. experienced the same "popping sensation" when she was lifting her son from the back seat of her car. She experienced severe back pain and was on bed rest for the following two months. Her pain has persisted ever since.

Physiotherapy treatments, visits to chiropractors and medication have been tried for years, with only short-lasting periods of relief. She had been taking about 100 Tylenol No. Three every three weeks for the past twelve years.

At the time of admission to the program, Mrs. J. reported a continual ache in the right hip region, and monthly flare-ups of lower back pain lasting five to six days. The pain had affected Mrs. J.'s lifestyle to the point that previous coping patterns within the family were no longer effective. Because she was rarely well enough to participate in family outings, Mr. J. had assumed much of the caretaking responsibility. Being left alone was increasingly frustrating for Mrs. J. and reinforced her self-perception as a mother who had failed. In addition, Mr. and Mrs. J.'s sexual relationship had become virtually non-existent due to Mrs. J.'s reduced desire as a result of the pain and Mr. J.'s fear of hurting her even more. This also resulted in increasing Mrs. J.'s feeling of failure as a wife.

During the first week Mrs. J. was seen individually by the social worker and then jointly with her husband and children. The social worker contributed to the orientation to the program while eliciting relevant information for the psychosocial assessment. The resulting effect was that Mr. and Mrs. J. became less anxious about the admission and hopeful about benefiting from the program. Mr. and Mrs. J. expressed a desire to explore the effects that Mrs. J.'s chronic pain had on their marriage. Given the time available in the program, they felt that concentrating on their marital relationship would be more beneficial than involving the whole family.

The couple was assigned a task to be accomplished during the patient's first weekend visit back home. They were to observe themselves during routine activities and interactions around the home. Mrs. J. and her husband subsequently reported that their "observations" were beneficial because they increased their sensitivity to each family member's behaviour and its effect on other family members. Mrs. J. noted that her sons now routinely picked up their clothes and toys without being asked and this activity elicited feelings of uselessness and failure in her. In allowing herself to recognize that her sons were at an age where this could be a reasonable task as members of their family, she was able to attribute a more positive meaning to their helpfulness.

Mr. J. recognized that each time his wife commented on a task to be done or her limitations on completing a task he would immediately complete the task himself. He indicated his need to learn how to distinguish when his wife needed assistance with a particular task from when she just needed to feel understood and appreciated. The marital counselling also focussed on their sexual relationship, Mrs. J.'s social isolation and the couple's feelings about Mrs. J.'s narcotic addiction.

Effective social work intervention also took the form of concrete, practical assistance. Due to reduced contact with her children and extended family during the Program, Mrs. J. was assisted with obtaining free access to a telephone so she could be in touch with her family twice a week.

The social worker exchanged information on a regular basis with team members in order to monitor Mrs. J.'s overall progress. Ongoing contact with team members also assisted the social worker in introducing updated information during the marital therapy sessions, together with remaining consistent with the interventions of the other team members and the overall objectives of the program.

The social worker scheduled the family conference near the end of the program. Along with the reports from the other team members, the social worker reported on the progress made by Mr. and Mrs. J. and the impact the changes were having on their children and extended family.

The social worker did not need to make referrals to the community where the J. family lived. It was already established that Mrs. J.'s family doctor would remain involved. One of the nurses on the unit agreed to act as the link to the program. The social worker continued to monitor the progress made by the family through the questionnaire sent out after three and six months.

At the time of discharge both Mrs. J. and her husband felt that they had made some gains in managing the chronic pain more appropriately, and in recognizing how the "real" work was just beginning for them.

References

Bandler, R. and Grinder, J. (1982). *Reframing: Neuro-Linguistic Programming and the Transformation of Meaning.* Moab, Utah: Real People Press.

Bonica, J. J. (1973). The management of pain. (Symposium Issue) *Postgraduate Medicine, 53,* 56-57.

Corey, D. (1988). Chronic pain: Is it time to change our perspective? *Rehabilitation Digest, 18,* 3-6.

Corey, D. & Solomon, S. (1988). *Pain — Learning How To Live Without It.* Toronto: Macmillan.

Ford, C. V. (1983). *The Somatizing Disorders: Illness as a Way of Life.* New York: Elsvier Biomedical.

Gordon, D. (1978). *Therapeutic Metaphors: Helping Others Through The Looking Glass.* Cupertino, CA: Meta Publications.

Hartman, A. & Laird, J. (1983). *Family-Centred Social-Work Practice.* New York: The Free Press.

Hibler, M. (1988). When the pain won't stop. *Legion,* 6-8.

Hudgens, A. L. (1977). The social worker's role in a behavioral management approach to chronic pain. *Social Work in Health Care, 3*(2), 149-157.

Marcus, M. (1986). Chronic pain: A social work view. *The Social Worker/Le Travailleur Social, 54*(2), 60-63.

Merskey, H. & Spear, F. G. (1967). The concept of pain. *Journal of Psychosomatic Research, 11,* 59-67.

Payne, B. & Norfleet, M. A. (1986). Chronic pain and the family: A review. *Pain, 26,* 1-22.

Roy, R. (1981a). Chronic pain and family dynamics. In D.S. Freeman & B. Trute (Eds.), *Treating Families with Special Needs* (pp. 219-229). Ottawa, Ontario: A.A.S.W. & C.A.S.W.

Roy, R. (1981b). Social work in chronic pain. *Health and Social Work, 6,* 54-62.

Roy, R. (1982a). Marital and family issues in patients with chronic pain: A review. *Psychotherapy and Psychosomatics, 37,* 1-12.

Roy, R. (1982b). Pain-prone patient: A revisit. *Psychotherapy and Psychosomatics, 37,* 202-213.

Roy, R. (1985a). Chronic pain and marital difficulties. *Health and Social Work, 10,* 199-209.

Roy, R. (Ed.) (1985b). The Family and Chronic Pain. (Special Issue). *International Journal of Family Therapy, 7*(4).

Roy, R. (1986). A psychosocial perspective on chronic pain and depression in the elderly. *Social Work in Health Care, 12*(2), 27-36.

Sternback, R. A. (1968). *Pain: A Psychophysiological Analysis*. New York: Academic Press.

Turk, D. C. & Stieg, R. L. (1987). Chronic pain: The necessity of interdisciplinary communication. *The Clinical Journal of Pain, 3*, 163-167.

Wolff, B. B. (1985). Review: Ethnocultural factors influencing pain and illness behavior. *The Clinical Journal of Pain, 1*, 23-30.

Chapter 26

SOCIAL WORK PRACTICE IN A MULTI-DISCIPLINARY PHYSICAL REHABILITATION SETTING

Carolynn Campbell, MSW
Zora Jackson, MSW
Libusa A Jeglic, M.SW

Abstract

Rehabilitation is the process whereby a person with a physical disability seeks to gain or regain independence and autonomy in different areas of functioning. At the Rehabilitation Centre in Ottawa, efforts are made by various disciplines, including social work, to help the disabled person achieve this goal. The primary social work task is to help the client and family achieve their optimal level of psychosocial functioning and help them return to a fuller quality of life in the community. There are separate medical programs each with a specialized multi-discipline team. Social work practice roles assessment, orienting the client to the rehabilitation process, counselling, education, advocacy/resource provision, discharge planning, teaching, research and team building are described. Escalating health care costs, deinstitutionalization and a desire for the disabled to live at home point to community outreach as the major potential for role development in the future.

SOCIAL WORK PRACTICE IN A MULTI-DISCIPLINARY PHYSICAL REHABILITATION SETTING

THE CLIENTELE

The Rehabilitation Centre was opened in April, 1981 with the purpose of serving and providing rehabilitation to physically disabled adults in the Eastern Ontario Region. This mandate is carried out through in-patient and out-patient services in a 77-bed, bilingual, multi-disciplinary setting that is part of the Health Sciences Complex of the University of Ottawa. In addition, there is a mobile clinic that visits outlying areas and provides consultation, education and some services to the rural communities. Our clientele is served by the following in-patient programs: 1) spinal cord, 2) stroke, 3) neurolocomotor, 4) amputee, 5) respiratory, 6) adolescent and 7) chronic pain.

In addition, there is a follow-up and out-patient program that includes clientele from the above disability groupings and also specialized clinics such as: multiple sclerosis, muscular dystrophy, cystic fibrosis and spina bifida. Brief descriptions of these client groups follow.

1. The spinal cord client is one who has suffered spinal cord trauma and damage that has resulted in either paraplegia, quadriplegia, paraparesis or quadriparesis. The latter two diagnostic categories are not as permanent and allow various degrees of recovery. The patient in this category was usually involved in an accident; e.g., motor vehicle, diving, industrial, stabbing, shooting, self-infliction, cancer or viral infection. The limited hand and arm movements of quadriplegics make them dependent in activities of daily living such as dressing, feeding, transferring, toileting, etc.

2. Stroke clients have suffered cerebro-vascular accident. Depending on the severity of the stroke and the areas of the brain affected, they have left- or right-sided paralysis or left- or right-sided weakness in addition to speech, cognition, balance and vision problems, swallowing disorders and emotional instability. Clients with good cognitive function, even though they have limited physical abilities, are likely to be able to again live reasonably independently.

3. The neurolocomotor program serves clients with multiple sclerosis, muscular dystrophy, burns, joint replacements, rheumatoid arthritis, cerebral palsy, amyotrophic lateral sclerosis and those with multiple injuries from motor vehicle accidents. Some of these debilitating conditions are chronic and progressive. The rate of progressive deterioration cannot always be predicted and therefore it is difficult for these clients and families as they have to make ongoing adjustments in their lives.

4. Amputee clients have limb loss as the result of injury, cancer or cardio-vascular problems associated with diabetes, .

5. Respiratory clients are usually elderly people with emphysema, bronchitis, asthma or a combination of the above. Smoking and environmental conditions such as dust, extreme cold or heat affect them. Respiratory illness is chronic and progressive. Clients have difficulty breathing, especially through exertion, and this affects their personal functioning.

6. The Adolescent Program serves young people from the age of eighteen to twenty-six with various neuro-muscular deficits and/or cognitive deficits. Some of these conditions are congenital while others are the result of an illness or accident. This is a group with unique requirements for vocational training and transition to adult living.

7. The chronic pain program, an intensive, six-week in-patient program, treats clients with severe chronic pain that cannot be medically eliminated. Rehabilitation focusses on learning to live constructively with pain.

Each of the above programs has social workers assigned to them. The social worker facilitates the rehabilitation process wherein a person with a physical disability seeks to gain or regain independence and autonomy in the various areas of her/his functioning. This facilitation process takes place on various levels:

1) with the client;
2) with her/his family;
3) with the medical team and
4) with the community.

The social worker addresses the areas of psychosocial functioning and helps client and family move from a situation of uncertainty, anxiety and dependence on others to a position of confidence, hope and autonomy, including resumption of control over one's own life and destiny.

The social worker meets with clients and families whenever possible and tries to understand the client's environment and her/his strengths and weaknesses in terms of adaptation, flexibility, confidence, assertiveness, resourcefulness, etc. It is important that the goals clients want to reach are realistic and mutually agreed upon. The social worker might help verbalize these goals and negotiate them with the appropriate system. An important component of social work is also planning appropriate discharge and facilitating funding for:

a) equipment,
b) possible home or work site modifications and
c) job retraining.

The social worker knows the available community resources and educates the client and the family accordingly. Sometimes there are limited services in the community and the social worker will advocate to bring them about. The social worker presents as many options as possible to the clients so that they are able to choose for themselves.

PRACTICE ROLES AND RESPONSIBILITIES

I. Assessment

Social workers in a rehabilitation setting share the team goal to maximize physical recovery and autonomy for clients. This often requires marked psychosocial re-adjustment. Grounding in systems theory prompts social workers to expand the view of their client to include the extended family and the community support network of the identified client. An added role is to identify for the rehabilitation team the reverberating impact of the disability on all parts of this network necessitating grief of the functional loss, adjustment of family and employment roles, learning of new skills, provision of emotional and financial resources and adaptation of physical environments. The primary role is thus assessment of the client's macro-system to determine how the medical diagnosis is affecting all of its component members, how well it is spontaneously marshalling its resources to adapt and what resources are needed to supplement these efforts to effect optimal rehabilitation. Assessment is the social workers' first point of intervention.

II. Orienting the Client to the Rehabilitation Process

While gathering assessment information, the social worker also orients the client and family to the rehabilitation team and its process. The rehabilitation process is distinct from traditional medicine wherein the patient is the passive treatment recipient at the hands of the expert doctor. Some clients are initially hesitant to take a more active role in negotiating their functional goals with their therapists. On most teams within the centre, clients attend team meetings to review their progress and re-evaluate their treatment goals. Coaching clients on the use of these meetings and preparing families for admission and pre-discharge family conferences where treatment is explained and problem solving occurs is also a social work responsibility. The emphasis here is to teach clients and families to live with the rehabilitation philosophy.

III. Counselling

Counselling is a central aspect of the social work role. The problem solving that must be done to ensure adaptation of the client and her/his network to the disability occurs best once diagnosis is accepted. Family members need to be provided an opportunity to hear and understand one another's concerns and to build on their strengths in a caring context. The social worker facilitates this process. Effective problem solving is slowed when the reactions of denial, anger and depression have not been respectively worked through by the client, family and/or friends. The meaning attributed to a particular disability is different within each family system. Thus, the family is helped in exploring these meanings and in expressing their feelings about the change brought on by the disability.

McColl and Skinner (1988) reported that social support is positively correlated with health outcomes. Specifically, they defined a social support as having three major components: perceived emotional nurturance; physical assistance and resources and education. One of the most imporant areas of social support is family support. Other support deficits could substitute one for another but nothing could substitute for deficiencies in family support. Often, however, adding material resources, home services and education could relieve the fears of potential family caregivers and bring them closer to their disabled loved-one. Supporting the family increases their willingness to support the identified client. The rehabilitation social worker intervenes through the counselling process to elevate the actual level of social support and her/his client's perception of that support.

Major adjustments are required in how a family divides their time, labour and support. For example, an adult child may take on the role of caregiver to a post-stroke parent. Perhaps a breadwinner is no longer able to work full time. A spinal-cord-injured male may have to give up the dream of having children. Nursing home or chronic care placement may become a startling reality to the client who has no family, or whose family cannot provide the required level of nursing care. One may have to deal with giving up the family home in favour of a more barrier-free environment. Then there are always the existential questions of "Why me?", "Is life worthwhile now?", "How do I find renewed purpose?" The hopes and fears for the present and future are the core of counselling in individual, couple and family therapy.

IV. Education

Education of clients, their families and other health professionals in order to increase the social support of rehabilitation clients is a major aspect of social work. This entails communicating information about the disabilities and also teaching coping mechanisms for clients and their families. The informed client and family usually sheds unrealistic fear about their future. This work is done both individually and in groups. Education on accident prevention and lifestyle counselling to the client and community is another facet of social work. For example, a social worker is often called on to speak to self-help groups in the community. Conducting educational lectures for health professionals in rural clinics of the region is another educational role of social workers who travel with mobile rehabilitation clinics. This outreach operation is extremely supportive of rural clinicians working in isolation, often on limited budgets.

V. Advocacy/Resource Provision

Advocacy is a role familiar to every social worker. The goal is to lend support and knowledge of governmental and voluntary services to the client for the short-term while they learn the skills of self-advocacy.

More specifically, the rehabilitation social worker is responsible for assisting her/his client to locate wheelchair accessible housing, arranging nursing home placements or securing funding to renovate their previous housing. S/He acts as an information broker and liaison in obtaining disability pensions, social assistance, wage loss insurance payments, etc. S/He facilitates provision of home support services such as adapted public transportation, homemaking, attendant care for personal hygiene or respite placement so that family caregivers may have a restbreak. S/He helps the client locate community self-help groups such as the Multiple Sclerosis Society, the Muscular Dystrophy Association and the Canadian Paraplegic Association. As The Rehabilitation Centre is situated very near the Ontario-Quebec boarder, social workers must guide their clients through the health and social service programs of either the provincial government or federal government. One finds that most clients are readily able to use their own autonomy once knowledge of these social and health care systems is provided.

The social workers in the Centre are also active in second-order advocacy. They have presented reports that prompted the hospital administration to lobby for needed reform to income maintenance for the disabled. We continue to serve on volunteer community boards for agencies providing housing, transportation, attendant care and vocational/recreational opportunities for the physically disabled in the Ottawa-Carleton region. Political action to redress service gaps is one additional important mandate. Further, representation on the various in-hospital, administrative committees is an avenue whereby one represents the client's and community's interests.

VI. Discharge Planning

The role of discharge planner has become contested territory as Ontario hospitals comply with legislation to instate job evaluation and pay equity. Every discipline on the rehabilitation team can legitimately claim a part in preparing the client for discharge, as each contributes through therapy to his or her increased independence.

The social worker views discharge planning not as a role in and of itself but rather as a composite end product of many of her/his previously discussed roles. A client is adequately prepared for the transition from hospital dependence to community living as a result of effective assessment, counselling and resource provision. The clinical vignette, Helen's story, which follows, illustrates the bolstering of the social support system in order to achieve the most efficacious discharge plan. Further, one needs to blend a psychosocial family focus with a familiarity with community resources in order to foster adjustment of the client's network to her/his disability. The instrumental planning done by team colleagues is thus an adjunct to the more holistic discharge plan carried out by the social worker.

VII. Teaching and Research

Client treatment is the core aspect of The Rehabilitation Centre's tri-fold mission in the community. However, it also is a teaching and research facility. The department participates in the clinical training of community college and university social work students. As well, it orients medical students to the psychosocial ramifications of the illnesses and injuries they will encounter in their future practices.

Research is a key to our on-going professional development. The department has been involved in two research projects. An exploratory study has just been completed on the family environment of physically disabled adolescents and young adults. The second is exploring the impact of physical disability on six major variables of family functioning. The objective is to fine tune assessment and treatment interventions in order to improve quality of client care.

VIII. Team Building

The above synopsis of social work roles and responsibilities has highlighted practice in a context where the rehabilitation team provides service. The skills of the social worker are frequently used in co-operation with other disciplines to provide team-building services to their members. Each team is a highly diverse group of multi-disciplinary specialists. The rehabilitation team consists of eight, and sometimes nine, disciplines. Each has their own knowledge base, skills and process, the foundation from which it assesses, formulates goals and directs intervention. Each, therefore, brings a differing focus to the client families who again have their distinct perspective. There must be consensus on goals and treatment methods or energy-wasting confusion results. The social worker's comfort with group dynamics facilitates arrival at such desired co-operation.

Inevitably, instances arise when a client, family and/or professional team do not meet the agreed upon goals. For example, the disease process may gallop. Perhaps there are entrenched psychological patterns one cannot break that support maladaptive behaviour. Further, insufficient services may exist to provide the required discharge environment where the client lives. At these junctures team morale generally plummets. As well, sometimes there may be anger or tears from clients and families. Staff who work closely with them may feel the brunt of recrimination. Sometimes there are blaming words impugning co-workers skills or commitment. These latter events, though human, are destructive to team cohesion and long-term efficacy of client care. At times of goal problems the social worker is one healer within the team itself. The disappointments must be de-personalized; the focus turned toward team process and program development. A specific example from one team in the centre illustrates this.

Through the spring and summer of 1988, this team experienced a string of disappointing cases. An initially medically stable patient developed congestive heart failure. A diagnosis of chronic pain proved to be metasticized bone cancer. A client with a psychopathological overlay sabotaged his treatment. A man needing routine physical treatment presented with severe dementia, undisclosed by his family physician. He could not respond to treatment. In another case, a crucial family member became terminally ill making it impossible for a patient to go home. There were many simultaneous successes, however team morale was noticeably slipping.

During a regular administrative meeting, the social worker requested a team-building retreat. A day was set aside. A multidisciplinary planning committee was recruited to develop the agenda. Each planning meeting was thus a preliminary occasion to hone interactional skills. When the planning committee met, the first period of each encounter focussed on venting of anger and blame. The social worker respectfully listened and then modelled a move away from fault finding toward each team member taking individual responsibility for changing their interactive process, rather than insisting co-workers make changes. The reader will recognize this method as integral to marital counselling strategy.

Over several meetings an agenda was devised and the labour divided so that each discipline had responsibility for a portion of the days program. This assured commitment to attainment of a shared goal by all participants. Many of the problems were hence worked through before the retreat!

The retreat day was broken down into small discussion groups and plenaries. All members had a chance to express their gripes and ideas collectively, having already diffused some of the destructive anger in the preparatory meetings. Just enough of that anger was saved for an honest, respectful interchange. In the plenary session, the team as a whole decided how to implement reform.

From the retreat came two positive innovations. The team now has a bi-monthly educational lecture at the administrative monthly meeting. Each discipline, by rotation, explains an important aspect of, or new development in, their work. The goal is a more thorough understanding of one another's skills and challenges as they contribute to the work of the team as a whole. The second innovation is a quarterly clinical review of two cases selected at random from the previous three months. This provides occasion for each therapist to reflect in private on her/his treatment goals, interventions and outcomes. A collective evaluation follows; how the team has worked together, the dynamics, the inter-communication, the mutual understanding of one another's expectations and limitations and suggestions for remedying problem areas. It provides the occasion for congratulatory feedback on a job well done. The improved climate can only increase the calibre of client care.

POTENTIAL FOR ROLE DEVELOPMENT

Many of the roles described in the previous section will continue to be necessary in the years ahead. However, given the nature of a multi-disciplinary setting, and the expertise required to work with many types of systems throughout the health care network, the potential for role development in social work seems favourable. Also, due to various societal factors, the nature of the health care system, and the great flux in the field of rehabilitation, new opportunities for social work may become available.

It is our view that the traditional casework role will continue to be important although new approaches will probably need to be developed. For example, because of greater public awareness of the psychosocial aspects of disabilities, it is anticipated that there will be more demand for social work services. Thus, assessment and intake procedures will need to be streamlined and levels of intervention defined in terms of specific client needs (Ell, 1985). Further, strategies will need to be developed to facilitate client change and to maintain achieved levels of functioning and prevent health deterioration. Because of the growing movement toward specialization, expertise will need to be developed by individual social workers in given fields of rehabilitation (e.g., spinal cord injury, stroke, head injury, etc.) or in given treatment modalities (e.g., family therapy, group therapy, marital therapy, etc.). At the same time, workers will need to be generalists (Browne, Watt, & Kirlin, 1981), able to carry out a number of different roles as the need arises (e.g., casework, vocational counselling, advocacy, etc.). Since every client, family and community situation is different, a broad range of interventive skills on the part of the social worker will be required.

In recent years, often due to financial restraint, governments have encouraged the disabled to live at home rather than enter large institutions. This trend will demand of social workers an increased awareness of the community and its resources, together with skills in working with new and different types of agencies (e.g., para-medical services, housing co-operatives, centres for independent living, groups for the disabled, etc.); so that client and family needs can be matched to what is available. With the appearance of new technologies and innovative resources (e.g., in self-care and mobility aids, transportation, accommodation, etc.) the situation of the disabled will become extremely complex. All of these different aspects will require social workers who are able to work autonomously and who have casework skills enabling them to intervene in a variety of ways. Although therapeutic counselling and support will continue to be needed, there will be an emphasis on working together with service consumers and helping them to establish their own support networks (e.g., putting newly disabled clients and/or families in contact with others who have successfully adapted to the same disability).

An important role of the social worker in this centre is education (Romano, 1981); i.e., teaching the patient, family, staff and community about the psychosocial aspects of disability, both in terms of specific disabilities, and also about disability in general. This also includes the teaching of preventative factors related to disability; e.g., teaching diving precautions to avoid spinal injury or educating families and employers of clients with respiratory conditions the importance of a smoke-free environment. The social worker will be expected to participate in community forums, multi-disciplinary workshops, in-service programs, etc., and be responsible for sharing with others their particular expertise. This will continue to be an area of role development for social work practice.

As well, consumers of health care services have become more sophisticated. They want to participate more fully in their treatment and rehabilitation and want to know more about the psychosocial aspects of disability and how to cope more effectively. Although the medical model with its focus on therapy and treatment will continue to have its place, there will be more emphasis on the educational aspects of rehabilitation. The social worker in a rehabilitation setting will continue to be a counsellor and therapist, but the role of teacher and educator will be enhanced. It is anticipated that this will be an important role for social work and that it will give new focus to working with different types of groups, e.g., patient groups, family members, self-help groups and community groups.

Social work research, though presently limited (Browne, Watt & Kirlin, 1981), will have potential for growth as well, both in clinical areas (e.g., family therapy intervention), and in non-clinical ones (e.g., program evaluation). Consumers want to know more about the psychosocial aspects of disability. Furthermore, they want this information to be scientifically based and to be both valid and reliable. They also want to receive treatment programs that have been proven effective. Research will thus become a very important social work role.

Decentralization of services may also hold a special role for social workers trained in rehabilitation and in multi-disciplinary approaches. In recent years, a major trend in hospital and rehabilitation centre has been to extend their services outside the institution into the community. Various outreach programs for the disabled have for their purpose the delivery of professional services to the local areas where the client lives. At this centre, for example, the mobile clinic (see description in previous section), a multi-disciplinary team of rehabilitation professionals, including social work, visit the outlying community hospitals to provide the disabled with services that would not otherwise be available. The role of the social worker is one of liaison with community agencies and providing case consultation, referral and education. In a similar way, satellite clinics of the centre might be established where social workers experienced in working with the disabled might be able to offer direct counselling to disabled persons and their families and provide consultation to other health care workers.

A related area that shows potential for future role development is that of community development. Many persons who are physically disabled seem to benefit greatly from having the opportunity to share their experiences with others who have the same disability. Self-help groups, such as the Ottawa Stroke Association, seem to satisfy this need (Ell, 1985). The rehabilitation social worker, aware of the psychosocial aspects of a given disability and of group process, may play a valuable role in terms of support and consultation to such groups (Katz, 1981). Other community organizations, composed of disabled, and/or non-disabled, whose purpose is to work on behalf of specific or general disability groups (e.g., the Ottawa Handicapped Association) may also benefit from professional help provided by the social worker; e.g., municipal sub-committees in charge of providing adapted services to the disabled (e.g., housing, transportation). Various other agencies in the private, voluntary and governmental sector that provide services to the disabled (e.g., housing co-operatives, attendant care, etc.) will find social work consultation helpful. It is anticipated that as more disabled demand to live in their home environment, this community development role of the social worker will become particularly important.

Another social work role that shows potential for development is that of political activist or advocate. In recent years the campaign for the rights of the disabled (Eisenberg, Griggins & Duval, 1982) and the Independent Living Movement (Dejong, 1983; Ell, 1985) have altered drastically the self-perception of the disabled and their expectations of service providers. The disabled want to live independently in the community and are asking society to provide the necessary means for them to do this. The focus is no longer on the disabled person and the difficulties of integrating into society. Rather, the new emphasis is on society and its inability or unwillingness to provide the resources and opportunities that would enable the disabled person to take a rightful place in society. People with disabilities are now called upon to be more assertive in claiming their rights and the social worker is invited to take a role alongside the disabled person to advocate on their behalf. An issue that the social worker may be involved in is helping to reduce the barriers of discrimination (Browne et al., 1981), such as in jobs and schooling, that prevent the disabled from obtaining their full potential. This will demand that social workers sustain their social action role at the municipal, provincial and federal levels of government. Adopting a leadership role and creatively challenging and influencing rehabilitation policies so that they meet the needs of the client (Browne et al., 1981) will be required. It will require continued requests of hospital administrators, physicians and others to lend their support as regards specific projects or legislation. Social workers will be asked to join and/or support various committees and organizations that will lobby for the disabled and their rights. There will also be a demand for participation of social workers in social action groups run by the disabled themselves. The growing crisis in health care and concerns about spiralling costs makes this role of the social worker particularly vital in order to ensure that emerging services needed by the disabled will be developed and that government programs already in place will not be eroded.

In summary, the potential for role development for the social worker in the field of rehabilitation and, in particular, in a multi-disciplinary setting is very favourable. The present crises in health care and the trend toward decentralization of services to the community offers opportunities to work with the physically disabled in ways that could not be envisaged only a few years ago.

CONCLUDING REMARKS

In the decade of the 1990s, the evolving demands on the social worker in rehabilitation will require a certain flexibility and fluidity in carrying out one's various roles. The worker will have to be able to perform a number of activities simultaneously or in quick succession. Thus, one may have to act as therapist with a client and family while being an advocate at the same time. With the advent of computerization, patient care systems will become more standardized with team members collaborating much more closely in assessing the different areas and levels of functioning of clients. This will demand social workers sharing some of their own professional autonomy, expertise and accountability. This may also demand using a more standardized language for the purposes of assessment and recording while retaining a therapeutic approach with one's clients. With the emphasis on the streamlining of health care services, new models for rehabilitation social work, outlining specific goals and outcomes (Champeau, Greene,

Apedaile and Jackson, 1989), may also need to be developed.

A final comment directs the social worker to the responsibility to practise self-care. The job is physically and emotionally stressful. Regular exercise, careful attention to mental and physical health and relaxing recreational activity inoculate against burnout. Ongoing professional development gives a sense of growth and renewed confidence to meet our work challenges. The encouragement given to and received from colleagues in the social work department and our rehabilitation teams, together with the satisfaction of clients and their families, is a powerful anti-stress elixir. When social workers practise effective self-care they become better caregivers.

CASE EXAMPLE

This is the case of Helen who was the youngest child of four siblings. She was three years of age when her forty-two year old pregnant mother died of a stroke at home. The ages of her brothers at that time were five and thirteen and her sister was eleven. The father, aged thirty-eight, remarried six weeks later to a woman who had a fifteen-year-old son. Helen remembers the stepmother as being abusive to the children, and that her sister, eight years older, attempted to be a surrogate mother to her. The Children's Aid Society was also involved. When Helen was seventeen, her nineteen-year-old brother was killed in a car accident. The oldest brother had some difficulties with the law. Her parents' relationship was stormy, with the stepmother leaving the family three times. She returned just before Helen's marriage but left shortly after with many of the household belongings. Helen married at age twenty-one. Her father died at age fifty-nine of a stroke when Helen was twenty-nine.

Helen had been medically (essentially) well. At age twenty-nine she bore her first child, a daughter, and five months later Helen had anaesthesia for the removal of her teeth. The day after she developed the symptom of dragging her left leg. Helen associated that the multiple sclerosis (MS) was brought on by the anaesthetic. However, she related earlier episodic symptoms in her hands and legs. Due to these symptoms she had been referred to a psychiatrist but Helen proudly told me she knew how to answer all the questions and he agreed that as she had everything in control she did not need his services.

Multiple sclerosis was definitely diagnosed during a short hospitalization in an acute-care hospital and two years later her family doctor referred her to the MS self-help group where I met her.

The initial impression I had of Helen was that she was threatened by seeing me. This, she explained, was due to her early childhood fears of having a social worker from Children's Aid visit the family to check on the condition of the children. She recalled she was told to say nothing and to run and hide when the social worker arrived.

My impressions of Helen were as follows: she walked with an ataxic gate, had limited use of one hand and had vision problems; she was guarded in her relationship with me; she was bright, concerned about her health, future, physical loss of independence and she carried many unresolved emotional issues.

I saw Helen on an irregular outpatient basis, as she didn't attend the MS group frequently due to distance and transportation. One day, she came to see me with a specific problem. Helen was pregnant; it wasn't planned and she spent several weeks deliberating on a decision whether she should have an abortion. Her family doctor and husband opted for it and, whereas Helen would have liked another child, the husband was quite adamant and the abortion took place.

Eventually, Helen became an in-patient at the Rehabilitation Centre for a three-month period. She came from an acute-care hospital where she was hospitalized following an exacerbation of her condition. The exacerbation had taken place while she was residing with her older sister after impulsively leaving her own home. Helen had had a minor disagreement with her husband and left him a note simply stating she was leaving him and their six-year-old daughter. She was forty-two years old at that time.

While at the Rehabilitation Centre, Helen made comparisons with the services and those of other hospitals. She decided she would discharge herself. Her sister's home was available but there were too many architectural barriers.

The three-month hospitalization was fraught with difficulties for the team and Helen. She often used her power as a patient positively calling her own conferences inviting all team members, where she read out reactions and feelings from a typed script she worked on in occupational therapy. The main themes were her struggle between dependence and independence and the question of her future with the underlying theme of her struggle in accepting her losses: physical, emotional and familial.

The usual routine of meeting with the family and including them in the team meetings was stymied. Staff were not able to meet with the husband as he didn't visit and Helen did not give me permission to phone him for an appointment for an assessment interview.

How does one plan a patient's discharge when most of the patient's belongings are in the home she has abandoned, when she doesn't want to claim any of her personal belongings or household effects or ask her husband for any money? She requested only a "spartan" room and would rely on a very small Canada Pension. Helen did not want any supplementary help from welfare if the agency would involve her husband. To help this patient under her terms was most challenging. An assertive manoeuvre was required.

I told Helen there was no choice but that I had to phone her husband to explain to him what services were available. If their problems could be discussed, I could possibly help them in coping with their marital difficulties. Helen listened attentively, knowing that she had admitted she acted in an impulsive way when she left her husband and daughter over a small argument. But she was too stubborn to meet with him and he, in turn, hadn't attempted to reach her or reconciliate with her. With reluctant permission Helen stated, "Go ahead, phone him, but you'll find he won't talk to you, he has no time for people intruding in our private affairs." The husband was initially guarded on the phone but he responded. It became clear that he didn't like hospitals and that he had a possible fear of her illness. He stated that if Helen hadn't walked out, he may have conceivably left her. He felt it was easier for her to leave than have him leave with the daughter and he may have left the country, but was vague. He felt Helen made it very difficult for their daughter who was often in tears from being reprimanded. Although he chose not to be involved in discharge plans because Helen needed to be independent, the lines of communication between the couple were opened.

With Christmas approaching, Helen's mood became more positive. She was beginning to think in a thoughtful way about her relationship to her husband and the daughter. She could express this in a Christmas card thanking me for my patience and sticking by her in a critical time in her life. "I have come a long way in understanding myself and seem to be headed in the right direction for making amendments to my family. With your guidance we will become a family once again. Social workers can be beneficial to those who allow them to perform their job. The last three years have been a struggle for me, but only because I have made it so. The last three months have changed from a struggle to something of a hopeful nature...thanks for everything."

Helen, however, did not make it possible to see her together with her husband, and she was discharged home with Home Care support services. Contact with me was sporadic on an "as need-ed" basis.

Four months later Helen's condition exacerbated; she found it difficult to walk and was re-admitted to the Rehabilitation Centre. Various stresses continued to affect Helen. These included her continued physical losses, her concern about herself for the future and her role as mother which, she saw in jeopardy.

Helen was also concerned about the possibility of needing a wheelchair as MS is a progressively debilitating disease. Indeed, the team argued she required one but Helen feared that her husband would have difficulty accepting it. However, she refused to allow me to see her husband on this matter, despite a remark made by him about the wheelchair while transferring her to the car. Helen interpreted this as her husband's rejection of the chair and categorically stated shortly thereafter, that she was no longer going home. Helen's refusal to be discharged to her home aroused sympathy in some members of the team, who viewed the situation only through the clients point of view; her husband was the brute, he was uncaring and unaccepting. This counter reaction in some ways reinforced some secondary gain in Helen and the continued dependence on the Rehabilitation Centre.

There were two major unresolved discharge problems: housing and financing for an electric wheelchair. Applications were sent to various housing agencies. Some hadn't any vacancies and the others required legal separation from the spouse and the division of property (home owned by Helen and husband). Helen would not consider legal separation. Another option was a boarding home, but she would require private attendants for transfers and this could not be provided without verifying whether her husband's insurance would pay the costs. Helen refused to have the husband contacted. The MS Society was contacted to finance the wheelchair. Due to their policies, they could not offer assistance if she was eligible for general welfare assistance.

A conference was set up with the team to examine the options.

A community social service worker advised the team that a nursing home bed had just become available. The worker knew the pressure of discharge — the patient's progress had plateaued and the team generally considered her ready to leave. Helen visited the nursing home a day later with a nurse as she was beginning to break her relationship with me (just as impulsively as when she had broken her relationship with her husband!). She felt I, too, was letting her down and she stopped talking to me.

Following the visit to the nursing home, Helen returned distraught and angrily sought me out in the office. "You should have given me a gun instead," she announced and stalked out. Staff on the ward were convinced that she was possibly suicidal but I maintained this reaction was not a threat to her life. Rather Helen needed to vent her anger.

By staying as long as she had in the Rehabilitation Centre, Helen had many dependency needs met. All avenues toward living independently in the community were thwarted by Helen. She viewed the nursing home as the end — the ultimate in being dependent.

Having only one option, Helen took a paradoxical stance and announced several weeks later that she was, after all, returning home. It was the lesser of two evils to choose what she saw as a fragile relationship with her husband with whom she didn't or couldn't communicate, where she deemed she would be more independent than choosing a nursing home where she would be dependent. To understand Helen's actions one has to examine the psychosocial factors involved.

Losses started early for Helen when her mother suddenly died when she was only three. The stepmother didn't fill the void and the relationship was corrosive and filled with several disruptions by the stepmother leaving. This provided little atmosphere for a healthy ego development. Helen may have felt she also lost her father with his new marriage and blended family. Any affection he could have given her was divided amongst many. Her adult relationship with him was also only tolerable. At the age of seventeen she lost her nineteen-year-old brother, and sibling nearest in age to her, in a car accident.

The loss of self-esteem from a debilitating disability and functional body loss was also difficult for a person as proud as Helen. Her young daughter didn't understand why her mother was different, had difficulty walking and was embarrassed by Helen coming to her school. Helen's unresolved relationship with her mother and stepmother got in the way of Helen's relationship with her daughter. On an unconscious level she emotionally deprived her daughter. Just as she had been abandoned by her forty-two year old mother dying, she too at the same age of forty-two walked out on her husband and daughter. This had occurred in the same month following the anniversary of her mother's death. Here we have an anniversary reaction which is symbolically augmented by Helen and her daughter, who celebrate the same birth date and look alike.

Loss for Helen and the circumstances around the mother's death was shrouded with mystery and unacceptance. Her sister upon visiting her at the Centre found Helen angry and yelling that their mother committed suicide. Was this a fear of her illness and an angry projection onto mother?

In continuing to speculate that Helen never resolved her mother's death and abandonment, knowing that she never accepted her stepmother, we see her as having come through childhood, adolescence and now adulthood without essential nurturing and without a positive role model for the wife and mother roles. How did she cope?

She had coped by being bright, liking people in a guarded fashion but, never having had a reciprocal ego-building relationship, she found it difficult to relate to people intimatel; ie., her husband, sister and brother. She wanted positive nurturing relationships but also fought them.

She also coped by being capable and independent. A discharge plan that included a nursing home elicited fears of dependency. Helen reacted and impulsively rejected the nursing home. She simultaneously rejected her social worker and their long-standing relationship. Though Helen's chosen plan of returning home surprised us in its timing, her move toward independence quietly pleased us all.

This independence/dependence theme together with the unresolved feelings of loss made Helen vulnerable, angry and an impulsive person. However, she was also a fighter who strove to be as independent a client as possible. Helen tested out the viability of a team, she corroborated the need for family/couple assessment and counselling where psychosocial issues are often painful, she used the rehabilitative process in directing her own conferences and advocacy/discharge plans and confronted various systems in the community and, in so doing, had the ultimate power.

References

Browne, J. A., Watt, S. & Kirlin, B. A. (1981). Conclusion: A challenge for change. In J. A. Browne, B. A. Kirlin & S. Watt (Eds.), *Rehabilitation Services and the Social Work Role: Challenge for Change* (pp. 348-362). Baltimore, MD: Williams & Wilkins.

Champeau, T., Greene, G., Apedaile, M. & Jackson, Z. (1989). *An Outcome Goal Oriented Model for Social Work Intervention with Rehabilitation In-patients and their Families.* Ottawa, Ontario (Canada): Department of Social Work, The Rehabilitation Centre, Royal Ottawa Health Care Group.

Dejong, G. (1983). Defining and implementing the independent living concept. In N. M. Crewe, I. K. Zola & Associates (Eds.), *Independent Living for Physically Disabled People* (pp. 4-27). San Francisco, CA: Jossey-Bass.

Eisenberg, M.G., Griggins, C. & Duval, R. J. (Eds.), (1982). *Disabled People as Second-Class Citizens.* New York: Springer.

Ell, K. (1985). The role of social work in rehabilitating people with disabilities. In E. L. Pan, et al. (Eds.), *Annual Review of Rehabilitation: Vol. 4* (pp. 145-177). New York: Springer.

Katz, A. H. (1981). Self-help and rehabilitation. In J. A. Browne, B. A. Kirlin & Watt (Eds.), *Rehabilitation Services and the Social Work Role: Challenge for Change* (pp. 177-186). Baltimore, MD: Williams & Wilkins.

McColl, M. A., Skinner, H. A. (1988). Concepts and measurement of social support in a rehabilitation setting. *Canadian Journal of Rehabilitation, 2*(2), 93-107.

Romano, M. D. (1981). Social worker's role in rehabilitation: A review of the literature. In J. A. Browne, B. A. Kirlin & S. Watt (Eds.), *Rehabilitation Services and the Social Work Role: Challenge for Change* (pp. 13-21). Baltimore, MD: Williams & Wilkins.

Chapter 27

DISCHARGE PLANNING AND THE ROLE OF THE SOCIAL WORKER

Mary Ciotti, MSW, CSW
Susan Watt, DSW, CSW

Abstract

This chapter examines the role of social workers in the planning and execution of discharges from a general hospital setting. Attention is paid to the groups of patients who need assistance and the kind of care they need following hospitalization for acute illness or trauma. The therapeutic, facilitator, broker, advocate and case manager aspects of the role are discussed from the perspective of the patient, the health care team, families and the community. It is argued that social work is the most appropriate profession to fulfil this role. A case example that demonstrates the complexity of discharge planning concludes the chapter.

DISCHARGE PLANNING AND THE ROLE OF THE SOCIAL WORKER

For the hospital, the patient is both the target of its activity and a necessary inconvenience to its operation. When the patient stays in the hospital beyond the time absolutely necessary to repair a "broken part," inconvenience becomes aggravation. From the hospital's point of view, it would be so much easier if the broken part could be brought into a repair shop or depot, worked on and returned to the owner, preferably without a money back guarantee.

The analogy to the broken part and the service centre may be amusing, but also points to the central problems of the health care system; both the cost effectiveness and the human problems of staff-patient and staff-staff interaction. To simply bring the broken hip, rather than the frail, "little old lady," to the hospital to be fixed would save weeks of care on the part of hospital staff, weeks of boredom, worry, and frustration on the part of the patient and her/his family and would avoid, most of all, the problem at the end point — how to get this broken hip out of the hospital.

Families would no longer have to debate the relative merits of two-storey houses, portable commodes, visiting homemakers, or dispensing three medications each on a different time schedule from the other. No one would have to find excuses why her/his brother should take mom to his house rather than send her to a sister. Family members would not have to argue with the hospital about discharge dates and arrangements, nor would they have to cajole the patient into accepting less than optimal plans for care, nor beg the hospital into changing the arrangements of the system to meet pre-existing commitments such as family or work. Hospital staff would no longer complain about under-utilization of their skills and could achieve the ideal, interdisciplinary team model of combining multi-disciplinary skills without serious debate about the human elements of patient care. In short, communication would become direct, functional and largely non-contentious and non-existent. Stress for all concerned would be reduced and the job would be done.

But Orwell's 1984 has come and gone and, despite many advances in the technology of medicine, society has not achieved the goal of separating the person from the illness, or medicine from other human needs. People bring to the hospital the hopes and expectations, the problems and dilemmas, the relationships and grievances of the world outside. They do not check these needs, these biases, these human dilemmas in the admitting department and, hence, not only their medical conditions, but also their other issues conspire to create a wide range of situations in which thoughtful, careful and creative discharge planning is required by patients, their families and hospital staff. In this chapter we will explore the role of social workers in discharge planning in the general hospital including the present responsibilities and potential developments.[1]

THE CLIENTELE

The goal of the hospital is generally to treat acute medical problems. In many senses, the general hospital has become a production line measured by the volume of medical interventions or services performed. Thus, it is critical to keep the flow of patients moving through the system; to keep acute care beds available for the treatment of acutely ill patients. Therefore, in the broadest sense, the clientele for discharge planning in a general hospital is potentially anyone admitted to the hospital.

Most people who are admitted to a general hospital in Canada have a clear plan prepared well in advance of their discharge, complete with housekeeping, child care, babysitting, meal preparation and home health care, in an attempt to have control over variables and outcomes in their own lives. This type of planning helps reduce the usual anxiety experienced by individuals who must temporarily loose control over their day-to-day activities, their work and family lives, their privacy and their health and well-being as a result of coming into hospital.

But there is never a "convenient emergency," as people come to hospital often on an unplanned basis. Once in the hospital, the course of illness and treatment is not always predictable. All the careful planning becomes inadequate to meet the new circumstances. For example, a mother of three small children has been scheduled to have her gall bladder removed in two months time. She and her family have made plans for child care and her personal care during her recovery. But, late on Saturday night, she suffers from an acute gall bladder attack and is rushed to hospital for emergency surgery. Suddenly, a new plan is needed that requires the same careful attention to detail that,, over time, she thoughtfully had primarily constructed.

Social work becomes concerned with discharge planning when patients, for whatever reason, are not able to formulate an adequate discharge plan on their own. There may be many reasons why an adequate discharge plan requires the intervention of a social worker including the patient's lack of resources to make one, a previous discharge plan that is no longer adequate, the absence of the necessary social or emotional supports for formulating or executing a discharge plan, patients with unplanned admissions,, or complicated illnesses.[2] These patients are considered to be "at risk." Unless adequate discharge plans are made, these patients may need to be re-admitted to hospital because the patient is unsafe or deteriorating in the community. In very real terms, inadequate discharge planning may lead to serious complications that compromise recovery and may result in protracted care at home, re-admission to hospital, permanent and unnecessary disability or even death.

In Canada, social workers are called upon to work in any inpatient unit of a hospital from neo-natal to chronic-care wards. The patient could be a child in paediatrics, a woman in obstetrics or a person undergoing surgery, cancer treatment or psychiatric care. The Emergency Room, Intensive Care Unit and the Cardiac Care Unit, because of the nature of service, usually provide an urgent element to the discharge plan, with the result that social workers are asked to formulate, within hours, plans that are acceptable to the patient and family, meet medical needs, can be delivered through community resources and would have taken weeks to make left to the devices of the family alone.

A variety of conditions exist in which a social worker will assist with discharge. Underlying all of these is the understanding on the part of the social worker that the patient cannot formulate or carry out the plan unassisted. Some examples of situations are

1) the patient is demanding to leave hospital immediately and often against medical advice and a plan is needed to ensure the patient's safety;
2) the medical staff unexpectedly informs the patient that they are discharged and a plan is required to ensure follow-up and medically safe care in the community;
3) the patient must leave because the bed is needed for a more seriously ill patient and a plan that provides comparable community-based care is necessary;

4) the patient cannot return home either because of her/his level of functioning or need for care, and an appropriate bed needs to be found elsewhere or

5) the patient does not want to leave the hospital and a plan needs to be developed to provide care and reassurance outside hospital sufficient to overcome the patient's resistance to leaving.

Patients are of every age and stage, from birth to death, and from every socio-economic group and social strata. They require varying types of health care from acute intervention (e.g., asthma, myocardial infarction, acute infection, overdose, heart attack, etc.) through rehabilitation (e.g., arthritis, amputation, motor vehicle trauma), to chronic care and palliative care in the community or in alternative institutional settings.

The problems that patients present are as unique as the patients themselves, requiring special plans for each individual circumstance. For instance, a tiny baby, recently taken off of a respirator, will need round-the-clock care at home, informed parents who can provide that care or others to help them, special equipment, portable oxygen, perhaps financial assistance, a plan for coping with inevitable emergent situations and a host of other resources combined to form a manageable and safe plan for this child outside an institutional setting. Similarly, a child who must adjust to treatments for cancer needs the family to understand the treatment regime, the necessity of such treatment and be willing to help the child adjust to severe physical limitations that her/his illness will bring at home. An abused child who leaves hospital with limbs in casts may need the supervision or protection of the Children's Aid Society. A trauma victim who has sustained burns or a head injury may need long-term rehabilitation both in the hospital and in the community. The high-risk pregnancy patient sent to bed for the remaining 16 weeks of pregnancy, in addition to needing considerable assistance with physical care, also requires help in coping with the social and emotional consequences of this form of treatment and the anxiety that the threat of losing the pregnancy inevitably causes. A patient with AIDS seeks help to live with the knowledge that, at this time, there is no cure for this fatal illness and that the course of the illness includes a decreasing ability to function in a variety of spheres, including paid employment, and an increased need for assistance with basic activities of daily living such as bathing, dressing and eating. A patient with chronic schizophrenia also needs assistance in meeting basic tasks such as finding housing, employment and recreational outlets.

Social workers function in a variety of ways to help meet the discharge planning needs of hospitalized patients starting with ensuring that the information flow between the patient and the treatment team is adequate to respond to the patient's needs. Explaining options is an ongoing process for a social worker who provides a link for the patient with the treatment team with the goals of attempting to ensure that appropriate information flows to and from the team, sorting out information the team has not understood and helping patients formulate the questions they want to ask.

The social worker may also facilitate information flow between the patient and outside resources such as government departments or the legal system (e.g., helping the patient complete Vocational Rehabilitation Eligibility forms, involving the Public Trustee in securing the estate of an elderly, incompetent patient, advocating with the municipal housing authority for subsidized housing, advocating for special assistance from Regional Social Services for special equipment or drug benefits, etc.)

To serve this clientele, the social worker functions as a member of an interdisciplinary or multi-disciplinary team that provides services to clients to enable them to function outside hospital. The service provided starts with a psychosocial assessment of the patient in the context of significant others in her/his life. The worker then must develop a treatment plan that takes into account the medical and psychosocial needs of the patient and includes a concrete discharge plan.

The social worker involves whomever the patient has in her/his network. For example, relatives, friends or neighbours may be important sources of information in coming to understand how the patient functioned in the environment prior to coming to the hospital and are central to predicting how the patient will function after discharge. This task must be accomplished within a critical time frame, usually under pressure from one source or another, (i.e., family does not want an elderly person to go home, or the patient is refusing to return to the family, or the hospital needs the bed) with dwindling community resources and significant institutional pressures added to the equation.

Whether obtaining referrals from the attending physician, other team members, patients themselves or by case finding, social work discharge planning services are usually confined to the hospital. However, with the growing number of patients without relatives or friends, coupled with limited community resources and increasingly complex medical, social and psychological needs, social workers increasingly are involved with patients as a link to the future following discharge from the hospital.

PRACTICE ROLES AND RESPONSIBILITIES

The primary role of social work in a general hospital is discharge planning (Watt, 1977). Some hospitals have discharge planning departments that are dissociated from social work services and, hence, do not take into account the social and psychological factors/needs of patients central to the discharge plan that social work would endorse.

Social work uses an ecological perspective in viewing discharge planning including the individual, family and community resources in developing appropriate discharge plans. In other words, social workers try to get the best person-environment fit to meet the needs of patients.

In preparing a patient for discharge, the possible outcomes can be viewed on a continuum from the most favourable, i.e., a discharge to a place the patient eagerly requests; to the least favourable, i.e., a discharge to a place to which the patient is reluctant to go and certainly would not have considered prior to hospitalization. The task of preparing the patient on the continuum may be relatively straightforward and easy, or extremely complex and time consuming, involving working through the feelings of sadness and loss over leaving one's home, spouse, memories, perhaps a loved pet and most of all one's independence. Patients leaving the general hospital go either to their own home, the home of a friend or relative or to a facility in the community that will provide care (e.g., a lodging home, retirement home, home for the aged, nursing home, chronic hospital or hospice).

To arrive at a plan for discharge, the process ideally begins as soon as the patient is admitted. Patients who are "at risk" for discharge planning problems are most often identified by nursing or medical staff and a referral is made to the social worker connected to that medical service. Sometimes the patient or her/his family contact the social worker directly or request a referral. This situation often arises when the patient or family are facing immediate difficulties resulting from the person being admitted to hospital (e.g., child care, spouse care, income loss) or anticipate discharge planning problems (e.g., when a relative has been coping marginally in the community prior to the admission). On other occasions, social workers identify situations that can be anticipated to be problematic for discharge planning (e.g., a confused elderly person living alone with no family in the immediate area). In such situations, the social worker is undertaking a case finding activity.

Once a patient has been identified as being in need of service, the social worker must complete a thorough psychosocial assessment of the patient/family needs including a focussed social history. This assessment pays particular attention to the person's previous ability to cope in the community and the resources that may have been used to support her/his functioning.

Patients are asked to anticipate what issues may arise when they leave hospital and what resources they may bring to bear on their own situations. It is important for the social worker to examine the personal strengths of the individual so that an appropriate plan can play to the strengths of the individual rather than unnecessarily expose their limitations, hence putting them at risk. As a part of this aspect of the assessment, the social worker must determine the ability of the patient to understand her/his own medical needs and the implications of the illness on her/his ability to cope after hospitalization. Family members are consulted, with the permission of the patient, to determine what role they may play in providing for the patient after hospitalization.

Sometimes this assessment includes determining the mental status of the patient and the patient's ability to make decisions in her/his self- interest. Consultation with psychiatric staff may be required when the mental status of the patient suggests that the patient's competence has been compromised.

The information from this assessment and the social worker's formulation about the patient and her/his discharge planning needs are communicated to the treatment team in a variety of ways including charting, patient care conferences and direct contact with key team members. It becomes part of the team's considerations in planning treatment and determining an appropriate discharge time.

The social worker then draws up a treatment and discharge plan based on the combined assessments of all the health care professionals and modifies the plan whenever necessary depending upon the changing medical, nursing and social needs of the patient. When further care is required beyond acute care hospitalization the social work assessment, in combination with medical and nursing assessments, is used to make a decision about the level of care the patient will need at discharge (e.g., home care, lodging home, nursing home, chronic care, palliative care).

While working with the patient/family, the social worker enters into a contract with them specifying the purpose and goals of intervention. A family conference sometimes is used to bring all the members of the health care team together with the patient and the family to discuss treatment plans, discharge plans, and any changes or modifications. Until a family conference occurs, the patient/family usually sees only one member of the team at a time and may hear conflicting plans, thus the conference permits a forum in which the team tries to provide a unified picture of issues to the patient and family while getting their perceptions of the situation and the plan. Further, it provides an opportunity for misinformation to be corrected and misunderstandings to be set straight.

There may be a variety of reasons why the ideal plan cannot be enacted, including a lack of personal resources (e.g., absence of a substitute caregiver, lack of money, unsuitable housing), the absence of resources in the community (e.g., no convalescent beds, absence of 24-hour homemaking services, inadequate transportation, lack of day programs), patient or family resistance to the plan, pressure on acute-care beds, which can scuttle the best plan at any point, or disagreement about the plan among treatment team members.

When the ideal plan is compromised by any of these factors, an alternative discharge plan must be developed. Part of the role of the social worker is to identify for the team those patients and families who are "at risk" if discharged according to the revised plan. The social worker is then left with working on the obstructive forces that caused the plan to be compromised. This may entail tackling the team, to increase their understanding of the issues faced by the patient, or helping the family come to terms with the limitations of community resources or addressing the fears and disappointments of the patient highlighted by the discharge plan.

The social worker's treatment skills are called upon to work with the patient and family in an effort to come to terms with the issues that are blocking discharge. Illnesses often elicit old conflicts and problems that people believe they had resolved or at least buried. It is in the context of discharge planning that many of these unresolved matters emerge in the form of disagreement with the discharge plan or the inability to support the plan in any meaningful way.

Skilled intervention requires not only an understanding of the ideal discharge plan but also the mechanisms within the individual and family that make it impossible for them to either agree with it or carry out their responsibilities within the plan (e.g., the family who can "never find time" to explore the recommended nursing homes for auntie). In short, a full range of social work intervention skills with individuals and families may be called into play to help operationalize the discharge plan.

Therapeutic intervention is often used to help the patient and staff adjust to what is available versus what the patient would like or what staff feel the patient should be given. Help is given to the patient to adjust to what is both appropriate and available.

Therapeutic intervention involves helping a patient get used to the idea of discharge; i.e., getting into staged Activities of Daily Living (ADL) with less intervention and more independence on a Leave of Absence (LOA) over the weekend. For example, patients who are very ambivalent about giving up their homes to live in a home for the aged can use this staged adaptation to ADL to take an LOA at the home of their choice for the weekend, and providing they like it, can take longer L.O.A's to make the transition from hospital to community as smooth as possible. The social worker at this stage will assess how the patient does on the LOA's and play a facilitative role with the patient while playing an interpretive role to the team members — explaining to them what is going on.

Discharge plans often require the co-operation of community resources to be enacted. Specifically, the social worker may become a patient advocate when those community resources required by the patient are unwilling to fulfil their mandates (e.g., advocating for the admission of your sometimes confused patient who needs to be turned during the night with a nursing home that prefers lighter care patients who are competent). Advocacy may extend to specific team members who are unable or unwilling to do their part in the discharge plan or who put their own personal value set ahead of the needs of the patient.

The role of broker is central to the discharge planning function of social work. The social worker provides a link between the patient and the institution, and the community and its resources. The role may also be enacted between any of the elements within the hospital and the patient and her/his family. The goal is always to have the right resources available to the patient, at the appropriate time, in a form that is useful.

There are some underlying assumptions and myths that need to be addressed to make this goal possible. It is extremely hard for some health care team members to recognize and admit the following:

1) that all patients who are bright and alert may not be financially and/or mentally competent, a fact that is important in the patient's future;[3]
2) that all family members who profess to want their relative home with them may not be guided by the best interests of the patient and rather may have other motives such as guilt or greed, which may pose a threat to the patient's safety;
3) families sometimes give clear but indirect signals that they do not want the responsibility of care for their relative and other plans will have to be made despite the conviction on the part of the team that home is where the patient should go;[4]
4) that patients who are dependent upon frail, elderly spouses for care are putting themselves and their spouses at risk;
5) that information given by patients or families with memory impairments cannot be taken at face value and needs corroboration before being used as baseline data for an assessment and
6) that the weak and infirm may be being abused, neglected or taken advantage of and if this goes unheeded in hospital, we are returning the patient to a dangerous environment.

When social workers assess patients, it is abundantly clear to them that the hospital wants the patients out. At the same time, it is also very clear to them which patients are "at risk." Although there is an absence of solid research, the profession has known clinically for some time that the high risk group that needs professional discharge planning assistance includes the following constellation cited by the Ontario Association of Professional Social Workers (OAPSW, 1982):

  – abuse and/or neglect (physical)
  – isolation (physical, social) and/or transience
  – psychiatric history and/or severe behaviour problems
  – financial implications — loss or interruption of income
  – placement — need for continuing care

- treatment implications — non-compliance to treatment
- implied change in lifestyle, education, employment, family role
- change in self-image
- family behaviour adversely affecting patient or staff
- legal involvement
- frequency of admissions
- alcohol or drug abuse.

In addition, other high risk factors include patients admitted to hospital a long way from home, failure to thrive, or decreased functional ability as a result of trauma or illness.

Assessment and intervention have to be viewed together as including

1) the mobilization of patient's resources along with the mobilization of external resources and
2) advocacy within the team and the community and follow-up to see that resources have arrived and to reassess further needs and/or readaptation of medication.

POTENTIAL FOR ROLE DEVELOPMENT

If social work abdicates responsibility for discharge planning, the profession will be left with discharge planners who are "body movers," who have little regard for, or understanding of, the human systems dilemma. Patients who require discharge planning assistance are not a homogeneous group, yet discussions on discharge planning often wander into abstract treatises on "those patients" and more particularly "those old people" — removed from our own experience and entangled in a statistician's cat's cradle. One disentangling effort was made by Hall and Bytheway (1982) when they tried to develop an understanding of what the British system call "the blocked bed." They found little agreement about the nature cause, or cure for the "discharge planning problem." They concluded that,

The blocked bed, far from being a relatively easy thing to identify and count, turns out to be something shaped by a particular view of what a hospital is and does. From an observers point of view, its attraction and interest lies in the way it highlights and encapsulates anomalies in the treatment of elderly patients. While the definitions offered are apparently non-controversial, the term itself is full of affective content. (Hall and Blytheway, p. 1984)

As the population ages, as medical technologies expand their claims to amelioration and cure, it is possible that a recognition will be needed that "people just don't die the way they once did." Indeed, stays in hospitals will become part of the expected life experience rather than an exception. Institutional care for some part of life may become the norm rather than a failure of the medical system to cure, and discharge planning will become an increasingly significant role for social workers in health care settings.

The advocacy role may extend outside the hospital into the community in informing policy-makers and resource planners as to what services are needed. Social workers may influence policy development by monitoring, documenting and publicizing needs to the appropriate political bodies.

The profession needs more empirical and theoretical research to provide it with "High Risk Predictor Scales" for patients in hospitals. Perhaps with such hard data the work of the discharge planner could be more easily understood, since social work has known for quite a while what is meant by the best person-environment fit, but at best this is taken idiosyncratically on the basis of the personal reputation or personality of the social worker making such a claim. Clinically, one knows who are the high risk elderly, who are the high risk children and who are the high risk infants and parents. The profession needs to translate practice knowledge into published and disseminated literature that can be used to teach other health care professionals the importance of these data in making appropriate intervention plans.

Also, increasing interest has been shown in the development of the case manager role for social workers as an extension of social work's commitment to discharge planning. As the health care system, both institutional and community based, becomes more complex and is inextricably bound to the social service system with its hurdles and pitfalls, the need for professional guidance increases. The individual ventures into a booby-trapped maze of rules, regulations, eligibility clauses, exemptions, prohibitions, limitations, time-lines and disjunctures all obscured in a snowstorm of forms each requiring another professional opinion and at least two signatures. For the individual there is no single place to get information, and rarely one right answer.

In the health care system, the social worker is the professional with the knowledge and training to guide the individual (and indeed other team members) through the maze, pointing out the pitfalls as they are encountered without getting bogged down and without misleading the patient. For example, patients frequently are unaware of the benefits packages provided through the workplace, including short-term disability benefits, or they may be unaware of the obligations that they have to apply for those benefits that are available, within a given time period. A part of good discharge planning takes into account the financial resources, including disability income, that is at the disposal of the patient.

CONCLUDING REMARKS

Until a comprehensive discharge plan that meets the needs of the patient is developed and enacted, active treatment hospitals and professional personnel cannot claim to have completed their jobs. Therefore, no matter what the circumstances, corporate president to welfare recipient, electively admitted or rushed to intensive care, headed for complete recovery or destined to live in an institution for her/his life, the patient is entitled to help with the discharge planning process, which will ultimately influence the health of that individual, her/his family and the community.

It is important that hospitals provide quality care including quality discharge planning. The better the hospital, the more sensitive it is to discharge planning, to its meaning for patients and their families and to the resources committed to the process.

CASE EXAMPLE[5]

You have been called by the nurses in the Cardiac Care Unit (CCU) to see Mr. A. because he is worried about his wife who is staying temporarily with his daughter and her family in another city six hours drive away. When you arrive, the nurses tell you that the daughter is here with her mother and wants to speak with you. They also indicate that the patient's wife has Alzheimer's disease.

When you go to see that patient you find a 78-year-old frail man on a cardiac monitor. His wife and daughter are in the room and you decide to have them remain. You have great difficulty in getting him to answer any questions about lifestyle and causes of stress. Mrs. A., also 78, fidgets with her hands, smiles and does not seem to be able to understand questions asked of her.

The patient has had a severe heart attack and is describing his living situation as close to ideal. He has a few regrets in his life but does not want to discuss them with you since he does not see them as important. Occasionally his daughter interrupts his narrative and reminds him that his story is not quite accurate. He asks her for clarification, considers what she says, and replies that he is not sure what has happened but if his daughter says it happened, it must be so. He adds that his memory is "not what it used to be." The daughter is unable to hide her shock on learning that her father is still driving since the family doctor had asked him to stop two months ago. The patient doesn't remember being asked.

You quickly learn that the couple has only one daughter who is married with school aged children; she lives and works full time in a city six hours away. There are no other relatives.

Since Mr. & Mrs. A. sold their rural home of 40 years, a hobby farm, and moved into an urban retirement village six months ago, there are few friends nearby. They are now living in a small one-floor cottage chosen because the patient loved to garden. Gardening had been his mainstay since his retirement at age 65 on a fixed, non-indexed pension. It had been his major form of relaxation and exercise; it had made him feel useful. His wife had been a homemaker; she was never employed outside the home and has no source of independent income except Old Age Pension.

In the past year Mr. A. could not manage to leave his wife alone for more than a few minutes at a time as she would get lost and frightened. He could not pursue his gardening on the farm and could not keep up with the household chores his wife used to do. Since living in the cottage, Mr. A. has been rather depressed, his gardening never amounts to more than 1-1/2 hours a day and the rest of the day he is not free since his wife is afraid to go out and cannot be left alone. She cannot perform her homemaking role so Mr. A., at age 78, is learning to do the housework, to do the washing and to prepare meals.

This history is presented by the patient in a rather off-handed fashion with no indication that, in light of his heart attack, the situation at home might have to change. He seemed not to have considered any alternative care for his wife and generally gave the impression that they would just continue to muddle on as they had been doing.

With the patient's consent, and away from the patient and his wife, you discuss discharge planning with the daughter. She quickly identifies many issues including the following:

1) no one is monitoring a complex set of medications at home and both Mr. and Mrs. A. have several medications, which Mr. A. is having increasing difficulty in remembering either for himself or for his wife;

2) the mother's diagnosis of Alzheimer's disease has never been communicated to the daughter and she wonders where the nurses learned the diagnosis and if it is true;

3) she feels that the family physician is keeping her mother sedated to relieve her father of pressure, but is not addressing the basic problem; i.e., Mrs. A. needs institutional care since she is a behavioural problem, not oriented to time or place and is deteriorating;

4) Mr. A. is fully responsible for all household tasks plus 24-hour-a-day care of Mrs. A. who has lately become quite anxious, argumentative and unreasonable; she will not bathe, change her clothing or have her clothing washed and

5) Mr. A. refuses to discuss the possibility of nursing home placement for Mrs. A. since all their finances went into buying the new cottage and he does not want to be separated from his wife when he believes she needs him most.

The daughter stated that her father has been making decisions for himself and his wife for years and did not consult the daughter before the recent move. She knows that he needs to feel useful and in control and she has been reluctant to interfere. Now she regrets that she did not stop the move, although she does not know what she might have done.

She is unfamiliar with the resources for seniors in this community and so are her parents. As well, the parents see seniors' groups as old people's social clubs rather than informed, peer resources. They have never been "joiners." The daughter is eager for any help and wants to arrange for care for both her parents as she sees both of them being at risk if the home situation does not change and her father does not get help to deal with her mother. The daughter's help can only be temporary; she is able to take time off work to care for her mother while Mr. A. is in hospital, but cannot sustain this plan for long.

Carefully, the root problems (the mother's increasing incapacity, the lack of long-term planning) were broached with the daughter resulting in the understanding that a formal psychiatric assessment of Mrs. A. needed to be done and that the daughter should make this request of the family doctor. She further understood that placement of her mother in an appropriate institutional setting could reasonably be assumed to be the outcome of such an assessment. However, appropriate institutional resources were scarce and placement could take up to two years. Since finances were tight, a facility with multi-layers of care needed to be found so that both parents could live together under one roof.

In the meantime, the patient would probably be discharged home within a week. Mr. and Mrs. A. had a number of immediate needs including a careful mental status examination for Mr. A., resources in place to help care for Mrs. A. on an adequate and predictable basi, and to have Mr. A. recognize the needs of both himself and his wife for resources and be able to accept what was available.

The community-based resources that you identify as needed by Mr. and Mrs. A. include a case manager in the community, a nurse to monitor medication, a homemaker for laundry and meal preparation on some days, meals-on-wheels for other days, visitation services for Mrs. A., community psychiatric assessment for Mrs. A., a contact at a Seniors Centre to facilitate socialization, peer support, and additional resource information, and an application for disabled transportation services so that Mr. and Mrs. A. can get to appointments without Mr. A. driving.

References

Bolaria, B. S. & Dickinson, H. D. (1988). *Sociology of Health Care in Canada*. Toronto: Harcourt Brace Jovanovich.

Hall, D. & Bytheway, B. (1982). The blocked bed definition of the problem. *Social Science in Medicine, 16*, pp. 1985-91.

Kane, R. A. (1975). Discharge planning: an undischarged responsibility? *Health and Social Work, 5*(1), pp. 33.

Novak, M. (1988). *Aging and Society: A Canadian Perspective*. Scarborough: Nelson Canada, 1988.

Schlesinger, E. G. (1985). *Health Care Social Work Practice*. St. Louis: Times Mirror/Mosby College Publishing.

Shapiro, E., Noralou P. R. & Kavanagh, S. (1980). Long term patients in acute care beds: Is there a cure? *The Gerontologist, 20*(3), pp. 342-49.

Watt, S. (1977). *Therapeutic Facilitator: The Role of the Social Worker in Acute Care Hospitals in Ontario*. Doctoral Dissertation, University of California, Los Angeles. Ann Arbor: Dissertation Abstracts, 1977.

Endnotes

1 There is no single model for discharge planning in general hospitals in Canada. In some hospitals discharge planning comes under the general responsibilities of Departments of Social Work, while in other facilities it is the responsibility of a separate "Discharge Planning Unit" which may or may not be administratively responsible to social work. Sometimes a lone discharge planner, often a nurse, serves the whole hospital. In other facilities, no discharge planning function is clearly associated with a staff position.

2 Complicated illnesses include all major traumas, illnesses that are often fatal (e.g., major cancers), those involving loss of functional abilities (e.g., amputations, strokes) and the presence of two or more major psychiatric illness are also included in this category, as are a variety of debilitating chronic illness (e.g., rheumatoid arthritis).

3 If incompetency is detected, special safeguards must be put in place to ensure the safety of the individual and her/his property.

4 Some of the indicators include lack of visits or phone calls, the inability to carry out necessary preparations such as securing a hospital bed or wheelchair and the raising of a full range of reasons why any proposed date for discharge couldn't possibly be accommodated by the family.

5 This case study is a composite of situations presented in practice. Any resemblance to a single individual is purely coincidental.

Chapter 28

DISCHARGING PATIENTS FROM AN ACUTE-CARE HOSPITAL

Margaret A. Dimond, MSW, ACSW
Theresa Jansen-Santos, RN, MSN, MA

Abstract

One of the major components of social work in hospitals is the responsibility to provide post-hospital planning to patients and their families. Discharge planning involves many client variables, environmental constraints and resources, in addition to hospital professionals working toward optimum patient recovery. Examples will be used as a guide in grasping the enormity of a social worker's role in health care both today and in the future.

DISCHARGING PATIENTS FROM AN ACUTE-CARE HOSPITAL

THE CLIENTELE

The acute-care hospital in a metropolitan area can range in size from 100 to 1,000 beds or more. The authors' frame of reference for this chapter is Henry Ford Hospital in Detroit, Michigan. This is a 900 bed inner city teaching hospital where clientele include the frail elderly, who populate the immediate geographic area, together with many ethnic and socioeconomic representations of society, living in the city, the suburbs and the outlying areas of the state. Health care staff also represent large concentrations of diverse ethnic populations. The emergency room is a major trauma centre and as many as 50% of the admissions to the in-patient hospital are unscheduled and emergencies in origin. Substance abuse (alcohol and drugs) is a major problem within the immediate neighbourhood with consequent high populations of trauma injuries related to violence.

Contrary to the emergency patient population are those patients and families attracted to Henry Ford Hospital through the world wide reputation of its physicians. Because of the teaching sector of this acute care centre and the medical experts whose reputations in many specialties elicit clients from throughout the USA and abroad, a large percentage of patients travel such distances with a specific need hoping to have their life threatening condition alleviated.

All of the clientele come with a problem unique to their own situation. Within the 900 bed acute hospital there is a demand for a team of social workers assigned to specific areas (e.g., critical care, neuro surgery, etc.) depending on patient acuity and needs. In Henry Ford, social workers are in a multi-disciplinary department with registered nurses. Social workers and registered nurses with community health background are teamed to "cover" a specific area of the hospital. Daily, they communicate and collaborate on assignments, using the expertise of each discipline to assist clients and staff with the most appropriate discharge plan. The hospital is also a centre for transplant surgery (cardiac, liver and kidney) in the area. A very specialized role of counselling and discharge planning is played by the MSW, dealing with these clients adjusting to major life-threatening situations. Problems encoun-

encountered by clients served in this setting can best be illustrated by a few specialty case examples:

a. *Trauma Surgery*: A 22-year-old female is admitted through the emergency room with a gun shot wound to the abdomen. When the patient stabilizes, she describes her situation: she is homeless and has been living in abandoned buildings. She steals food from grocery stores and prostitutes herself to obtain money for drugs. Her family lives in another state and she is divorced from an abusive husband. A child was taken from her by the courts two years ago, due to neglect. The physician refers the patient to social work for post hospital planning.

b. *Neuro-surgery*: A 32-year-old male is admitted because of headaches that cause him to have a temporary loss of vision. The patient is confident that after further testing, a medication can be prescribed to alleviate his painful headaches. After thorough testing, this patient is diagnosed with a brain tumour. The neuro-surgeon explains to the patient that the outlook is bleak and that surgery would only have a 30% chance of success. The patient has been married four years, has children, aged three and one, and just bought a home last year. His job does not provide disability or death benefits and he does not have a life insurance policy. Patient and family are in a state of shock.

c. *Kidney Transplant*: A 40-year-old male presents to the nephrology service with end stage renal disease. The patient has been on dialysis for eleven years, but is deteriorating rapidly. The patient's only hope is for a kidney transplant. He has been on the waiting list for four years, but has not been successfully matched with a donor. The patient has a brother living in Germany. His brother is the only possibility for a living related donor. The patient has not seen or spoken to his brother since their father's death eighteen years ago, when they had "a falling out" over money. The patient is reluctant to contact his brother, and knows the expense to fly from Germany to the United States will be exorbitant. The patient is losing more strength every day. A social work consult is made for psycho-social intervention.

The above reflect a case diversity present in most urban medical facilities. Specifically, clients may be admitted as a result of a psychosocial or emotional crisis, combined with somatic complaints. Hence, a singularly medical model is insufficient in evaluating both the complexity and comprehensiveness of the patient/family assessment and post hospital planning. As Rock

(1987) stated, "Discharge planning is a psycho-social process involving life choices for patients. It is thus at the core of a problem-solving approach to psychotherapy."

The patient's needs may range from needing help in coping with illness, to the patient's inability to remain independent, thus requiring an alternative to returning home. There are some patients who will be recognized as "high risk" at time of admission:

> High risk patients are those patients who are automatically noted at hospital admissions with a presumption that discharge planning will be needed. These patients include those who have attempted suicide, are elderly, and/or confused, have numerous chronic illnesses, are without family or support systems, or may refuse medical treatments. (Mullaney & Andrews, 1983)

PRACTICE ROLES AND RESPONSIBILITIES

Prior to the onset of insurance reimbursement changes in the United States, and an increased popularity of HMO's and managed care, discharge planning was a function that social work education did not recognize as critical. Counselling patients around adjustment to illness issues was the primary function of hospital social workers. However, the outlook for the 1990s in medical social work is that good discharge planning skills are a means of delivering comprehensive services to the patient and family, and the key to job security.

Discharge planning is no longer an option, it is a necessity in hospitals. Many health care professionals need to be involved in the post hospital planning process, with the social worker acting as collator of the information and liaison to patients/families.

There are two organizational imperatives in the delivery of quality discharge planning services. First, one department, discipline, or division must be designated as the co-ordinator of discharge planning for the institution. Second, discharge planning must be conceptualized as a total organizational effort involving all clinical departments and the hospital administration.

I. Elements of Discharge Planning

Before a social worker in the health care setting can embrace discharge planning as an integral job function, the multiple aspects of the process need to be examined. The American Hospital Association states that discharge planning "is an interdisciplinary hospital-wide process that should be available to patients and their families in developing a feasible post hospital plan of care. The discharge planning main principles outlined by the AHA include: indication of the patient's preferences for post hospital care, evaluation of the patient's capacity to care for themselves, an assessment of the patient's living conditions, identification of health or other community resources needed to assure continuity after discharge, and counselling of patient and family to prepare them for post hospital care" (AHA, 1984).

The fundamental aspects of preparing a discharge plan can be broken down into five major categories: screening, assessment, planning, intervention and follow-up.

1. Screening

The way in which discharge planning screening is implemented varies from hospital to hospital. The ideal way to screen patients is prior to admission (e.g., for an elective surgical procedure). With the emphasis on shortened lengths of stay, and increased pressure to avoid delays in timely discharge, many hospitals have developed a screening tool used at the time the patient is admitted. The necessity for a screening tool to identify high risk categories of patients, assists nurses to recognize the need for a referral to the Department of Social Work and Discharge Planning. Such an instrument is presented in Figure 1.

Figure 1. *A Screening Tool Discharge Planning Used at Henry Ford Hospital*

DISCHARGE PLANNING SCREEN - ADULT   DATE:_____
HENRY FORD HOSPITAL   NAME:_____
ADMISSION DATE:_____   MRN:_____

Please check any and/or all criteria appropriate. If a patient meets any of the criteria, generate a consult to the Department of Social Work and Discharge Planning.

__ Patient with a dependent family

     ember or questionable support.

__ Evidence of difficulty coping with illness – in need of social work counselling.

__ Suspected abuse or neglect.

__ Homeless or financial crisis.

__ Admitted from a nursing home or needing nursing home placement.

__ Injury resulting from violence. _

__ History of mental illness– retardation.

__ Other

__ Unscheduled readmission within 2 weeks.

__ Followed by home care nurse prior to admission.

__ Patient dependent for ADL's – no capable caregiver in the home.

__ Age 80 or over.

__ Patient/family non-complaint with medical regimement.

_ Skilled nursing needs after discharge (i.e., diabetic teaching, care of wounds, catheters, feeding tubes, teaching use of meds, mobility problems, cast care, nutrition teaching, monitoring of unstable vital signs.

__ Equipment needs in the home– hospital bed, wheelchair, commode, etc.

DISCHARGE PLANNING CONSULT:

__ No consult indicated; date: _____   Signature:_____

__ Consult initiated; date: _____   Signature:_____

515

The staff nurse, prepared to conduct an admission assessment, is the primary link to social work, as the first information is communicated from the patient and/or family to the admitting nurse during the admission assessment interviews (Pearlman, 1984).

> Data collection for discharge planning begins at admission: the admission history form includes pertinent questions. The nurse assesses the patient's living environment, how well the patient has been coping at home, and who is available to assist after the hospitalization. With the assistance of other team members, collecting data, assessing needs, planning for home care and following up continues throughout hospitalization. Consequently, last minute "panic planning" has decreased. (Clausen, 1984)

The key questions that need to be raised when screening patients are multi-faceted. Some examples include:

1. What is the patient's admitting diagnosis, and/or other complications? Will the illness hinder optimum recovery (e.g., patient admitted with a stroke, neurologic functioning affected)?
2. Is the patient in a high risk age group (e.g., 70 and over) for discharge planning needs?
3. What is the patient's family and home situation; is there a lack of support?
4. Can the patient perform functional (ADL's) activities independently (e.g., arthritic patient, states she cannot cook for herself due to her arthritic hands)?
5. Will the patient need skilled or personal care upon discharge (e.g., visiting nurse or home health aide)?
6. Is patient or family having difficulties adjusting to illness?
7. Does family need information regarding medical legal issues (guardianship or power of attorney)?
8. Will patient need linkage to community resources and agencies upon discharge (e.g., cancer society support group, home delivered meals)?
9. Does patient/family have a realistic view of any lifestyle changes that illness has mandated? Do they need ongoing education or monitoring (e.g., heart attack victim needing to change diet and exercise patterns)?
10. Has patient had a major change or loss in her/his personal life in the last year (death of spouse)?

in the last year (death of spouse)?
11. Are patient coping mechanisms intact?

2. Assessment

The next step in identifying the patient's needs is direct contact with the patient and family by a social worker or discharge planner in order to formulate her/his impressions of the situation and provide a clinical assessment for other health care professionals. Often, the assessment of problems and issues is utilized to better plan for post hospital options (e.g., a hospital social worker may often be asked to assess a mother's ability to care for her multiple-needs child hospitalized for surgery). The initial discharge planning interview with the patient or family will give direction to the remainder of the intervention needed. The interview should cover:

1. General background information on patients: social/emotional demographic, financial and support networks.
2. Anticipated needs of the patient at the time of discharge (physical, emotional, financial and social).
3. Ability of the patient and family to meet these needs.
4. Available support and resources.
5. The patient's wishes regarding his care after discharge.

The social worker draws on crisis and systems theory and explores the patient/family's ego functioning to assess the impact of illness on the patient/family matrix. This assessment is also an indicator of the patient/family's ability to make realistic decisions around patient care issues.

This assessment also includes discharge planning subject matter. The role of the medical social worker includes looking at patient/family financial, psychosocial and lifestyle alterations that will result from the hospitalization.

3. Planning/Intervention and Follow-Up

According to the American Hospital Association's *"Guidelines of Discharge Planning,"* the following must be considered when looking at medical social work intervention:

> The psycho-social and physical assessment and counselling of patients and families to determine the full range of needs upon discharge and to prepare them for the post hospital

stage of care is a dynamic process. This process includes evaluation of the patient's and the family's strengths and weaknesses; the patients condition, understanding the illness and treatment; the ability to assess the patient's and family's capacities to adapt to changes, and where necessary, to assist the persons involved to manage in their continued care...in complex situations...the plan should ensure follow up with the patient, the family and/or community services providing continued care to determine the discharge outcome. (AHA, 1984)

In this context, the social worker may be analogous to an orchestra conductor. It is essential to ensure that all pieces of the post-hospital plan come together in a timely and harmonious manner. Further, the social worker may have to be the change agent for major decisions faced by the patient and family. Conjointly, the social worker walks the delicate line of adhering to the patient's right to self determination, while simultaneously assessing the feasibility of the patient's plans and wishes. This process is most easily termed informed consent.

A primary goal of health care decision making is to respect and enhance patient autonomy by protecting the patient's rights to self-determination. From this principle flows the fundamental doctrine that the competent adult patient has a right to make informed choices and decisions about medical care, treatment and placement in health care facilities. Neither a competent adult, nor his duly authorized representative must accept treatment based on someone else's belief that treatment would be in the patient's "best interests." (AHA, 1987)

Hence, the patient must remain at the helm of all decisions on post hospital options. The primary responsibility of the medical social worker is not only to present the patient with all possible options and consequences, but also to respect the decision the patient has made, whether or not the social worker agrees with that decision.

Bear in mind that individual and institutional health care providers are not responsible for arranging the ideal discharge; instead they must only take steps to do what is reasonable under the circumstances and to eliminate those risks that may have a foreseeable negative impact upon the patient's health or medical status. (AHA, 1987)

The theories around a client's right to self determination taught in social work programs are employed regularly by medical social workers. It often becomes the responsibility of that professional social worker to weigh ethical, legal and practical dilemmas when developing a discharge plan for a multiple needs patient.

Some examples of discharge plans ranging from simple to complex are as follows:

1. The patient is discharged home to the same environment from whence he came. Many patients who return to their own homes after hospitalization need no social work/discharge planning department intervention. Although all patients need discharge teaching, the floor nurses and the physician traditionally have addressed these needs with the patient. For patients whose condition would indicate a need for a home-care nurse to assure follow-up of care, a home-care referral is processed to an agency of the patient's choice, assuring the patient and family that a professional nurse will visit on the day following discharge to carry out physician's orders.

2. Mary Brown, a 60-year-old single female, lives alone in a single family dwelling. She has severe arthritis, is unable to leave the home unassisted and is a newly diagnosed diabetic. She is obese and has never followed any regular eating pattern. Efforts by the nursing staff to educate her concerning her diabetes and insulin administration while in the hospital have been somewhat effective; however, because Mary is a slow learner, there is some doubt about her readiness to be discharged from the hospital. A referral is made to the Department of Social Work and Discharge Planning.

The social worker learns from the patient that she has no siblings or close friends who could help her at home. Her income is such that she cannot afford to hire anyone to help her or to obtain help from the Department of Social Services. Mary agrees to have a visiting nurse stop by early in the morning on the day following discharge to assist her with insulin administration and then continue teaching her diet therapy. The social worker sends a referral to a home-care agency of the patient's choice and the patient is able to leave the hospital safely. The visiting nurse makes several visits and gradually Mary is able to manage her care independently.

Mary's is an example of a routine social work assessment and home care referral. More complex needs of patients can also be met in the home if there is a strong enough support system; that is, family members who are willing and able to learn the care with the help of the home care resources available. It is not uncommon for cancer patients to return home to the care of their families, who manage the pain control with small medication pumps, and to rely on visiting nurses and social workers in the home to assist with care of the terminally ill.

As exemplified in the case of Mary Brown, the first responsibility of a medical social worker is to determine the multitude of needs a patient may present an admission. However, to think the job is completed at that point would be a fallacy. It is necessary to look beyond the surface, and into the care of social work tasks and roles within the acute care setting.

POTENTIAL FOR ROLE DEVELOPMENT

The health care system in the United States appears to be in an ongoing state of flux. Cost saving measures affect both hospital workers and patients. Downsizing bed size and lay-offs are headline material for articles involving acute-care topics. Where, then, is an overhead expense department such as social work in the future blueprint of a community or teaching medical facility?

Such a discussion must include an introspective review of inherent social work attributes. The following are a list of assumptions related to skills integral to comprehensive-care delivery:

1. Social workers have the skills and knowledge necessary for discharge planning.
2. Social workers are committed to helping patients make informed choices.
3. Social workers collaborate with other professional colleagues in discharge planning.
4. Discharge planning occurs within a prescribed time frame that has an impact on decision making. (Blumenfield & Lowe, 1987)

Timely and effective post hospital planning is of utmost importance, as hospitals move toward capitated payments from HMO and government health insurance.

The charge of discharge planning has been given to social work departments in most American hospitals. This responsibility creates exciting new changes and challenges for the medical social creates exciting new changes and challenges for the medical social work role, some issues that are essential to integrate for the future are

> Emphasizing the importance of discharge planning screening at the time of the patient's admission, and devising mechanisms to ensure the completion of screening. In many settings, social workers are hampered and frustrated by large caseloads and limited time. Because of this, screening and/or early involvement with those suffering from catastrophic illnesses is essential to continuity of care from admission through discharge and follow up....The social worker can facilitate communication with the physicians and medical staff or aid the family in understanding hospital procedures. (Blazyk & Canavan, 1986)

Social workers may utilize other health care professionals to assist them with early screening and identification of patients with psychosocial or post-hospital needs. Rounds with staff nurses and residents can be a routine function. Admission screening criteria and case finding will be key for future early case referrals.

Social work departments joining resources with other professions will be an option in the future. At Henry Ford Hospital, nurses and social workers work in the same department and utilize each other's expertise in order to develop comprehensive post-hospital plans. A case management approach has recently been implemented, which teams a registered nurse discharge planner and a social worker to a specified unit.

Social workers in medical settings must be prepared to be adaptable in defining their future roles and responsibilities. However, that does not mean negating the multi-faceted talents and potential that social workers possess and have to offer in hospital systems.

CONCLUDING REMARKS

To the social work student, who is in the process of defining interests and choosing a specialty, the field of medical social work may seem somewhat listless. Sigmund Freud, Murray Bowan and Virginia Satir never included the electrifying aspects of medical social work in any of their publications. Jane Addams may have passed up exciting discharge planning opportunities at a Chicago area hospital in order to start Hull House. Further, discharge planning has never been one of the top rated responsibilities in the social work field.

However, discharge planning is a dynamic process. It includes the theoretical aspects of crisis intervention, problem solving, ego-centred therapy, systems approach, and grief/loss counselling. The job role is never stagnant, and the medley of clientele is an exciting challenge.

The interaction with other disciplines in a hospital setting can diversify the social work role and strengthen the social work identity as a health care team member. Physicians, nurses and allied health therapists look to social workers for their expertise in many areas. Social workers are educated to see the continuum of care, and treat the patient in a holistic manner. The initiative and innovation of social work talent cannot be duplicated easily by any other profession.

Post-hospital planning is just one aspect of the broad spectrum of opportunities a medical social worker has. The future of this field in the future is one of unlimited potential.

CASE EXAMPLE

Esther, a 67-year-old black female, was seen in Henry Ford Hospital's emergency room on November 13, 1988 because of severe respiratory distress. She was admitted to the hospital Intensive Care Unit and placed on a ventilator. After extensive testing she was found to have Amyotrophic Lateral Sclerosis (ALS) also known as Lou Gehrig's Disease. ALS is a progressively degenerative disease of the muscles usually affecting the arms and legs initially and progressing to the respiratory muscles and those of swallowing as the patient becomes more debilitated. Esther's case was somewhat atypical since she had use of her upper and lower extremities, but minimal use of respiratory muscles. A referral was made to the Department of Social Work and Discharge Planning four days after admission. It read as follows, "Pleasant, alert 67-year-old black female presented as respiratory insufficiency/hypoventilation. Work-up is positive for ALS. Patient can only breathe short periods off of ventilator. She will need home vent for survival. No family, limited resources. Please evaluate."

The discharge planning nurse from the department of social work and discharge planning visited Esther in the ICU on the day that the referral was received. Because of Esther's inability to speak due to shortness of breath, and the insertion of an endotracheal tube, a tablet and pen was provided. In an effort to make an assessment of Esther's resources in the community, the worker asked for some vital information. (i.e., names of family or friends who could be reached to assist Esther and the nurses in planning for Esther's future needs after she is well enough to leave the hospital.)

It was learned that Esther is an unmarried retired nursing aide who lives with an elderly confused aunt in a two-storey home near the hospital. Her income is$ 650 per month (combined pension and social security income). Her home is paid for, and with the additional income of her aunt's monthly social security check of $500, Esther was managing comfortably prior to her illness. She has no brothers or sisters, has a rather close relationship with a second cousin (Erma) and is a member of a Baptist Church Community. Esther gave the telephone number of her cousin Erma by memory. The discharge planning nurse was able to set up an appointment with Erma and Esther while Esther was still a patient in the ICU. Esther verbalized (in writing) her understanding of the seriousness of her illness and the fact that she would be on a ventilator for the remainder of her life and would probably become progressively weaker. Esther adamantly expressed the desire to return to her own home on a ventilator with home care visits by nurses, social workers and therapists. The physician felt that placement in a nursing home was the only option because of the need for 24-hour supervision and assistance with personal care.

Within a few days, Esther was transferred out of the Intensive Care Unit; a permanent tracheostomy was performed and a portable ventilator (on a bedside movable cart) was attached by way of tubing to Esther's permanent tracheal opening. The physician stated Esther was medically stable and ready for discharge. While the worker in the social work department explored the possibility of placement in a nursing home, cousin Erma (respecting Esther's somewhat unrealistic wishes to return to her own home) explored all the possibilities of finding a 24 hour live-in companion to care for Esther and her aunt in their home.

Nursing homes that care for ventilator patients in the Detroit metropolitan area charge over $300.00 per day for patient care.

Medicare (federally funded health insurance for people aged 65 and over) pays less than one third of that cost. Unless Esther had the savings to pay for that care the only avenue open to her was to apply for Medicaid (a state funded welfare program for indigent people). After numerous calls to the experts on financing nursing home care of ventilator patients, it was learned that Esther would not be eligible for Medicaid until a certain number of Medicare hospital days were "used up," resulting in the hospital losing over $50,000.00 if the patient were to remain in the hospital until she were eligible for Medicaid.

Cousin Erma was unable to care for Esther because she is already raising four toddlers while her two daughters work. However, Erma's daughters are willing to assist their mother in relieving a primary care giver if one could be found. Because of the nature of Esther's illness and the continued dependence on a breathing machine, numerous (otherwise eager) live-in caregivers turned away not wanting to take on such a responsibility. After two weeks of searching the community with telephone calls and want ads, the Baptist pastor knew of a woman who was a new member of his congregation who was looking for a place to live. Esther and her cousin interviewed the woman, checked her references and made an agreement with her for free housing and meals and a few hundred dollars income per month.

The prospective caregiver agreed to be taught the care of the ventilator while Esther was still in the hospital. She spent several hours during the week in the patient's room of the hospital until the respiratory therapists assessed that she could safely care for Esther at home. Cousin Erma and her daughters also learned the procedure of caring for the tracheostomy and the ventilator. The visiting nurse who would be providing follow-up care in the home also met the caregiver in Esther's presence and the respiratory therapist reviewed the post-hospital care required with the entire team.

Esther's insurance paid for the cost of the home care team to make intermittent visits in her home as medically indicated and paid for the cost of the equipment needed.

Esther returned to her home, had minor safety adaptations made in her environment, was linked up with senior community resources for "Meals on Wheels" and home maintenance programs by the community health team and today is continuing to live with her aunt in her own home.

She walks with her ventilator at her side, has received speech therapy and has regained the use of her speech. She knows that some day her disease may dictate nursing home placement, but she is grateful for every day that has been made possible for her to live in her own home. A card on a plant in her living room (sent to her by the discharge team) says its all, "Welcome Home."

References

American Hospital Association. (1987). Discharging hospital patients: Legal implications for institutional providers and health care professionals. *Report of the Task Force on Legal Issues in Discharge Planning*. Chicago, Illinois.

Blazyk, S. & Canavan, M. M. (1986). Managing the discharge crisis following catastrophic illness or injury. *Social Work In Health Care, 11*(4), 30-31.

Blumenfield, S. & Lowe, J. I. (1987). A template for analyzing ethical dilemmas in discharge planning. *Health and Social Work, 12*(1), 49.

Clausen, C. (1984). Staff RN: A discharge planner for every patient. *Nursing Management, 15*(1)1, 59.

Evashwick, C. J. & Weiss, L. J. (1987). *Managing the Continuum of Care* (pp. 365-382). Aspen Publications: Rockville, MD.

Mullaney, J. W. & Andrews, B. F. (1983). Legal problems and principles in discharge planning: Implications for social work. *Social Work in Health Care, 9*(1).

Pearlman, I. R. (1984). Discharge planning: The team is behind you. *Nursing Management, 15*(8), 36-38.

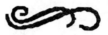

SECTION III
Community-Based Practice

Chapter 29

SOCIAL WORK PRACTICE WITH FAMILY CAREGIVERS OF FRAIL OLDER PERSONS

Ronald W. Toseland, PhD
Charles M. Rossiter, PhD

Abstract

This chapter begins with a review of the major issues and concerns facing family caregivers of frail older persons. Described next are generic social work roles and responsibilities, together with consultation, co-ordination and management, three specific social work roles that are commonly used in work with family caregivers and frail older persons. Opportunities for social workers in outreach, supervision, co-ordination and delivery of services, particularly as they relate to the needs of underserved family caregivers are also described. The chapter ends with three case examples illustrating the three previously discussed social work practice roles.

SOCIAL WORK PRACTICE WITH FAMILY CAREGIVERS OF FRAIL OLDER PERSONS

Family caregivers represent a large and growing clientele whose needs for social services will increase dramatically in the coming decades. In America it is estimated that nearly 5.1 million older people living in the community need assistance with some aspects of personal care or home management activities (AARP, 1986). These needs range from occasional assistance with specific tasks, such as shopping or household chores, to around-the-clock monitoring of serious health problems. Because chronic and acute health problems increase in frequency and intensity with advancing age, and as the population itself ages, the number of older people needing assistance will increase dramatically in future years and family caregivers will provide most of this care.

THE CLIENTELE

Close family members, particularly spouses and adult daughters, are the most likely to assist frail elderly with physical and emotional needs. Shanas (1968) suggested that the decision about who will provide care follows a "principle of substitution." If a spouse is available, he or she is most likely to provide care. If a spouse is unavailable, an adult daughter is most likely to become the primary caregiver. In the absence of adult daughters, daughters-in-law, sons, sons-in-law or other relatives, neighbours or friends are most likely to provide care.

A recent national survey (Stone, Cafferata and Sangl, 1987) has provided helpful data about family caregivers. Most caregivers are female and between the ages of 40 and 65. Their average age is 57.3 years. One third are over 65. Many have some chronic health problems themselves. Most are wives (29%) or adult daughters (23%). Most are white, although 20% are non-white. A majority (57%) report low or middle incomes, and nearly a third (31.5%) report income at poverty or near poverty levels.

The average age of the frail elderly who are the recipients of family care is 78. Twenty percent are over 85. The majority (60%) are female. About half are married (51.3%), but many (41.3%) are

531

widowed. Only 11% live alone. The remainder live with spouses, children or other family members.

I. The Effects of Caregiving

The effects of providing care for a frail older family member are many and complex, yet caregiving can be a rewarding and fulfilling experience. Whether done out of love, a sense of responsibility, perceived obligation to restore equity in interpersonal and intergenerational relationships, compassion, guilt, the expectation of reward or a complex combination of reasons, caregiving can have a variety of beneficial effects.

Caregiving provides a meaningful role and an important purpose for some caregivers. There is often a heightened sense of self-esteem and self-worth because caregivers feel they are "doing the right thing," and are doing it with altruistic motives. Caregivers take pride in their efforts and feel good about being able to help. Pride and satisfaction are enhanced when caregivers are praised for their efforts by family members, friends and others whose opinions they hold in high regard.

At the same time, social workers should be aware that caregiving can be extremely demanding and extremely stressful. Caregiving often involves a long-term commitment, which taxes the resources of the caregiver. The average caregiver devotes four hours each day to caregiving. Twenty percent of all caregivers in the previously mentioned national survey provided care for five or more years, eighty percent provided care seven days a week and virtually all spousal caregivers reported daily caregiving (Stone, Cafferata & Sangl, 1987).

Caregiving demands can create stresses that overburden caregivers and endanger their well-being. Stress is "a relationship between the person and the environment that is appraised by the person as taxing or exceeding his or her resources and endangering his or her well-being" (Lazarus & Folkman, 1984, p. 21). A number of elements of the caregiving situation contribute to the stress experienced by family caregivers.

Uncertainty is a major factor. Frail elderly needing care are usually in a condition of declining health. As the care receiver's health status worsens, new demands are made on the caregiver that, in turn, often necessitate changes in the relationship between the caregiver and the care receiver. For example, an adult child may have to learn new ways to relate to an increasingly dependent parent. Spouses may have to learn to live without some pleasurable aspects of their marriage relationship that ailing partners can no longer provide. To be effective in working with caregivers, social workers in health care settings should be sensitive to the shifting dynamics of the caregiver-care receiver relationship and the profound psychological adjustments that have to be made as the care receiver's health status changes.

Middle-aged women, a group that includes the majority of caregivers, are particularly vulnerable to the stresses of caregiving (Brody, 1981; Fengler & Goodrich, 1979). In addition to the changing nature of their relationship with the care receiver, adult children often have to cope with the demands of work and their own family. Many caregivers are employed outside the home either full time or part time (Stone, Cafferata & Sangl, 1987; Toseland, Rossiter & Labrecque, in press). Employed caregivers must make adjustments in their work schedules to fulfil their caregiving responsibilities. Stone, Cafferata and Sangl (1987) found that 9% of caregivers quit their jobs in order to provide care, and over half said the demands of caregiving required them to reduce the hours they work, to rearrange their work schedules, or to take time off without pay.

Stress from caregiving can have a negative effect on caregivers' psychological, social and physical well-being. Depression, the most frequently cited symptom of caregiver stress, has been estimated as high as 52% (Sanford, 1975). In addition to depression, some caregivers are troubled by anxiety, anger, frustration and excessive guilt and self-blame. In a recent study, when caregivers were asked what problems resulting from caregiving troubled them the most, psychological problems were mentioned more than twice as often as any other type of problem (Toseland, Rossiter, Labrecque & Beckstead, 1988).

The sources of emotional distress for caregivers are complex. Many caregivers feel guilty about how they are performing their caregiving duties. They believe they are not doing enough for the care receiver. Others feel guilty about the feelings they have about caregiving. For example, they may feel anger or frustration because of demands made by the care receiver and then, later, feel guilty for their anger.

A general sense of anxiety and worry often permeates the caregiving situation (Hasselkus, 1988). Caregivers worry about the health of the care receiver. Little changes, such as the development of a small sore, or refusal to eat a meal, can be frightening, as any small change may be an early warning of further decline in the care receiver's health. Caregivers worry that a decline in their own health might interfere with their ability to fulfill essential tasks for a frail family member. Social workers can help caregivers reduce their feelings of worry and anxiety by enabling them to ventilate their concerns, to sort out realistic and unrealistic fears and to develop plans for coping with emergency situations that may arise.

Caregiving can also contribute to social and interpersonal problems. Leisure and recreational activities are often restricted. Caregivers frequently feel socially isolated, lonely and trapped (Farkas, 1980). Conflicts with other family members about caregiving responsibilities are common (Cantor, 1983). For example, some caregivers express resentment toward siblings for "not doing their fair share." Others experience interpersonal conflicts with their own children or spouses as increasing demands are placed on their time by a deteriorating care receiver. Caregivers sometimes express this latter problem to social workers by stating that they are in a "no win situation," caught between the competing needs and demands of different family members while feeling that they have no time for themselves. At such times, it can be helpful for social workers to suggest one or more family meetings in which concerns are shared, conflicts are de-escalated and family members are helped to work together to improve problematic aspects of the caregiving situation.

Disturbance of normal sleep patterns, lack of appetite and psychosomatic complaints are also frequently experienced by over-burdened caregivers (Golodetz, et al., 1969). In addition, lifting, transporting and other physically demanding aspects of certain caregiving situations can cause physical injuries. Many caregivers have little or no prior experience in providing care and are not aware of the most effective or efficient home care techniques. Social workers can assist caregivers with the physical demands of caregiving by encouraging them tp

1) develop a plan for taking better care of themselves;
2) obtain periodic respites from caregiving;
3) acquire the knowledge and skills necessary to perform home health care tasks without endangering their own health and
4) utilize available home health care resources to supplement their own caregiving efforts.

PRACTICE ROLES AND RESPONSIBILITIES

Social work practice roles and responsibilities with caregivers are similar to those engaged in with other client groups. For example, social workers establish therapeutic relationships, assess needs and plan, implement and monitor intervention plans as they would with other client groups (Pinkston, et al., 1982; Rubin, 1987). However, specific adaptations in these roles and responsibilities are needed when serving caregivers.

I. Engaging the client

Making initial contact with caregivers is sometimes difficult. Caregivers are often reluctant to ask for help. Some believe it is their responsibility to provide care and that relinquishing that responsibility would be like abandoning the person for whom they are caring. This is particularly true in certain ethnic groups where family bonds are strong and normative expectations prescribe family caregiving as a duty. Caregivers may never have had to ask for help before and pride may become an obstacle. In other situations, it is the frail older person who resists or refuses "outside help."

For all these reasons, it is important for social workers to engage in active outreach efforts that make information about services and resources for family caregivers available throughout the community. In-person telephone contacts with health, social service, religious and civic organizations, press releases, newspaper stories, appearances on talk shows, public service announcements on radio and television and educational forums and workshops sponsored by community planning agencies are all useful ways to reach out to caregivers (Toseland, 1981).

Social workers must be particularly careful in designing outreach strategies for particular groups of caregivers. For example, black and Hispanic caregivers rarely respond to traditional avenues of publicity used in recruiting participants (Toseland & Rossiter, 1988). Extensive personal contacts through established and trusted religious and service organizations in the community are a much better approach to engaging this client group (Garcia-Preto, 1982; Roberts, 1987).

Male caregivers are also difficult to reach. Davies, Priddy & Tinklenberg (1986) found that even though men from a larger caregiver program had requested a smaller, male-only support group, these men were only willing to participate when they were told that the group was part of a pilot program to test a new intervention. They were unwilling to join the group for the sole purpose of gaining help for themselves as caregivers.

II. Establishing a Relationship

Once initial contact has been made, the primary job of the social worker is to develop a trusting and supportive relationship with the caregiver. Research suggests that many caregivers are reluctant to admit to difficulties with caregiving, even though they may be nearly overwhelmed by them (Toseland, Rossiter, Labrecque & Beckstead, 1988). We have interviewed caregivers who break down and cry during interviews and say they have not slept well in weeks. Yet when asked about their stress levels, these same caregivers say they experience "a little" stress. Many caregivers would rather bear their burdens in silence than risk being seen as complaining or uncaring. To make it possible for caregivers to acknowledge and accept their thoughts and feelings about the caregiving situation, social workers should be attentive and empathic listeners.

Caregivers have a strong tendency to believe that those who have never been in their situation cannot possibly understand what they are going through. If the worker has had direct experience with caregiving, appropriately timed self-disclosures can be helpful for universalizing the experience and for increasing trust and promoting client self-disclosure.

In addition to providing an opportunity for ventilation, the worker should be a supporter and an enabler. As a supporter, the worker provides encouragement and validation. Many caregivers are unnecessarily critical of themselves. They believe that they are not doing all they could do in the caregiving role. They also tend not to take as good care of themselves as they could, foregoing their own needs for those of the care receiver and other family members. As a supporter, the worker applauds any indication that the caregiver is taking better care of herself or feeling better about how well she is providing care. The worker also validates and elucidates more fully the caregiver's experiences, so that the caregiver can better accept "negative" feelings such as anger or frustration with the care receiver.

As an enabler, the worker encourages change by helping the caregiver to become motivated to mobilize social resources to improve a problematic situation. To function effectively as an enabler, the worker must be aware of available community services that caregivers and care receivers are likely to need. The worker should also be aware of eligibility requirements and other difficulties in accessing services. The worker may help a client complete necessary paperwork to obtain services, or go to an agency with the client to provide support and assistance during the application process. In some situations, the worker may also act as an advocate for the client, helping her to obtain services that are not readily available.

III. Assessing the Situation

As the caregiver discloses information about herself and her situation, the worker assesses her needs. Assessment of the caregiving situation includes not only understanding the caregiver and the care receiver but also their relationship to each other, to other family members and to the larger society. Ideally, social work assessments should include a thorough examination of the current physical, psychological, emotional, social, financial and environmental status of the caregiver and the care receiver and their life situation. Any pertinent historical data bearing on the current situation should also be ascertained. For a detailed discussion of comprehensive assessment techniques for the frail elderly see Kane (1985) or Kane and Kane (1981).

In many health care settings, it is important for social workers to co-ordinate their assessments with allied health personnel. For example, important information about the course of a specific illness, the effects of medications, and the physical limitations and abilities of the care receiver may be provided by doctors, nurses, and physical therapists. For this reason, comprehensive assessments of the caregiving situation are sometimes best made by a health care team.

As team members, social workers may be expected to focus their assessment on certain dimensions of the caregiver or care receiver functioning. For example, the social worker may be the member of a team who is responsible for gathering pertinent data about the caregivers' social support networks. To gather such data, the social worker might inquire about the individuals who comprise the caregivers support network and the quality of existing relationships with these individuals. The social worker might also assess the extent to which the caregiver is satisfied with existing informal social supports and whether the caregiver is motivated to reach out for additional support. The social worker uses this information, with information obtained from other team members, in the development of a comprehensive assessment of a caregiver's situation.

IV. Developing an Action Plan

Based on the needs and desires of the caregiver and the care receiver, an intervention plan is developed. A major decision in developing an action plan is what mode of intervention would be most beneficial. For caregivers with very high levels of psychological stress, those with very personal issues or those who are not ready to share their experiences with a group, individual counselling may be most appropriate. In contrast, family or couple counselling may be most appropriate in situations where interpersonal tensions and conflicts predominate (Gallagher, Lovitt, and Zeiss, 1989; Horowitz, 1985). Recent research indicates that support groups may be particularly useful for reducing feelings of loneliness and isolation and for increasing social support (Gallagher, Rose, Rivera, Lovett & Thompson, in press; Green & Monahan, 1987; Montgomery, 1988; Toseland, Rossiter, Labrecque & Beckstead, 1988). Participation in a support group helps caregivers to feel understood and supported by others in similar situations.

Another important decision when developing an action plan is determining the most appropriate role to take in a particular situation. A social worker may play three primary roles: consultant, co-ordinator; and manager. Each of these roles requires different actions and responsibilities on the part of the caregiver and the worker, which are summarized in Table 1.

Table 1

Social Worker Roles And Responsibilities When Working With Family Caregivers

Selected Decision Criteria	Consultation	Co-ordination	Management
Type of Caregiver	An independent, responsible, dedicated, informed caregiver with time, energy and competence to cope with the situation and to meet the care receiver's needs	A competent caregiver seeking assistance because she is becoming overwhelmed with duties and responsibilities and needs help on a regular basis	Unable to fulfill many caregiving duties; e.g. caregiver out-of-town and unable to take care of many of the day-to-day needs of the care receiver
Need for Outreach	Greatest	Intermediate	Least
Responsibility For Care	Primarily with caregiver	Shared between caregiver and social worker	Primarily with social worker
Assessment	Caregiver plays a major role by providing information about the care receiver's condition	Social worker and caregiver jointly assess situation	Social worker plays a major role in determining accuracy of information
Development of Action Plan	Caregiver in consultation with social worker	Social worker in consultation and collaboration with the caregiver	Social worker responsibility in consultation with caregiver and care receiver
Implementation of Action Plan	Social worker maintains occasional contact on an "as needed" basis	Social worker provides some services and helps caregiver and care receiver to utilize other community services as needed	Social worker delivers or arranges for the delivery of services to the care receiver
Monitoring Action Plan	Caregiver monitors situation and requests support, information and help gaining access to services as needed	Caregiver monitors care plan day-to-day, social worker maintains regular contact monitoring situation and the delivery of services	Social worker monitors day to-day situation of care receiver, co-ordinates services and arranges for services as needed

Table 1 was developed to distinguish and highlight the differences in the three roles. In actual practice, in many health care settings social workers are expected to move comfortably from one role to another depending on the changing needs and evolving health status. At one point in time, the worker may act as a consultant. Later, the worker may act as a manager. With some family caregivers, the social worker may actually play different roles with the same person. For a particular concern, a family caregiver may only need consultation to be able to cope with or resolve a problem. However, for another concern, the caregiver may need the social worker to act as a co-ordinator.

V. Consultant Role

The social worker should consider adopting the consultant role in situations where the caregiver is an independent, responsible, dedicated person who

1) prefers to take primary responsibility for the care receiver's needs without deferring to outside help;
2) is coping effectively and
3) has been assessed by the social worker as in need of relatively little assistance.

When deciding on whether the consultant role is most appropriate, the social worker assesses the caregivers' capacities and abilities, together with their current level of functioning. The social worker should also assess the client's willingness to ask for help when needed. Because of heavy caseloads, social workers may not be able to contact the client very frequently. Therefore, before assuming a consultant role, social workers should assess whether or not they can rely on the client to acknowledge a need and request appropriate help.

The worker must also consider the ethical issue involved in deciding whether to adopt the consultant role or a more active role. Ethical issues often arise when, in the worker's judgment, clients could benefit from more help than they think they need. A general practice principle that applies in this situation is that, unless caregivers or care receivers are in jeopardy of endangering themselves or some other third party, the clients request for autonomy should be respected. The worker should also guard against adopting a consultant role because of caseload considerations.

Because caregivers who are independent and competent feel the least need for assistance, active outreach is often needed to inform them about community resources and services that may be helpful to them in their current situation, or in the future. But no matter how this group of caregivers comes into contact with social workers, Table 1 clearly indicates that the responsibility for providing care and ensuring the well being of the care receiver remains primarily with the caregiver.

When social workers adopt a consultant role, the caregiver is expected to play a major role in the assessment process. The worker recognizes that the caregiver is intimately familiar with the situation and can provide information about the care receivers' functioning in a variety of areas. Because caregivers in this category are responsible and competent, they are relatively reliable and accurate sources of information on which the social worker heavily depends.

As a consultant, the social worker may be asked to help the caregiver and the care receiver with a wide variety of environmental, social, behaviourial and emotional problems. Tonti and Silverstone (1985) indicate that some of the more frequent are helping with

1) the nursing-home placement decisions;
2) adjustments in living status such as when a frail older person moves from her own home to her daughter's home;
3) behaviourial and emotional problems;
4) resistance to some aspect of what the caregiver believes is in the best interest of the care receiver;
5) alcoholism and
6) mental impairments such as Alzheimer's disease.

When developing and implementing action plans, social workers who are acting as consultants rely heavily on caregivers' input. For example, a caregiver requests information about a day care centre that the worker had mentioned during a previous contact. When the worker provides the information, the caregiver indicates that she will contact the centre and enrol her mother. As consultant, the social worker supports the caregiver and informs her that she is available should any obstacles be encountered when attempting to obtain the service.

Social workers may adopt a consulting role following a period of more active intervention. In the consultant role, social workers sometimes maintain occasional contact to assure that the situation remains stable, to offer information and advice or to help the caregiver connect with needed services. At other times, workers respond on an "as needed" basis with information, advice and other help that is requested by the caregiver.

VI. Co-ordinator Role

Because of the care receiver's situation, or the caregiver's ability or willingness, more assistance may be needed than can be provided by a consultant. Some caregivers have provided care for many years without the need for the assistance of a co-ordinator, but then become overwhelmed by their duties and responsibilities. The care receiver's physical or mental condition may deteriorate, or the caregiver's abilities may become diminished by health problems or increased responsibilities at work or at home. For caregivers who are overburdened and finding it difficult to cope with increasing stress, the social worker should consider adopting the role of co-ordinator.

Table 1 indicates that outreach efforts can be a little less active with this group of caregivers than with those who can benefit from consultant services only. Stress resulting from feeling overburdened is more likely to motivate caregivers in this group to seek services for the care receiver, or for themselves. Another reason why outreach does not have to be as active with this group of caregivers is that they are more likely to be receiving services, and referrals from health care and social service providers are likely to be more frequent.

In the co-ordinator role, the worker and the caregiver share responsibility for ensuring that the care receiver is receiving needed services in a well-planned fashion. In assessing the situation, social workers should gather as much data from the caregiver as possible. However, they are more likely when acting as a consultant to make independent assessments of caregivers' and care receivers' abilities.

In the co-ordinator role, the social worker may provide needed services such as individual, family or group counselling. For example, the worker might provide brief family counselling to reduce conflicts about caregiving responsibilities in the family and to develop a more complete and co-ordinated plan of care.

The social worker helps to arrange for whatever services the caregiver needs by being an enabler, a broker or an advocate. The worker also helps the caregiver to arrange for services for the care receiver. This might include helping the caregiver to develop a written schedule of informal and formal services (Toseland, Derico & Owen, 1984). Such a schedule could be posted on a refrigerator or a bulletin board so that appointments for different services will not be confused or improperly scheduled.

Once the services for the caregiver and the care receiver are in place, the worker generally maintains regular contact with the caregiver. However, the caregiver continues to take the day-to-day responsibility for the functioning of the care receiver and for the appropriate provision of services. As co-ordinator, the worker makes sure that any difficulties the caregiver is having in fulfilling these responsibilities are resolved during their regular meetings.

Since the caregivers and care receivers with whom a worker might function as a co-ordinator differ greatly in their levels of stress, capabilities and needs, it is important for the worker to consider each caregiver's short- and long-term needs. For example, if the caregiver is an older person who has chronic health problems, the worker might need to maintain more frequent contact than with a caregiver in better health.

VII. Management Role

The management role is differentiated from the co-ordinator and the consultant role by the degree to which the caregiver is involved in the plan of care for the care receive, and in the implementation and monitoring of that plan. When caregivers are unable to fulfill duties and responsibilities necessary for the care of frail older persons in their family, social workers who are managers ensure that proper care is provided.

As Table 1 indicates, there is frequently less need for outreach with this kind of caregiver and care receiver because many are already in contact with health and social services for chronic health problems before their need for management arises. In other situations, acute medical problems bring older persons who are unable to care for themselves into contact with medical social workers.

In the management role, the worker takes primary responsibility for helping the care receiver live independently in the community. After gathering information from the caregiver and the care receiver, the worker makes independent assessments of the condition of the caregiver and the care receiver and determines what services, if any, are needed. To whatever extent possible, the practitioner involves the caregiver and care receiver in the development and implementation of the action plan. The social worker then either provides the needed services or obtains whatever services are needed and sees to it that these services are administered in a timely, efficient and effective manner.

As a manager, the social worker is expected to

1) develop a comprehensive assessment of the client without relying solely on the judgments of a family member who may not be able to fully provide what the care receiver needs;
2) develop a comprehensive plan for the care of the frail older person whose needs cannot be fully provided for by a care receiver;
3) implement the plan by providing and co-ordinating health and social services to meet the needs of the caregiver and the care receiver and
4) monitor the situation to ensure that the caregiver and the care receiver are receiving services that are appropriate (Steinberg, 1985; Steinberg and Carter, 1983; Johnson and Rubin, 1983).

In the management role, workers maintain frequent and regular contact with care receivers to make sure their needs are being met. Continuous monitoring is important because, unlike in the co-ordinator or consultant role, the manager can't rely on a family caregiver to monitor the day-to-day situation or to take appropriate action should problems arise in the delivery of services. As manager, the worker either provides all needed services for the care receiver or ensures that they are being provided by informal caregivers or by professional health care and social service providers.

POTENTIAL FOR ROLE DEVELOPMENT

There is great potential for the development of social work with family caregivers, particularly in the following areas:

1) home health care;
2) collaborative work with peer helpers;
3) outreach and
4) the development and management of caregiver support programs.

544

The anticipated increase in the elderly population, particularly the old-old, in the next forty years, means that there will be a greater need for home care services in the future. Social work services are an important component of comprehensive home care. Therefore, as the population ages, the social work role in home health care should increase dramatically, unless social work services are performed by other professional helpers. This is a real possibility as nurses and psychologists trained in community work are now performing many of the tasks traditionally considered to be a part of the social work domain.

Working with peer helpers is a second expanding area for social workers. There are thousands of self-help support groups for caregivers sponsored by organizations such as the Alzheimer's Disease and Related Disorders Association. Working with peer helpers requires a relationship that is based on mutual respect. Social workers can build such relationships by reaching out to peer helpers and developing a relationship with them. Ideally, these should be based upon social worker's appreciation of the experience that peers can bring to the situation, the therapeutic benefit of self-help efforts for both the person giving help and the person receiving help and a respect for the autonomy of peer helpers.

There is a also a need for innovative outreach and culturally sensitive intervention programs in minority ethnic communities. Cultural differences may influence how minority caregivers respond to efforts to inform them about services and also how they respond to intervention efforts (Haber, 1984; McGadney, Goldberg-Glen & Pinkston, 1987; Taylor & Chatters, 1986). Therefore, development of appropriate, culturally sensitive outreach and intervention programs is an important, albeit neglected, role for social workers.

Fourth, there is an expanding role for social workers in the development and management of caregiver programs. In future years, there will be an increasing recognition of the importance of family caregivers to the welfare of frail older persons. With this recognition, social workers will be called upon to develop and implement programs of support to assist caregivers. This, in turn, will require social workers to be familiar with the array of administrative, supervisory and direct service skills that are necessary to develop and manage a social service program.

CONCLUDING REMARKS

The typology of social work roles outlined in Table 1, and described in this chapter, is intended as a heuristic device to elucidate the range of social work practice roles in health care settings with caregivers of frail older persons. In actual practice, the roles may not be so clearly differentiated. The changing needs of caregivers and care receivers, the availability and receptivity of different referral sources, the degree of emotional burden experienced by caregivers in relation to specific caregiving tasks and responsibilities and a host of other factors often necessitate the use of a mix of roles and practice strategies in a particular situation. Still, the typology that has been presented should serve as a useful guide for social work practitioners deciding on the most appropriate mix of roles and strategies to employ in the complex caregiving situations they confront in many health care practice settings.

CASE EXAMPLE

Social Worker as Consultant

Marie, at 43, is energetic, capable, well educated and in excellent health. She works as a freelance artist and has a self-defined work schedule. Her husband, Earl, owns a small business and his responsibilities allow him to take time off from work when necessary. Since he works only five minutes from home, he is available to respond to emergencies that may arise at home.

Marie's mother, Theresa, aged 83, had lived at Marie's brother's house for 7 years. While visiting Marie during her son's annual winter Florida vacation, Theresa experienced stomach pains, and was taken to the nearby hospital where she was diagnosed as having cancer. Following an operation, which was not able to remove all of the cancer, she moved to Marie's home to be closer to the hospital and to the rest of her family.

The immediate family was highly supportive. Marie's older brother and sister lived approximately a half hour away. Each volunteered to provide respite for Marie and Earl and each visited with Theresa at least one or two half-days per week while she was in the hospital.

Prior to discharge, the hospital social worker talked with Marie, Theresa and other family members about Theresa's situation. Marie's brother agreed to look after the paperwork, which Theresa had difficulty doing, regarding medical insurance and hospital bills. Marie agreed to have her mother continue to live with her but inquired about a service to "look in on Theresa" should she suddenly take a turn for the worse.

With the hospital social worker's help, Marie made some phone calls and arranged for services from a local hospice program. After contacting the hospital social worker and receiving a formal referral, the hospice team initiated regular contact with Theresa. The hospice program continued to provide services to Theresa, who remained mentally alert and able to ambulate with the assistance of a cane, until she died at home six months later.

Social Worker as Co-ordinator

Julie is an 82-year-old black women who is in poor health. Her husband, Jim, has advanced heart disease, diabetes, hearing loss and severe arthritis. The latter problem worries Julie, who fears that Jim will try to move about when she is not home, will fall down and hurt himself. Julie has always taken care of Jim and would not consider placing him. Their only child died 5 years ago in an automobile accident and there are no other immediate family members who live close enough to provide care for Jim. However, Julie has a close friend, Ann, who sometimes watches Jim and is a source of emotional support.

Julie was brought to the social worker's attention by Ann. When Julie refused to go to the community senior centre for their weekly card game, Ann went anyway. She mentioned that Julie seemed as if she was having an increasingly difficult time caring for Jim to a social worker who worked for an affiliated community health centre located directly across the street. The worker contacted Julie who said she was not feeling well and didn't think she had the strength to leave the house. However, since she knew the worker from previous visits to the centre, she agreed to a home visit. During several home visits over the course of a month, the worker concluded that Julie could use some help in caring for Jim. Julie reluctantly agreed to some help as long as she could remain in charge of Jim's care.

In assessing the situation, the worker determined that Jim's increasing deafness was an important problem. The worker consulted a non-profit agency for the deaf and through them arranged for Julie and Jim to acquire a telephone amplifier, a device to allow them to see captioning on television and a light hook-up on the doorbell so that Jim could see that someone was at the door when Julie was not at home.

The couple's financial situation was also problematic. Recently, they had incurred non-reimbursable medical expenses that their pension and social security checks did not cover adequately. Accepting any financial assistance was difficult for Julie, who had been brought up to believe that a person should avoid being "on welfare" at all costs. The worker explained to Julie that the taxes she had paid over the years entitled her to financial assistance now that she needed it. With the worker's help, Julie was able to re-frame her situation and realize that to refuse assistance might result in a deterioration of her own health condition, or that of her husband's. This, in turn, might cost society even more money in the long term. Therefore, she reluctantly decided to accept the worker's assistance and applied for food stamps and Meals on Wheels.

Convincing Julie to get out of the house and remain active was another issue that needed to be addressed. Julie's main concern was that Jim would fall down and hurt himself while she was out. The social worker recommended that Julie enrol in *Lifeline*, a program sponsored by a local hospital. They fitted Jim with a special device that hung around his neck and connected to the telephone, so that he could signal for help at any time.

Julie was also somewhat depressed about her situation. The worker, concluding that Julie was suffering from a mild reactive depression, helped Julie and her friend, Ann, who was also a caregiver, to enrol in a support group program for caregivers sponsored by a nearby family service agency. These sessions, and the other services that were arranged, proved to be very helpful, and soon Julie began going to the senior centre again. The social worker continued to monitor the situation by meeting with Julie at the senior centre on a regular basis, but provided no other active support for the three years she remained working for the agency.

Social Worker as Manager

Mary, aged 79, began living independently again after 32 years of hospitalization with a DSM-3 diagnosis of Bipolar Disorder, Depressed. In the early 1970s she was given a trial of lithium, which stabilized her mood swings.

Sarah, Mary's social worker from a social health maintenance organization (SHMO), first met Mary while she was an in-patient.

Together with the discharge planning team in the hospital, a small one-bedroom apartment was located for Mary with a landlord who had previously rented to former psychiatric patients and was tolerant if not sympathetic to their plight.

Sarah helped Mary to contact her niece, Gwen, who lived about a mile away, and who had not seen Mary in about 13 years. Gwen offered to assist Mary in any way possible, although it was clear that Gwen, who worked part time and had her own family, would not be able to provide a great deal of assistance.

Sarah helped Mary to pay bills and deal with other paperwork that Mary was not familiar with because she had lived so long as an inpatient. Gradually, Mary learned to handle most of her own affairs, except for complicated paperwork that she sometimes encountered when applying for or receiving health and social services.

Sarah encouraged Mary to enrol in a seniors-only day treatment program at the health centre. She also helped to arrange for transportation to and from the program. This arrangement worked quite well. Mary did not experience any difficulty until about 18 months after leaving the hospital. She stopped taking her lithium and soon became quite depressed.

Sarah, who had continued to see Mary on a monthly basis after setting up the day treatment program, went to see Mary in the hospital and arranged a plan with Mary and Gwen to keep Mary's apartment for one month until she could be stabilized and returned to the community.

Once Mary returned home, Gwen agreed to monitor Mary's medication. Every other day, Gwen stopped by to see Mary. She watched while Mary took her medication and she checked on the remaining pills to make sure that Mary was taking the correct dosage when she was not present.

Sarah arranged for Mary to have more frequent checkups to monitor her lithium blood level. She also arranged for Mary to attend the day treatment program again. As Mary's needs change, with Gwen's help, Sarah will continue to help Mary live independently.

References

AARP (1986). *A Profile of Older Persons: 1986.* Washington, DC: American Association of Retired Persons.

Brody, E. (1981). Women in the middle and family help to older people. *The Gerontologist, 21,* 471-480.

Cantor, M. (1983). Strain among caregivers: A study of experience in the U.S. *The Gerontologist, 23*(6), 597-604.

Davies, H., Priddy, J. M. & Tinklenberg, J. R. (1986). Support groups for male caregivers of Alzheimer's patients. *Clinical Gerontologist, 5,* 385-395.

Farkas, S. (1980). Impact of chronic illness on the patient's spouse. *Health and Social Work, 5,* 39-46.

Fengler, A. & Goodrich, N. (1979). Wives of elderly disabled men: The hidden patient. *The Gerontologist, 19,* 175-183.

Gallagher, D., Lovett, S. & Zeiss. A. (in press). Intervention with caregivers of frail elderly persons. In M. Ory & K. Bond (Eds.), *Aging and Health Care: Social Service and Policy Perspectives.* New York: Tavistock.

Gallagher, D., Rose, J., Rivera, P., Lovett, S. & Thompson, L. W. (in press). Prevalence of depression in family caregivers. *The Gerontologist.*

Garcia-Preto. (1982). Puerto Rican families. In M. McGoldrick, J. Pearce, & J. Giordino, (Eds.), *Ethnicity and Family Therapy* (pp. 164-186). New York: Guilford.

Golodetz, A., Evans, R., Heinritz, G. & Gibson, C. (1969). The care of chronic illness: The responsor role. *Medical Care, 7,* 385-394.

Greene, V. L. & Monahan, D. J. (1987). The effect of professionally guided caregiver support and education group on institutionalization of care receivers. *The Gerontologist, 27,* 716-721.

Haber, D. (1984). Church-based mutual help groups for caregivers of non-institutionalized elders. *Journal of Religion & Aging, 1,* 63-69.

Hasselkus, B. R. (1988). Meaning in family caregiving: Perspectives on caregiver/professional relationships. *The Gerontologist, 28,* 686-691.

Horowitz, A. (1985). Sons and daughters as caregivers to older parents: Differences in role performance and consequences. *The Gerontologist, 25,* 612-617.

Johnson, P. J. & Rubin, A. (1983). Case management in mental health: A social work domain. *Social Work, 28,* 49-55.

Kane, R. A. (1985). Assessing the elderly. In A. Monk (Ed.), *Handbook of Gerontological Services* (pp. 43-69). New York: Van Nostrand.

Kane, R. A. & Kane, R. L. (1981). *Assessing the Elderly: A Practical Guide to Measurement.* Lexington, MA: D. C. Heath.

Lazarus, R. S. & Folkman, S. (1984). *Stress, Appraisal and Coping.* New York: Springer.

McGadney, B. F., Goldberg-Glen R. & Pinkston, E. M. (1987). Clinical issues for assessment and intervention with the black elderly. In L. L. Carstanson & B. A. Edelstein (Eds.), *Handbook of Clinical Gerontology.* New York: Pergamon.

Montgomery, R. (1988). *Family Support Project: Outcome and Measurement Implications.* Paper presented at the annual conference of the Gerontological Society of America, Washington, D. C.

Pinkston, E. M., et al. (1982). *Effective Social Work Practice.* San Francisco: Jossey-Bass.

Roberts, R. (1987). The epidemiology of depression in minorities. In P. Muehrer (Ed.), *Research Perspectives on Depression and Suicide in Minorities.* Washington, DC: HHS-NIMH.

Rubin, A. (1987). Case management. In A. Minahan et al., (Eds.), *Encyclopedia of Social Work* (pp. 212-222). Silver Spring, MD: NASW.

Sanford, K. A. (1975). Tolerance of debility in elderly dependents by supporters at home: Its significance for hospital practice. *British Medical Journal, 3,* 471-473.

Shanas, E. (1968). *Old People in Three Industrial Societies.* New York: Atherton Press.

Steinberg, R. M. (1985). Access assistance and case management. In A. Monk (Ed.), *Handbook of Gerontological Services,* (pp. 211-239). New York: Van Nostrand.

Steinberg, R. M. & Carter, G. W. (1983). *Case Management and the Elderly.* Lexington, MA: D. C. Heath.

Stone, R., Cafferata, G. L. & Sangle, J. (1987). Caregivers of the frail elderly: A national profile. *The Gerontologist, 27,* 616-626.

Taylor, R. J. & Chatters, L. M. (1986). Church-based informal support among elderly blacks. *The Gerontologist, 26,* 637-642.

Tonti, M. & Silverstone, B. (1985). Services to families of the elderly. In A. Monk (Ed.), *Handbook of Gerontological Services* (pp. 211-239). New York: Van Nostrand.

Toseland, R. W. (1981). Increasing access: Outreach methods in social work practice. *Social Casework, 62,* 227-234.

Toseland, R. W., Derico, A. & Owen, M. L. (1984). Alzheimer's Disease and related disorders: Assessment and intervention. *Health and Social Work, 9,* 212-226.

Toseland, R. W., & Rossiter, C. M. (in press). Group intervention to support family caregivers: A review and analysis. *The Gerontologist.*

Toseland, R. W. Rossiter, C. M. & Labrecque, M. (in press). The effectiveness of peer-led and professionally-led groups to support family caregivers. *The Gerontologist.*

Toseland, R. W., Rossiter, C. M., Labrecque, M. S. & Beckstead, J. W. (1988). *The Effectiveness of Two Kinds of Support Groups for Caregivers.* Paper submitted for publication.

Chapter 30

SOCIAL WORK PRACTICE WITH HEAD INJURED PERSONS

Sabine Huege, MSW, CSW
Michael J. Holosko, PhD

Abstract

Head injury has been termed "the silent epidemic" and is presently the leading cause of death and disability among Canadians under the age of 45. Head injury rehabilitation involves the intervention of various health care professionals from initial trauma to a long-term recovery process. Social work practitioners have much to contribute to head injury rehabilitation. Traditional social work functions may be applied to this ever increasing and challenging client group in terms of the need for intervention not only with the client, but also with family members and the community at large. It is the community and family-based support services that will confront the profession as it evolves in serving the needs of this ever increasing group of persons.

SOCIAL WORK PRACTICE WITH HEAD INJURED PERSONS

Recent media attention has colloquially referred to head injury as "the silent epidemic." Each year approximately 50,000 (or 250 per 100,000) Canadians suffer from head injury (Vargo, Karpman & Wolfe, 1987). In Ontario alone, 44 residents daily acquire a brain injury serious enough to kill them or significantly alter their life style. Many more are recipients of a mild head injury that will result in long-term cognitive or physical problems (Ontario Head Injury Association, 1988). Recent reports by the Ministry of Health (1987) and Ministry of Community and Social Services (1987) indicate that traumatic head injury is the leading cause of death and disability to Ontario residents under the age of 45. Head injury is certainly not a Canadian phenomenon as Jennett & Teasdale (1981) found similar occurrences in Britain and the United States among the general population.

THE CLIENTELE

The causes of traumatic head injury are many and varied. The major cause is traffic accidents involving a motor vehicle (also motor vehicle and pedestrian, or motor vehicle and bicycle). The other primary causes ranked in descending order of occurrence include falls, sports injuries, assaults and work-related accidents (Annegars, Grabow, Kurland & Laws, 1980).

The highest "at-risk" group for traumatic head injuries are young, single males (aged 15 to 25 years) who account for approximately 70% of all occurrences. After such injury, it has been estimated that only 25 % or less from this group are able to return to normal work and daily living activities (Vargo et al., 1986).

Depending on the severity of injury, the specific area of the brain affected and injury type (for example, whether the injury was open or closed, and whether there was concussion, fracture, hematoma and/or other complications), a head injured person typically faces not only life threatening injuries, but a combination of physical, cognitive, psychological and/or social disabilities, some or all of which will never be fully restored to pre-morbid functioning.

As a result, rehabilitation needs are extensive and long-term, and range from acute in-hospital care to chronic care requiring social re-integration and adjustment. Six months to two years seems to be a benchmark figure for the major portion of basic recovery (Sbordone, 1984). However, it may take up to five years or longer for head injured patients to recover to an optimal level of functioning within the limitations of their residual deficits. Rehabilitation of the head injured person is a complicated and multi-faceted process that must take into account the various combinations of deficits the head injured person is left with.

Physical disabilities common to severe head injury are hemiplegia or hemiparesis. Further, poor balance, diminished eyesight, headaches and post-traumatic epilepsy are also common complaints (Jennett & Teasdale, 1981). In short, the head injured person not only faces the very real problems of adjustment to physical disability, but also must contend with specific and unique cognitive deficits.

General areas of cognitive disabilities resulting from head injury are short-term memory loss; loss of problem-solving abilities and rate of information processing; poor judgment and perception and communication disorders (Goldstein and Ruthven, 1983; Diller & Gordon, 1981; Ben-Yishay, 1981). Moreover, each of these cognitive disturbances adversely affects the head injured person's psychosocial adjustment. For instance, Priganto and Fordyce (1986) indicated there may be an unrealistic appraisal of self and others, inappropriate verbal and/or behaviourial responses to social situations and difficulty with organizational skills required in work or academic settings. As well, social/behaviourial problems occur if frontal lobe damage has occurred. These impairments have typically resulted in difficulties faced by head injured persons in the areas of return to work or school, family and social relationships and leisure activities (Newton & Johnson, 1985; Tyerman & Humphrey, 1984).

The emotional stress endured by head injured persons as a result of the above disturbances is widely discussed in the literature. For example, Newcombe (1982), Stevens (1982) and Carlson (1980), among others, identified psychological problems such as depression, anxiety, lack of motivation and low self-esteem resulting from emotional stress and the inability to cope with disability following traumatic head injury.

Not only does head injury have a potentially devastating effect on the individual, the family of a survivor of head injury also must cope with overwhelming stress. In addition to having to deal with the initial trauma of an accident/injury to a loved one, family members and significant others may be required to adjust to a lifetime with a decidedly and drastically changed family member, who in all likelihood will never be the same as before the injury. Moreover, rehabilitation may be very long-term and, in most cases, the family is left to cope with the head injured person on its own without continued support from the community or professionals. Burden and stress in such families have been well documented (Bond, 1984; Vargo et al., 1987), and "...rehabilitation services must now consider adopting the concept of the 'head injured family' rather than solely the head injured patients" (Brooks, 1984, p. 144).

It is apparent from the previous discussion that many health care professionals may be involved in the process of head injury rehabilitation. A multi-disciplinary team is required to deal with the various consequences of head injury — from acute-care trauma team to neurologist, physiatrist, neuropsychologist, rehabilitation nurses, speech pathologist, physiotherapist and occupational therapist.

Research also points to the need for intervention required in three areas of secondary (non-medical) consequences of head injury: psychological adjustment, emotional adjustment and social adjustment (Holosko & Huege, 1989). As well, the needs of the family must also be addressed. It is our view that social work practice is most relevant in this aspect of the rehabilitation process. In an effort to ensure a comprehensive rehabilitation program providing continuity of service progressing and continuing from the acute stage and throughout the chronic stage of head injury toward optimal functioning, the role of the social worker can accommodate this entire process.

Panting and Merry (1972), both medical doctors, addressed this concern by offering the same solution. They indicated the following:

> It seems to us that the greatest need is for a coordinator who would follow up the patient from the time of the acute accident to complete recovery and who, with full knowledge of the patient's history would be able to mobilize the appropriate resources. ...we feel that this coordinating function could be carried out best by a medical social worker...to whom (relatives) could appeal in difficulties. (p. 36)

It follows that much planning, co-ordination and working together by the many professionals involved in the rehabilitation of head injured patients is essential to achieve a positive rehabilitation outcome.

The role for social work is clearly identified in this process and should be an integral part of the rehabilitation of the head injured. Traditionally, social work has been involved in meeting human needs through assisting people in acquiring the necessary resources (both personal and environmental), to function to the best of their abilities within their own communities. In order to achieve this end, social work employs methods such as crisis intervention; individual, marital and family counselling; group work; social support and community networking. These basic methods of intervention fit perfectly to the rehabilitation needs of the head injured patient and family from early trauma to community re-entry (see Figure 1).

Figure 1. *Social Work Roles and Functions in Head Injury Rehabilitation From Early Trauma to Follow-Up Services*

Continuum of Care	*Roles and Functions*
Trauma Unit (Acute Care)	- Crisis intervention - Family support - Liaison with family and medical professionals

Rehabilitation Unit	- Patient and family education
	- Social assessments
	- Individual, marital and family counselling
	- Group sessions
	  1. patient's peer support group
	  2. family/significant others support group
	
	- Discharge planning (involves medical team, patient, and family)

Community Re-entry	- Referrals to and liaisons with Community Resources - Advocate for Community Resources (i.e., financial services, housing, legal services, insurance companies, assistive devices, home care, vocational services, schools and employers, local head injury associations)

Follow-Up and
Auxiliary Services   - On-going out-patient groups for patient
                              and family
                            - Advocacy for head injury programs
                            - Public awareness education
                            - head injury rehabilitation research

Specifically, in the emergency trauma unit, the social worker may offer comfort and support at a time of crisis to the family. Basic information as to what may be expected in the following days can be answered by the social worker when the medical team may be too difficult to contact. The social worker serves as a liaison between other health care professionals and family members.

In the rehabilitation unit, patient and family education about the long-term effects of head injury and how to cope with specific problems should be the first function of the social worker (Frye, 1982). Subsequently, through the use of psychosocial assessments and regular contact with both the patient and the family, it will become apparent to the social worker whether there is a need for more extensive individual and/or family counselling. Three major components of this phase of the assessment are

1) analysis of pre-morbid history of patient and family;
2) identifying the severity and potential duration of mental and physical deficits and
3) understanding signals from the family that would appear to reflect a need for intervention (Rosenthal, 1984, p. 233).

Aside from individual, marital or family counselling, social workers may also run group sessions for patients, which may serve as peer supports and provide an opportunity for patients to ventilate their frustrations constructively. Such groups for family and significant others are usually set up with the goal of information sharing and support.

Discharge planning is a traditional function of social workers in any health care setting. It is up to the social worker to involve all members of the rehabilitation team, which of course includes patient and family members, in the planning process to ensure the most appropriate course of action is determined. Adequate discharge planning for this population group is an especially challenging task as, at present, community re-entry services for head injury patients are few and very limited.

It is at this point of the rehabilitation process that the social worker requires expertise in, and knowledge of, community services and resources that may be accessed by the head injured patient and family. The social worker becomes much more than a referring agent and acts more in the capacity of liaison or advocate on behalf of patient and family in linking with legal services, insurance companies, financial services, housing, employers and schools. Approaching community service clubs for funding of assistive devices, e.g., transportation services, may also become necessary. Referrals to home-care services, vocational and employment training services and local head injury associations may also be made at this point.

Follow-up support services cannot be neglected in cases of head injury due to the long-term, continued support these persons require as they move toward their optimum potential and community re-integration (Holosko & Huege, 1989). One way of providing such support is by establishing ongoing group sessions for patient and family on an out-patient basis.

POTENTIAL FOR ROLE DEVELOPMENT

Much medical technology has been advanced in the past decade to both diagnose and treat head injured persons. For example, specialized mobile and institutionally based life saving trauma units and more sophisticated road-side techniques have consistently saved more lives than ever before. Although such statistics of head injury survivors are encouraging, it has been noted that survival of head injury is not without serious consequences.

The 1990s will see the development of further technological advancements and, with the establishment of more local trauma units, one may surmise that the number of head injury survivors will rise proportionately. In turn, this may result in an increased demand for specialized services for the head injured population. Presently in Canada, there are only a few hospitals offering specialized units for the head injured, these being mostly situated in large urban centres. However, as the health care system becomes more aware of the growing numbers of head injured persons and their needs for specialized yet comprehensive services, the role of social workers in this setting can only be increased.

Moreover, due to the long-term support needs of this client population, social work practice with head injured clients cannot be confined to the residential health care setting. As more special-ized community programs and services are established for this client group, social workers will be able to provide professional expertise in areas such as residential, life-skills and vocational counselling. As well, social workers have begun to branch out into private practice specifically dealing with head injury. They offer such services as psychotherapy to patients and families, case management services and consultation services. Therefore, as case managers and/or co-ordinators, the social work professional will be able to practise many aspects of social work methods and func-tions within any setting for head injury rehabilitation.

Effective role development for social workers involves the con-tinued stradling of practitioners between the hospital and commu-nity. Hospital technology and services for this patient group will inevitably increase and, as a result, social work practitioners in this field will be faced with both keeping abreast of the medical needs of these persons and developing creative and cost-effective community-based services. The implications for the latter include a whole range of new roles for social workers such as lobbying and advocacy at policy-making or funding levels, training or edu-cating the community about prevention, treatment and follow-up services, proactive networking with community services, fund raising, developing support networks for such persons, liaising with employers and job trainers and essentially marshalling avail-able support services in the community to help this group of per-sons. Certainly such roles will be both challenging and exciting for the profession.

CONCLUDING REMARKS

Head injury rehabilitation is a rapidly expanding field offering exciting challenges for social workers to creatively use their social work skills to assist head injured individuals toward a goal of community re-integration and optimum quality of life within the confines of their cognitive and/or physical deficits. Presently, two essential aspects of social work in the area of head injury are:

1) research and
2) advocacy on behalf of clients for more and specialized community programs.

As well, public education and awareness programs should be incorporated into the responsibilities of the social worker specializing in head injury. The public must be made aware of the causes, effects and long-term repercussions of head injury (even milder or minor head injury) in order to foster greater understanding and more acceptance and support of the head injured individual within her/his own local community.

Social work practice in head injury rehabilitation is essential in the health care setting; however, is not necessarily limited to this setting. Social work practice must include community-oriented, non-medical issues that challenge survivors of head injury on a daily and ongoing basis.

CASE EXAMPLE

D. is a 35-year-old single man who suffered a stroke four and a half years ago leaving him with mild left-sided hemiplegia and neurological damage resulting in poor concentration; distractiblity; poor short-term memory; slowed information processing capabilities and decreased math skills.

Pre-morbidly, D. had achieved a grade 11 education and had excelled at mathematics. After high school he began work and was trained on-the-job as a mould making technician. He thoroughly enjoyed this work and was an asset to his employer due to his superior abilities; thorough training of new workers and willingness to put in many hours of overtime. He worked steadily in this field for 13 years until the time of his stroke. After his stroke, D. was kept in the intensive care unit for two and a half weeks and then was transferred to a rehabilitation unit for four weeks.

D. made a quick recovery physically after the stroke, in that his hemiplegia was barely noticeable. At no time during his hospital stay was there mention of possible neurological deficits or what may be facing D. after discharge.

D. returned to his former employment four months after his stroke. At that time, D. was disoriented on the job, unable to concentrate and unable to perform the mental calculations that had been second nature to him. The exertion and stress of these circumstances caused considerable fatigue and irritability. His co-workers began to comment about his lack of productivity and called him lazy. Although the employer provided him with some adjustment time to the job, he was eventually let go.

In the subsequent two years, D. was hired and let go from several jobs as a mould-maker, each time for the same reasons.

Depression and bitterness set in. Friends and family were confused as to D.'s "sudden" lack of motivation and inability to keep a job. His family doctor also put down D.'s unemployment status as lack of motivation. No mention was made to D. of the effects of brain damage due to his stroke.

Nine months ago, D. was referred to Vocational Rehabilitation Services, and a thorough assessment (neurological and vocational) was conducted. The results of these assessments were discussed with D., and counselling regarding adjustment to his neurological impairments began. Over the period of a few months, D. came to accept his deficits and worked to minimize their effects instead of struggling against something he could not change.

Vocationally, he still wanted to return to his previous work environment. Contact was made with D.'s first employer. A meeting was arranged with the employer and two plant foremen in order to educate them regarding D.'s situation—his present limitations and strengths and generally how brain damage can effect an individual's functioning. With this understanding, and as D. had been a valued employee for so many years, the employer was willing to pursue a vocational assessment in order to determine if there was any work D. could perform up to standard within the company.

After a three month assessment, it was determined that D. could not manage any of his previous work functions; however, his manual skills were still acceptable and it was suggested that a work adjustment training begin in order for D. to practise and feel comfortable in performing jobs he had always considered beneath his skills and abilities. Again, counselling regarding acceptance of this outcome was necessary, and D. slowly came to the realization that he could still be a good employee and take pride in his work. Upon successful work adjustment, D. was hired on for full-time employment.

D. wants to work on improving his math skills and problem-solving. Referral has been made to a cognitive retraining program, and also to the local Head Injury Association support group meetings. At present, D. feels more accepting of himself as he is earning a living, has a better understanding of his situation and has some hope for the future.

References

Annegers, J. F., Grabow, J. D., Kurland, L. T. & Laws, E. R. (1980). The incidence, causes and secular trends of head trauma in Olmsted County, Minnesota, 1935-1974. *Neurology, 30,* 912-919.

Ben-Yishay, Y. (1981). *Working Approaches to Remediation of Cognitive Deficits in Brain Damaged Persons.* (Rehabilitation Monograph No. 62). New York: New York University Medical Center, Institute of Rehabilitation Medicine.

Bond, M. R. (1984). Effects on the family system. In M. Rosenthal, E. Griffith, M. Bond and J. D. Miller (Eds.), *Rehabilitation of the Head Injured Adult* (pp. 209-217). Philadelphia: F. A. Davis Company.

Brooks, N. (1984). *Closed Head Injury: Psychological, Social and Family Consequences.* Oxford: Oxford University Press.

Carlson, C. E. (1980). Psychosocial aspects of neurologic disability. *Nursing Clinics of North America, 15*(2), 309-320.

Diller, L. & Gordon, W. A. (1981). Interventions for cognitive deficits. *Journal of Consulting and Clinical Psychology, 49,* 822-834.

Frye, B. A. (1982). Brain injury and family education needs. *Rehabilitation Nursing, 7,* 27-29.

Goldstein, G. & Ruthven, L. (1983). *Rehabilitation for the Brain Damaged Adult.* New York: Plenum Press.

Holosko, M. J. & Huege, S. (1989). Perceived social adjustment and social support among a sample of head injured adults. *Canadian Journal of Rehabilitation.* 2(3), 145-154.

Jennett, B. & Teasdale, G. (1981). *Management of Head Injuries.* Philadelphia: FA Davis Company.

Ministry of Community and Social Services (1987). *Report on Head Injury Services in Ontario.* Unpublished report.

Ministry of Health (1987). *Report on Services for Residents of Ontario with Acquired Brain Damage.* Unpublished report.

Newcombe, F. (1982). The psychological consequences of closed head injury: Assessment and rehabilitation. *Injury: The British Journal of Accident Surgery, 14*(2), 111-136.

Newton, A. & Johnson, D. A. (1985). Social adjustment and interaction after severe head injury. *British Journal of Psychology, 25,* 225-234.

Ontario Head Injury Association (1989). *Public Provincial Hearings: The Status of Wellness Opportunities for Ontario Residents with Traumatic Brain Injury.* St. Catharines, Ontario.

Panting, A. & Merry, P. H. (1972). The long term rehabilitation of severe head injuries with particular reference to the need for social and medical support for the patient's family. *Rehabilitation, 38,* 33-37.

Priganto, G. P. & Fordyce, D. J. (1986). Cognitive dysfunction and psychosocial adjustment after brain injury. In G. P. Priganto (Ed.), *Neuropsychological Rehabilitation After Brain Injury* (pp. 1-17). Baltimore: John Hopkins University Press.

Rosenthal, M. (1984). Strategies for intervention with families of brain-injured patients. In E. T. Couture & B. A. Edelstein (Eds.), *Behaviourial Assessment and Rehabilitation of the Traumatically Brain-Damaged* (pp. 227-246). New York: Plenum Press.

Sbordone, R. J. (1984). Rehabilitative neuropsychological approach for severe traumatic brain-injured patients. *Professional Psychology: Research and Practice, 15*(2), 165-175.

Stevens, M. M. (1982). Post concussion syndrome. *Journal of Neurosurgical Nursing, 14*(5), 239-244.

Tyerman, A. & Humphrey, J. (1984). Changes in self-concept following severe head injury. *International Journal of Rehabilitation Research, 7*(1), 11-23.

Vargo, F., Dennis, S., Thomas. E., Wolfe, S., Mueller, H. & Brintnell, S. (1986). A social-vocational rehabilitation program model of closed-head injured adults. *Rehabilitation Digest, 17*(2), 7.

Vargo, J. W., Karpman, T. & Wolfe, S. (1987). Family adjustment to closed-head injury: Implications for rehabilitation counselling. *Natcon, 14,* 137-147.

Ylvisker, M. (1985). *Head Injury Rehabilitation: Children and Adolescents.* San Diego: College-Hill Press Inc.

Endnotes

We gratefully acknowledge the assistance of Brenda Watkin, Social Worker, Neurorehabilitation Unit, Parkwood Hospital, London, Ontario.

Chapter 31

SOCIAL WORK PRACTICE WITH MILITARY PERSONNEL IN A HEALTH CARE SETTING

Marvin D. Feit, PhD
Raymond D. McCoy, MSW, ACSW

Abstract

Providing social work services in a military hospital is based on its primary mission — maintaining the stability of the family unit. The number of social workers in the United States military is determined by the Department of Defense, and while they are administratively responsible for each social work department, their major treatment role is as a family advocacy representative. Military social workers work in conjunction with available community resources while upholding foremost the military responsibility.

SOCIAL WORK PRACTICE WITH MILITARY PERSONNEL IN A HEALTH CARE SETTING

The history of Naval Military social work dates back to 1973 when the first social worker was hired to work with returning prisoners of war and their families. Since then, the primary mission has been child and adult protective services. During the late 1960s and 1970s, society and the nation openly recognized a growing concern about child and spouse abuse. In 1966, all fifty states implemented laws requiring mandated child abuse reporting. By 1974 the Naval Bureau of Medicine organized child abuse programs in military treatment facilities and in 1979 included spouse abuse.

In 1980, the first active duty commissioned Medical Service Corps Social Worker, (Lieutenant Commander David Kennedy), was hired. In 1981, the Department of Defense issued a directive instructing all branches of the military to implement a "Family Advocacy Program" dealing with child and spouse abuse and neglect, sexual assault and incest. In 1984, the Secretary of the Navy issued a Family Advocacy Instruction, and in 1987 the Chief of Naval Operations issued a Family Advocacy Instruction. At this time, Family Advocacy is a primary medical/social work treatment program.

Since 1980, the ranks of Commissioned Medical Service Corps Officers with a specialty in clinical social work have grown to twenty worldwide. Clinical social workers in the Navy must be nationally certified by the Academy of Certified Social Workers or must be licensed by a state as a Licensed Clinical Social Worker before being commissioned. While the number seems small, for every Commissioned Social Worker procured, a health care related position must be closed out. Congress establishes the total number of officers permitted. Adding a new specialty to the military service corps must come from existing health care personnel or be "taken out of hide," as the Navy term indicates.

THE CLIENTELE

I. Organizational Structure

Similar to all military organizations, military medicine operates through the "chain of command." As a department within military medicine's ancillary services, clinical social work is organized as an independent department. The department is autonomous and it interfaces with all other health care departments. Military health care endorses many of the standards and organizational requirements delineated by the Joint Commission of Accreditation of Hospitals (JCAH) and their Ambulatory Care standards. The Social Work Department is expected to comply with such standards, within the content of its manpower resources and primary mission responsibilities. Some smaller health care facilities that serve only active duty personnel, and utilize military trained paraprofessionals (e.g., hospital corpsmen), may at times fall short of overall JCAH standards. With only twenty active duty social workers worldwide, and about one hundred civil service counterparts in military treatment facilities, social work services meeting national standards are not feasible in all military health care environments.

The Navy is the only branch of the United States military that has a formal policy for the mandated treatment of incest perpetrators. All branches of the military have mandated treatment for spouse abuse and other forms of child abuse. The rationale for such a policy is that the Navy values its highly trained personnel and desires to retain them if their clinical evaluation suggests they have a good prognosis for successful therapy outcome and they manifest future potential for worthwhile military service. It also desires to enhance the quality of life for its military family members.

The Navy is a unique system in that it operates as a total institution for its family members. This means that the responsibility between it and a family is a 24-hour job. Four major aspects of the Navy clientele will now be discussed. These aspects are the environmental context, the setting, the program, and client demographics. The environmental context provides an understanding of the effects of Navy life on a family. The setting describes the structure of military social work in a local command and the program provided in the setting. Finally, client demographics provide insight regarding the amount and the types of problems military social work is confronted with in the setting.

II. The Environment Context

Before therapists can understand their patients, they must understand how an individual fits in his or her environmental context. In the military, "the mission comes first," and "if they wanted you to bring a family with you, they would have issued you one in your duffle bag" are commonly referred to when describing how military family members "fit in." Current statistics reveal that over 50% of all active service members are now married, compared to only 17% several years ago (Military Family Resource Center Statistics, 1988). The endorsement that the military family is one of the Navy's greatest assets has never been more accurate. Job satisfaction and retention rates are often linked to family life satisfaction.

Family life in the military is unique. The processes of individualism and autonomy are in a constant state of evolutionary resolution. Family conflicts are related to previous developmental life experiences and unresolved psychological issues of its members, which are often exacerbated by the regimented and authoritarian leadership style required of a loyal and unconditionally responsive military organization. For example, "the mission comes first," is a complex statement that affects service men and their families. Some active duty service personnel "marry" into the service; i.e., they are adopted by their military extended family. This requires placing one's biological, nuclear and extended families in a different position of hierarchial importance. The new role of the military family becomes to support his role and commitment to the military organization. This "celebrated warrior syndrome" (Kaslow & Ridenhour, 1984) is necessary for the efficient functioning of the military organization. In most situations, extended and nuclear families are proud of their son or father's commitment to their country. In time however, the emotional toll is often too much for a family to tolerate, and when a service person's loyalty to a mission interferes with family stability and family life, conflicts emerge and may result in marital and family dysfunction, job dissatisfaction or both.

Individuals join the military for a variety of personal reasons and purposes. Problems arise when those expectations are not met. The marital couple usually does not understand the implications of frequent and long separations and the subsequent impact upon their relationship and family life experience. Fathers, who are out to sea for six to nine months, often fail to see the birth of their children and are not included in the bonding. Children initially do not know their fathers and both must adjust to new relationships while establishing effective attachments.

As well, the military lifestyle often creates a feeling of alienation within the civilian community. Usually a close network is established in the military community and gives a family a sense of "belonging" to a group that has many things in common. When the opportunity to bond with the military community is not accomplished, or does not occur for other reasons, the family may feel rejected, alienated and alone. Predispositions for emotional and psychosocial crises and instability are common in such families, especially during periods of stress.

There are additional conditions in the Navy that create stress on the military family. These common stressors include:

1) frequent transfers and short term location — the shortest lengths of time in a given location are reported by Marine Corps enlisted personnel and Navy Officers, with the longest by Air Force enlisted personnel and Officers;
2) Navy and Marine Corps personnel tend to spend more time separated from their families then do Army or Air Force personnel;
3) Navy and Marine Corps enlisted personnel find lower levels of job satisfaction than Army and Air Force enlisted personnel;
4) strict rate/rank and fraternization/social pressures;
5) lack of control over pay and
6) the constant fear of death (Doering & Hutzel, 1982).

A relatively new issue confronting the military is the increase in single parents. In America in1960, 1 out of 10 children were living with a single parent. By 1990, this figure is projected to be 1 out of 4. The military is already experiencing difficulties adjusting to this phenomenon, despite their efforts to enlist more women. A recent trend is one in which fathers assume single parenting and child custody roles. This has caused the military to deal with the whole single parent issue (Kaslow & Ridenhour, 1984).

III. The Navy Family Advocacy Program

It is important to note that the Family Advocacy Program is a military-wide program. Attention will be focussed on the implementation of this program in a local setting.

The Naval Medical Clinic, Norfolk, Family Advocacy Program received reports of 1,391 new incidents of child and spouse abuse during the year 1987. Of those, 218 were filed as physical child abuse; 135 were incest and child/sexual abuse; 236 were neglect and emotional child abuse and 802 were physical spouse abuse. These new cases were added to the existing caseloads.

The staffing pattern is large compared to other Navy Social Work programs. The Norfolk/Virginia Beach area is heavily populated with military from the Air Force, Army and Coast Guard, in addition to Navy and Marine Corps. This area is considered to have one of the largest, if not *the* largest, Navy population in the world. As one would assume, the family advocacy caseload is also considered one of the largest.

The Social Work Department Staff consists of two Navy active duty social workers, one of whom acts as the Department Head; three civil service (GS-11-185) social workers and one (GS-5) secretary.

The military Family Advocacy Program has probably the only reported unified policy implemented by any state or federal agency to provide organizational intervention and mandated treatment. The policy permits Commanding Officers to take direct action in conjunction with the Family Advocacy Representative's recommended treatment plan. It grants authority to mandate that the service member vacate his home and remain separated from his spouse or child until the therapist and/or the Family Advocacy Representative feel it is safe to reunite.

The rationale for this is quite different and enforceable intervention is based on two considerations. The first consideration is the structure of the military, an organization intertwined in all aspects of family life. The second consideration acknowledges the fact that studies reveal children who witness family violence have a much higher likelihood of becoming an abuser. Therefore, spousal abuse is often considered as child neglect when it interferes with the healthy development of a child who witnesses family violence. The request to remove the offender from the home is often justified in the interest of the healthy development of child and family.

When the family desires the return of the incest perpetrator, mandated treatment for at least twelve consecutive months of uninterrupted treatment is initiated and monitored. Practically all incest perpetrators are referred to civilian practitioners for treatment for reasons just mentioned. However, this treatment usually requires the reassignment of the sailor to a shore billet. This reassignment is a great inconvenience to the operational continuity of a command, as every sailor is considered invaluable and indispensable to the operation of that sea or air command. Therefore, acceptance for treatment is a serious undertaking in this program.

The Family Advocacy Program at the Naval Medical Clinic also provides group treatment for child sex offenders. At present, fifteen active duty servicemen are in treatment. A behavioural and psychodynamic approach is used to modify deviant cognitive projections and restructure their deviant sexual arousal into more socialized and non-deviant behavioural outlets. Treatment is always adjunctive to monitoring by Child Protective Services, Probation and the courts. Legal consequences, even if incarceration is suspended, is perceived to have a favourable influence upon treatment outcome and is always sought.

Staffing shortages do not permit individual treatment as it is too labour intensive and requires a consistent therapeutic structure. Due to the erratic staffing resources and large workload, comprehensive treatment is not feasible and case management has become the primary function. Thus, with limited staffing resources, one is able to manage and monitor more individuals in treatment than one can treat singularly.

The emphasis on case management does however present some problems for social workers. Job turnover, burnout and job dissatisfaction are major programmatic issues. Many social workers who meet the credentialing requirements for the ACSW and LCSW find little job satisfaction in the day-to-day "paper pushing," and desire clinical experience. Hiring case managers who have a bachelor's degree is being considered to improve staff morale. However, the additional personpower costs are a major concern.

IV. Family Demographics

Family violence is widespread in American society, and this problem is also reflected in the Department of the Navy (DON). Several early studies suggested that serious injuries resulted in over 50% of the child maltreatment cases involving military families, compared with only 27% for the entire sample (Johnson, 1974). The latest data indicate that military family violence incidents are comparable to that of the civilian sector. In 1987, there were 6,032 cases of child and spouse abuse maltreatment substantiated by Naval authorities. During that same year, twelve children and six adults in Navy/Marine Corps families died as a result of injuries caused by family violence (NMPC-663, 1988).

Family violence affects the stability of the family unit, the service member and the readiness of every Navy and Marine Corps Command. It is incompatible with the high standards of professional and personal discipline required of members of the United States Navy and Marine Corps (USMC). This statement is a reflection of the Navy's proactive concern. The "new" Navy must be "family" oriented, for over 50% of all active duty personnel are married, whereas ten years ago, only 17% were married. Presently, the total number of Navy personnel in active duty is 576,940. There are 291,825 spouses and 309,308 dependent children (Defense 1987, Almanac). While the military traditionally did not think "family," they do so now.

The goal of Naval social work is to promote a healthy and stable family. Family violence is a complex and multi-dimensional problem requiring a multi-disciplinary approach. The Department of the Navy has made great strides through its Family Advocacy Program in the areas of identification and intervention with child and spouse abuse. These efforts have been proactive rather than preventive in nature, as the latter is expensive, and it is hard to document beneficial outcomes.

It is roughly estimated that close to half of all child dependents raised in a military family join the military. As a result, the "military family tradition" is strong. How "strong" depends on present efforts to support military families, and enhance their quality of life. By regonizing the importance of promoting a healthy family, Naval social work works toward the stability of the military.

PRACTICE ROLES AND RESPONSIBILITIES

There are three major social work roles in the military. One is providing supervisory and administrative control in the family advocacy program. The second is to implement the tasks of the Family Advocacy Representative and the third is to provide services as a medical social worker.

I. Supervisory and Administrative Role

The primary military mission for the Naval social workers is to provide supervisory and administrative responsibility for implementing the Family Advocacy Program. This duty distinguishes the military social workers' duties in a military health care context from their counterparts in civilian health care settings. One additional difference is that the commissioned military social worker is on active duty, as are his patients. Both are trained for combat readiness and are on 24-hour call. Military medicine and the Medical Service Corps' purpose is to support the fleet and their military missio, and keep them operationally ready. Military social work must subscribe to this philosophy as well.

Almost all military social workers in the Navy also act as Social Work Department Heads. Because the ranks are small, it requires each commissioned Naval social worker to exercise administrative responsibility in addition to the clinical duties of a social worker.

Administrative responsibilities include the supervision of subordinates, including enlisted, civilian contract and Government Civil Service personnel. Program and policy development, budgeting and the management of direct services require leadership and management skills. All commissioned Social Workers receive Leadership Management and Education Training (LMET) upon their initial military training at Officers Indoctrination School and periodically throughout their career.

A military career is based upon one's capacity and competency as a leader and manager of men and organizations. Clinical orientation and treatment skills are initially required and admired; however, their value lessens as one's career progresses. The military motto holds that it trains and develops officers to lead men. This is true in both military health care and military social work.

II. The Family Advocacy Representative

While family advocacy is a primary duty, a key social work role is as Family Advocacy Representative. Other duties such as medical social work with its emphasis upon discharge planning are also important. Military social workers are also utilized in alcohol rehabilitation, health and physical readiness/stress management, and psychiatric social work; these roles are more recent and are discussed as areas of development. Serving the military family and the active duty service member to enhance their quality of life, and maintaining the service member's operational readiness from a psychological standpoint, remains the military's primary justification for commissioning active duty social workers.

The Family Advocacy Representative (FAR) is the Commanding Officer's expert advisor regarding child and spous abuse matters and invokes local prevailing laws with which all medical personnel must comply. The Family Advocacy Representative is usually the active duty social worker. When an active duty social worker is not present, and a civil service social worker is not available, a senior medical or nursing officer is appointed to this position by the medical treatment facility's Commanding Officer. Ultimately, it is this Commanding Officer who is accountable for the effective functioning of the Family Advocacy Program, in addition to all other aspects of medical care under his purview.

With society's concern increasing rapidly over the past decade to reduce and treat child and spous abuse, the military's Family Advocacy Program has become a highly visible and primary mission for most military social work departments. Naval social workers participate in a multi-professional team to assist the medical department with the identification and treatment of domestic violence offenders. Active duty service members who are identified as offenders are screened by the Family Advocacy Representative located within the military treatment facility's social work department. It is the Family Advocacy Representative's responsibility to provide, or obtain, a mental health assessment, a psychosocial evaluation and to develop a treatment plan for the offender, the victim and the entire family. The philosophy is that if the service member's family is not stable, the service member is not psychologically or operationally ready for service; hence, the term "family" advocacy, as family violence impacts directly upon military medicine.

By federal regulation, active duty service personnel are considered federal government property. Any medical or psychiatric, including clinical social work, treatment is not approved of by civilian resources, except with prior approval and authorization. Two reasons prevail: (1) documentation of illness or disease resulting in a medical/psychiatric disability must be "service connected" in order to be eligible for military disability benefits and (2) all aspects of health status must be available for military health care to judge an individual "fit for duty." This disposition is important in maintaining operational forces and combat readiness, and it also minimizes safety risks and military medical liability.

When active duty personnel are referred, efforts to utilize existing military resources are explored. If treatment is unfeasible within the military system, the Navy accepts its military obligation to "take care of its own" and will authorize the payment of treatment in the civilian community. In emergencies and in cases where any military treatment facility is not within access, the civilian medical facility and the active duty service member must contact his Command and request authorization for treatment by a civilian facility. The Office of Medical Affairs (OMA) within the region will authorize payment for appropriate treatment and will then monitor the treatment and make every effort to transport the service member to the nearest military medical facility at the most opportune time. Supplemental care funds provided by each Medical Treatment Facility (MTF) will then be authorized for treatment at the local level.

Advocating for defenceless children has been, and continues to be, a social work and medical mutual concern. The Family Advocacy Representative (FAR) works with the Department of Pediatrics in this respect. Treatment planning and discharge planning are some of the functions collectively performed. The FAR also acts as the community liaison between military social work and child protective services, providing a link to medical and nursing personnel regarding the mandated reporting laws, community resources and military health care resources available for dependent family members.

III. Medical Social Work

Providing health care to military dependent family members is offered if resources permit, and if such care does not compromise the provision of health care to active duty members. Almost 95% of the referrals for intervention with dependent family members are made into the civilian community under CHAMPUS (Civilian Health and Medical Program of the Uniformed Services). The social worker's responsibility becomes to provide information and referral resources and to be a case manager.

If stationed at a Naval hospital, the military social worker has responsibilities in addition to family advocacy. Discharge planning is the primary task. Since the implementation of hospital utilization reviews and diagnostic related group regulations (DRG), military medicine utilizes social workers to assist in the discharge planning for its patients. Crisis intervention and therapy related to grief and bereavment, chronic illness and chronic medical disability, such as AIDS, are two additional services provided by the social work department at a large naval hospital.

Discharge planning assures that patients have adequate follow-up health care to meet their medical and psychosocial needs. This enhances recovery and usually minimizes medical complications. Indeed, social workers have a proven track record in discharge planning secondary to their function as a knowledgeable community resource point of contact and their philosophy of helping patients adjust to their psychosocial environmental "fit" in the military.

POTENTIAL FOR ROLE DEVELOPMENT

The Navy has recently embarked on two major program areas in which social work has contributed its practice expertise. Alcohol and food addiction centres are keeping military personnel physically and mentally fit, while stress management deals with health and mental health readiness.

I. Alcohol Rehabilitation / Overeaters Program

The Navy is concerned with all aspects of health and physical readiness. Alcohol and food addiction are two areas of health care in which military social work has recently become interested.

Military standards demand rigorous physical and medical fitness to assure optimum performance and minimization of medical health care risks. Two such risks that are considered serious detriments to the overall well being of its service personnel are alcohol abuse and obesity. Both are treated through the regional Alcohol Rehabilitation Centers (ARC), utilizing a multi-modal behavioural approach. Educational awareness, physical exercise, group therapy and behavioural control are the counterparts to a dietary regimen that is suitable at home or onboard a ship. Social workers are utilized as group therapists and educators, and also program administrators in this regard. Service men and women who are unable to modify their alcohol addiction or obesity after this six week residential treatment program, and a prescribed out-patient follow-up program, may be discharged from the military.

II. Health and Physical Readiness / Stress

Management

The most recent addition in the utilization of social workers in an overall effort to improve physical and psychological readiness is stress management. Military regulations required all personnel to pass strength and endurance tests (1.5 mile run, pushups, sit ups) and to meet specific body fat/weight standards. Social work involvement is in the policy formation and implementation of a standardized stress management program. In addition to family advocacy and medical social work, stress management has the potential for beneficial results across a wide range of behavioural and performance-related activities. It contributes favourably to the overall functional capacity of the service member in conflict resolution in the family and also on the job.

In an occupational setting such as the military, with regimented authoritarian leadership, occupational stress often results in family violence and ineffective work-related performance. In turn, compromises in work performance can often result in safety hazards and security breaches. Working around military weaponry and installations that safeguard many military secret projects can also result in stress among its personnel. In the interest of national security and the safety of those who depend on accurate and dependable job performance, stress management is seen as an integral aspect of military social work's contribution to supporting operational readiness.

CONCLUDING REMARKS

When interpersonal issues become conflictual in any family relationship, triangulation is often used consciously, or unconsciously, to deal with one another. The military is usually the third party triangulated into such conflicts. Social workers dealing with military families during marital and family turmoil must remain objective and not identify with the individual by projecting blame onto the "unreasonable" military bureaucracy. It is likely that the conflict is related to the family's own development or is in the usual progression of its life cycle in the military. Such conflicts are likely to arise during the birth of children or through personal loss and family separations. The social worker would do well to help the military family re-focus their conflict upon themselves and assist them with their struggles to achieve individualism, separation and autonomy as a developmental life cycle process (Kaslow & Ridenhour, 1984). In this manner, their growth experiences can be better used for internal processing and will minimize projection and disillusionment with the military. The military is at many times hard and rigid, but it is often the only family some have. To influence their decisions and collude with their projection may result in rejection of the therapist, just like a rebellious teen who rejects a parent for not offering the structure and discipline required for a healthy development.

It is also important for the military social worker to analyse her/his own reasons and motiviations for working with military families, how they feel about the, and why they apply the therapeutic techniques and styles to help them (Kaslow & Ridenhour, 1984). Therapy with service families often engenders strong value judgments and counter-transference issues regarding conscious and unconscious prejudices concerning aggression, nuclear weapons, combat training and anyone committed to war. The social worker should allow individuals to make their own choices and mistakes and assist them by being a catalyst in their pursuit to resolve their ambiguities and personal struggles. While most families will want the military to change so that their lifestyle will be improved, this should not be the focus of treatment or intervention efforts. Changing the military system is beyond the capability of one person or family. Limitations set by military rigidity may also frustrate patients and therapists alike. Treatment expectations and unrealistic goals must be carefully evaluated. Client goals must be carefully evaluated. For example, asking for the return of a dependent wife's husband, who is deployed at sea, so he can be present for the birth of their child or during an operation or family crisis will most often not be granted.

Another health care related stressor is the lack of confidentiality. In most situations, privacy and confidentiality is maintained. However, all active duty personnel's medical, psychiatric or social work records are available for review in the course of an investigation to ascertain "fitness for duty." Any active duty service member can be "ordered" to undergo such evaluations in the name of military readiness and national security. This invasion of privacy must be justified by a legitimate "need to know" situation, which relates to a person's military performance.

Active duty service personnel are taught to depend on one another as a unit, but there is respect for individual values and responses and for shifts in job responsibility. Healthy families also operate in this fashion, maintaining a sense of the separate identity of each other and, at the same time, a commitment to the overall unit structure and its goal (Kaslow & Ridenhour, 1984). Healthy families in the military must find a balance between their identification with their military family, their civilian/social family and their cultural family of origin.

Certainly, the most difficult time for Navy families is just before, during and just after a long term deployment. The Navy is always at sea. Its ever-present appearance at strategic places around the world is part of the military balance of sea power and the struggle for control of important sea lanes for commerce and military operations. This is the life of the sailor, which then becomes the experience of the family. Even during shore duty, one is usually involved in training missions and frequent absences from home. While the Navy is well aware of the difficulties such long-term and frequent separations cause its Navy families, "the mission comes first," which is to man the ships and steam at sea.

Assisting the Navy dependent wife, who experiences separation anxiety and emotional difficulties when her spouse deploys, is a major function for the social worker. Once a level of satisfaction is achieved and exercised, conflict may then arise between the wife's new-found independent autonomy and her spouse's efforts to present his influence upon the family when he returns from a long-term deployment. A delicate balance in any marital relationship, between marital respect, shared responsibility and autonomy without the fear of engulfing one another in a power struggle is complicated by the constant separations and deployments. This reality has resulted in one Navy motto being "Navy Wife ... it's the toughest job in the Navy."

CASE EXAMPLE

Senior Chief Jones is thirty-eight years old. He is a highly respected senior enlisted electronics specialist. He has 16 years active duty military service and has been married for 14 years. It is both his and his wife's first marriage. He has three children ages seven, nine and eleven. His military performance record reveals he has been an outstanding sailor with no adverse legal or administrative actions. His Commanding Officer thinks highly of him as an outstanding performer who has potential for promotion and worthwhile Naval service. This individual was referred to the Family Advocacy Representative by his department head after his court hearing in a civilian court proceeding. He was accused of sexually molesting his nine-year-old daughter three years ago. The abuse consisted of oral and digital penetration of the child's vagina over a period of approximately six months. Abuse ceased when the daughter told her mother, but no one reported it to the authorities at that time. Mrs. Jones threatened to leave; however, Senior Chief Jones apologized, appeared remorseful and promised not to do it again. The child was six when the incestuous molestations began. There has been no remolestation since.

The daughter's disclosure came after her school had a puppet show about child sexual abuse. When the children were asked if they had ever been touched by a parent or relative in a wrong way, his daughter was one of several who described what had occurred to her three years ago. Her father was then investigated by Child Protective Services, Naval Investigative Service and the local police department. He pleaded guilty to the charges and since he was taking full responsibility for his behaviour, and did not attempt to deny or minimize his involvement, Child Protective Services felt he was a good candidate for therapy, and recommended to the Commonwealth Attorney's office that the sentence be suspended and treatment mandated. The court agreed and suspended a twenty-year incarceration and mandated therapy and probation. He also had to move out of his home until the therapist and Family Advocacy Representative and the Department of Social Services/Child Protective Services gave permission for him to return.

Senior Chief Jones was seen by a military social worker two months after the initial disclosure, and sentencing had already taken place. He was quite co-operative and highly motivated for treatment. The Family Advocacy Program was explained to him and his Commanding Officer. It was made quite clear that although the civilian courts had finished their legal procedures with the Senior Chief, the military could still recommend legal or administrative action, which could include court martial or administrative discharge. If approved for rehabilitation, the military also offered an opportunity of mandated treatment if the Commander, Naval Military Personnel Command, agreed that the individual had a good prognosis for successful rehabilitation and worthwhile Naval service.

The Family Advocacy Representative communicated with the Child Protective Services case worker and acquired the details of the molestation. Naval Investigative Service also provided their investigative evidence. Both consisted of interviews and statements made by the victim, the offender and all other family members. The reports were consistent with the offender's statements and he was judged by the Family Advocacy Representative to be a good candidate for rehabilitation under the aegis of the Family Advocacy Program. The case was staffed with the Family Advocacy Child Abuse Case Review Subcommittee. The subcommittee consisted of civilian and military social workers, military pediatricians, nurses and a chaplain. The group consensus was that the individual did indeed look like a good risk for treatment and a low risk for re-molestation. The basis for such a decision was made after a clinical evaluation was performed by the Family Advocacy Representative and a psychological assessment was performed by his civilian therapist. All agreed that he was not a fixated pedophile. His profile was consistent with heterosexual age appropriate psychological development until a period in his life where his marriage and marital sexual satisfaction became dysfunctional. This individual represented what Nicholas Groth refers to as a "regressed" child molester; an individual who may not exhibit primary orientation and sexual preference for children, but at a stressful point in the family's life cycle, regressed and offended with his daughter.

The report outlining the recommendation for retention and rehabilitation was forwarded to his Command and endorsed by his Commanding Officer. This packet was then forwarded to the Incest Program Manager at the Naval Military Personnel Command (NMPC). After three months of satisfactory therapy progress reports, this individual was officially "accepted" as a treatment candidate and his therapy was monitored for twelve consecutive months. He was transferred from his ship to a shore billet early in his treatment so as to remain available for consistent therapy. The Family Advocacy Representative forwarded quarterly therapy reports to his command and the NMPC. After twelve months of successful therapy and a statement by his therapist that he had utilized therapy well and achieved maximum therapeutic benefits, he was recommended for termination from mandated treatment and endorsed for regular naval reassignment. During his twelve months, he was not eligible for reassignment, and during his future career may not be eligible for overseas or isolated duty stations should his family accompany him. He will also be monitored by Family Advocacy for the duration of his Naval career and be required to participate in self help/group therapy.

References

Doering, Z. D. & Hutzler, W. P. (1982). *Description of Officers and Enlisted Personnel in the U.S. Armed Forces: A Reference for Military Manpower Analysis,*. (R-2851-MRAL). Santa Monica, CA: Rand Corp.

Finkelhor, D., Gelles, R. J., Hotaling, G. & Straus, M. A. M. (1983). *The Dark Side of Families.* Beverly Hills, CA: Sage Publications, Inc.

Gelles, R. (1987). *Family Violence* (2nd ed.). Beverly Hills, CA: Sage Publications, Inc.

Kaslow, F. W. & Ridenhour, R. (1984). *The Military Family: Dynamics and Treatment.* New York, NY: The Guilford Press.

Lagrone, D. M. (1978). The military syndrome. *American Journal of Psychiatry, 135,* 1040-1043.

Military Family Resource Center (1988). *The Military Family.* Office of the Assist. Secretary of Defense, Force Management and Personnel, 4015 Wilson Blvd., Arlington, VA.

Naval Military Personnel Command, (NMPC 663). Family Advocacy Program Manager, Washington, D. C. 20372.

U.S. Department of Health and Human Services (1980). *Child Abuse and Neglect Among the Military.* Publication # (OHDS) 80-30275, National Center on Child Abuse, Washington, D.C.

U.S. Government Printing Officer. (1987). *Defense Almanac '87.* Washington, D.C. 20402.

Endnotes

1   The views expressed in this article are those of the authors and do not reflect the official policy or position of the Department of the Navy, Department of Defense nor the U.S. Government.

Chapter 32

SOCIAL WORK PRACTICE WITH COMMUNITY-BASED DEMENTIA CARE

Roberta Y. Krakoff, ACSW
Lucy Esralew, MS

Abstract

A well-established group of consumers and providers with no direct service component identified a gap in services. Utilizing social work services, the organization developed a single-entry access to a continuum of care for victims of Alzheimer's disease and their caregivers. The project, now in its fourth year, is a unique and innovative approach to community-based dementia care.

SOCIAL WORK PRACTICE WITH COMMUNITY-BASED DEMENTIA CARE

There is an urgent need for services to Alzheimer's victims and their caregivers. Traditional services for this population are institutionally initiated and based. The Washington Heights and Inwood Council on the Aging (WHICOA — a fifty member consortium of consumers and providers in northern Manhattan) has made a unique contribution in this area by developing a model for single-entry access to a continuum of community-based care.

The project addressing the needs of this target population was initiated in 1984. At that time, recognizing the total absence of support services for Alzheimer's victims and their caregivers, WHICOA began to focus its attention on this deficit and the needs of this population. Its mission was to improve the life of 34,000 elderly in the area by encouraging the expansion and co-ordination of services. The area was perfect for the project having located within its boundaries such resources as Columbia Presbyterian, a nationally known teaching hospital, Yeshiva, a renowned university, Isabella, a prestigious geriatric centre with housing for the independent elderly and many fine senior centres and voluntary agencies.

The intent of the Council initiative was to provide leadership in addressing an identified gap in services. By adopting, centralizing and organizing dementia-related services, the Council fulfilled its role.

In less than three years, the Council has gone from the point of no organized services for individuals with dementing disorder and their caregivers, to a weekly Family Support group, a social respite program conducted in English and Spanish and a clearinghouse of information for referrals to services both within the community and citywide. The Council has been the hub for the organization and centralization of dementia-specific services within the community. Additionally, the Council has served as the conduit through which citywide services have flowed into the community, including Brookdale, ADRDA and the Visiting Nurse Service. With limited funding, drawing upon the in-kind services of its member agencies, the Council has succeeded in lessening the fragmentation and duplication of services to dementia victims and their caregivers. The Council has additionally proven the feasibility of co-operation of large and small agencies toward the accomplishment of a common goal.

THE CLIENTELE

The Council began in consultation with staff from the New York City Chapter of the Alzheimer's Disease and Related Disorders Association (ADRDA) and through observation of existing programs. The Council adopted a model for a Family Support Group (FSG) based upon one in effect at Einstein Medical Center where dementia victims were to be cared for while family members attended support group sessions. This arrangement enabled relatives to attend FSG meetings without worrying about substitute caregiving. The FSG was seen as a first step in alleviating caregivers' burdens. It provided information, support and a forum for the caregivers to give input into the community about what was needed to support families in their decision to maintain impaired relatives in the community.

The Council obtained the services of a consultant with expertise in the organization and delivery of dementia-specific services and experience in group leadership. The role of the consultant was to organize and run the FSG and to further identify gaps in services for this target population.

Through meetings with the Executive Committee of the Council and general membership of WHICOA, the consultant involved member agencies in the recruitment of clients for this project. Member agencies were asked to review their caseloads to identify clients who were caregivers of individuals afflicted with dementia and who could benefit from a weekly group meeting focussing on "caregiving." Agencies had the responsibility for initial preparation of the client, educating the client to the nature of this new service and helping to bridge the client from contact with the agency to contact with the consultant who functioned as the group leader.

The consultant conducted initial phone screenings and invited prospective group members for intake interviews. These interviews served to educate prospective members to the function of the group, enabled the group leader to establish a rapport with prospective members prior to their entry into the FSG. Both leader and prospective member were able to address expectations for participation and to collaboratively identify the areas in which caregivers needed assistance.

I. Home Visits

The consultant/leader realized in the course of conducting telephone screenings that most prospective members either would not or could not manage office visits and needed home visits. This opened a new dimension to our contact with caregivers. Most of the caregivers we contacted did not have a regular arrangement for substitute caregiving and were therefore unable to leave the impaired relative for an office visit. For several caregivers this was their first involvement with a community service addressing AD care. They evidenced some reluctance in making a commitment to the consultant, preferring to have the initial contact in their homes. The home visits were an unanticipated development which afforded valuable additional information, gained from the opportunity of observing caregiving on-site.

What emerged was that the caregivers were primarily spouses living on low or fixed incomes, who, in many cases, were suffering from personal physical problems. It became clear even in this early stage that families were in need of a range of concrete and psychosocial services to sustain both the dementia victim and the caregiver in an at-home caregiving situation.

II. Formation of the FSG

The Family Support Group represented a co-operative endeavour among WHICOA member agencies pooling their resources under the stewardship of the Council. The Council paid for the part-time services of the consultant/leader and reimbursed the cost of supplies. Other staff time was donated by agencies as in-kind service to the project. These workers were assigned to the project on a part-time basis in addition to their regular work responsibilities.

The FSG of Washington Heights was the first such group in New York City to be sponsored, organized and run as a community service. The group met once a week for an hour and a half and — consistent with the Einstein model — dementia victims were cared for in a separate space on the same site. A unique feature of this respite program was that in addition to a safe, supervised environment, a therapeutic activity program was provided for the participants.

All the members of the FSG were spouses, several of them were over eighty and suffering from various infirmities. Consequently, weather and the vicissitudes of both caregivers and their spouses' health, were obstacles in achieving consistent group attendance. Weekly telephone contact was maintained to remind caregivers of meetings and to follow-up with members when they did not attend. A common problem that affected attendance was the difficulty caregivers experienced in preparing themselves and their spouses for group sessions. Leaving the apartment, negotiating transportation and managing their spouses', at times, "difficult" behaviours became overwhelming for some members, which required assistance from the group.

The recreational sessions were particularly important. For many, they were the only social experience that was available to these impaired clients outside their homes. In the sessions, the impaired clients participated in a range of adult recreational activities geared to their cognitive deficits. This format proved to be valuable for caregivers and staff by allowing them to discover the abilities of the impaired individuals in such areas as socialization, task performance and relationship building. These sessions also served as a respite for caregivers, enabling them to have time away from their caregiving responsibilities, attend the FSG meetings and trust that other individuals could take care of their spouses during their absence.

There were many themes that emerged during that first program year. Caregivers needed information about the disease process and how to handle "difficult to manage" behaviours. They were mourning the loss of their spouses as healthy partners, looking for ways to form satisfying relationships based on changed circumstances, looking for ways to take care of their spouses without totally abandoning their own needs as individuals. They needed help in dealing with family members, friends, neighbours and physicians, along with obtaining assistance and support from these important others. Some of the members moved closer to the decision to institutionalize their spouses while others drew upon the group to support their decision to maintain impaired spouses at home for as long as possible. Clearly the group was diverse in both their caregiving experiences and needs.

In addition to the FSG it was clear that caregivers needed concrete services such as Meals-on-Wheels, financial and legal assistance, home care and medical services. Unlike other programs that functioned solely as support groups providing valuable information, the FSG provided referral to community service providers, entitlement assistance and counselling together with linking clients to social service agencies and other relevant resources. Indeed, in the second year of the program, the services of a social worker were secured to work particularly with group members on entitlements, refer clients to appropriate community and citywide resources and to conduct intakes for incoming FSG members. In response to caregivers' needs, more than one meeting a week was inaugurated.

"Respite" was a primary concern for caregivers. Recognizing this urgent need and the absence of such services in the community, the leadership of the Council approached the leadership of the Brookdale Center on Aging of Hunter College with regard to launching a co-operative venture in the Washington Heights-Inwood community.

Brookdale had already established a track record with several social respite sites in the City and was interested in expanding. Brookdale offered staff leadership for the program, staff assistance in recruiting clients, program supplies and volunteer training. Under the stewardship of the Council, member agencies pooled resources to enable the expansion of services. One member agency offered a site for the respite, another transportation. Lunch was available to participants at the Senior Center at a nominal fee according to guidelines set by the New York City Department for the Aging. Volunteers were obtained from a variety of sources including R.S.V.P. and the City Volunteer Corps administered through the Mayor's Office. The consultant served as Council co-ordinator for this project.

Member agencies were called upon to review their caseloads and to identify individuals who would be candidates for this service, to educate prospective clients to the nature of the service and to help clients bridge contact from agency to contact with staff for the new service. Referrals were solicited through phone contacts and by visiting senior centres to talk to staff and to centre members about this service.

The social respite had a dual focus. The program consisted of individuals who were suffering from a severe memory impairment. The intent of the program was to provide caregivers — family or paid — with planned time away from their caregiving responsibilities. Additionally, the program was structured to provide the memory-impaired client with opportunities for social contact and adult recreational activity. Our site was unique insofar as we provided transportation and lunch for our clients.

The Respite Program began in November of 1986. The staff leader assigned to the senior citizen centre site was bilingual because of the high concentration of Hispanic elderly in the Heights-Inwood.

III. Paid Caregivers' Education

An eight-week cycle of one and a half hour sessions started and was devoted to exploring the role of the paid caregiver. This cycle was in response to reports of difficulties in arranging and monitoring home care in addition to an interest in understanding what paid caregivers perceived as their issues and needs in providing service to dementia victims and their families. During this cycle, the consultant served as group leader, providing information about Alzheimer's disease and related disorders, and leading discussions on management of difficult behaviours such as resistance by clients to receiving care, rummaging and hoarding, wandering, and accusations by clients and their families of paid 'caregivers' negligence. The workers expressed particular concern about dealing with clients' paranoid behaviour, especially as it might affect family caregivers' trust of the workers. Workers also discussed how they became very involved with their clients, sometimes functioning as surrogate family. Paid caregivers were given release time by their clients to attend this program and were paid for their participation by their home care agency.

IV. Memory Disorders Clinic

During the second program year, a link was developed with the Memory Disorders Clinic — a joint venture of Columbia Presbyterian Medical Center and New York State Psychiatric Institute. The Memory Disorders Clinic was a valuable community resource to which one could refer individuals for evaluation; the Clinic also served as a potential referral base to our services. Differentiating dementia from other illnesses and syndromes that mask as dementia ensures referral to appropriate services.

V. The Restructured Family Support Group

By the third year of the program, the leadership of the FSG consisted of the pastoral counsellor and a social work student from Yeshiva University who combined the functions of co-leader and case worker. Staff had recommended that follow-up and assistance was best provided by a worker who was also involved in the weekly meetings. This modification of the model aided in the growth and consolidation of a core group and enabled the group to stay in contact with caregivers who were not able to attend FSG meetings on a regular basis but who derived support from their peripheral involvement.

VI. Expansion of Social Respite

In recognition of the success of the social respite program in Washington Heights and the potential for developing programming for Hispanic elderly, Brookdale obtained funding to support another program day; namely, one day of a social respite program conducted in Spanish and one day in English. In addition, the consultant worked with Brookdale staff to mount a special outreach to Hispanic elderly in the community.

PRACTICE ROLES AND RESPONSIBILITIES

During the several years of the project the consultant has served a multitude of roles, among them, direct service provider, educator, co-ordinator and case manager. What has been clear during this time is that case management/co-ordination is a key to the success of pooling together community resources and organizing and shaping such resources into a network of dementia-specific services. Case management/co-ordination is also essential if caregivers are to be spared the burden of negotiating with the myriad of agencies and are, instead, to have single-entry access to a network of organized services. Such access better ensures the smooth flow of clients along a continuum of care that includes evaluation and liaison to an array of relevant services and/or institutionalization.

An important function of the consultant has been to educate community professionals and older adults about the nature of dementia, related disorders and relevant services. This has been accomplished by touring senior centres and community groups to talk about memory disorders, clarifying the distinctions between normal and abnormal memory changes, identifying available resources and outlining possible steps in obtaining assistance for individuals with dementing disorders, and/or their caregivers.

To the extent that prospective clients and community professionals are aware of such issues, they are in a better position to appropriately identify clients for service and to better utilize existing services. Education is particularly important for senior centre populations and staff where a variety of individuals who cannot function in mainstream activities and whose behaviours may appear "difficult" or "odd" in such social settings are often mistakenly identified as having dementia. It becomes important, in developing appropriate programming, to differentiate the individual who is severely memory impaired from someone who is depressed or whose delirium is secondary to some other physical or psychosocial problem.

POTENTIAL FOR ROLE DEVELOPMENT

As the mission for social work services must increasingly move beyond institutional walls, particularly in health care settings, there are new implications for practice. The Community-Based Dementia Project demonstrated that flexible generic social work service skills work effectively and efficiently in helping this population. The professionals worked collaboratively in the community using outreach, counselling, linkage, information giving and referral services. The old adage that "we must start where the client is" was once again true.

In terms of role development, social work must learn to identify and create needed services rather than just implement them. The services must be cost effective and should then serve as a model so that other communities and populations can adopt the model. In other words, innovative approaches to practice must be documented so that models can be shared.

CONCLUDING REMARKS

The basis of the Community-Based Dementia Care model is that families caring for an individual with a dementing disorder have single-entry access to an array of social, medical, ancillary, supportive, home care and concrete services. These services represent a continuum of community-based care. A full-time case manager has responsibility for overall co-ordination of services serving as a liaison among small and large community agencies and ensuring the smooth movement of clients across this continuum of care. Building upon already existing services such as the Family Support Group, the social respite program, the Memory Disorders Clinic, Columbia Presbyterian Medical Center and Isabella Center for Geriatrics, the free-standing community model would add a social therapeutic day care program.

In the process of working on this model, a number of services were identified that could be shaped and organized into a dementia-specific network including home care, dental, psychiatric and rehabilitation therapies. The proposal served as a catalyst to mobilize support and interest of large and small agencies in pooling resources and meeting the diverse needs of this target population.

CASE EXAMPLE

Mr. and Mrs. N. were referred to the community-based project by the Family Support Group co-leader who had worked with the couple through pastoral service. At the time of the initial assessment in 1985, Mr. N., then 78, had been suffering from Alzheimer's disease for three years. Mrs. N., then 61, had sole caregiving responsibility.

Mr. N. exhibited a cluster of symptoms associated with the moderate-to-advanced stage of the disease: he was functionally dependent in all activities of daily living, he exhibited gross sensory and cognitive impairments, he wandered. Mr. N. needed 24-hour supervision. Mrs. N. was in good physical health but clearly stressed and visibly depressed. During the intake interview she expressed feelings of hopelessness and helplessness. The couple had been married for 25 years and were childless. They lived in an apartment in a deteriorating urban neighbourhood on Mr. N.'s pension.

Mrs. N. managed her husband's care without any assistance.

She was adamant about maintaining her spouse at home "as long as possible." An extensive intake including several home visits revealed that Mrs. N. had an idiosyncratic and unrealistic approach to her husband's care: she bathed, toileted, dressed and otherwise carefully attended to him until her resentment and hurt over her husband's incapacities overwhelmed her; when she felt overtaxed, she would totally forego attention to her spouse's routine needs. Mr. N.'s care was thereby determined by Mrs. N.'s mood and not by his requirements. The couple had no social contacts and the apartment was in disorder.

The worker determined that the stress of caregiving had exacerbated Mrs. N.'s personality problems, interfering with Mrs. N.'s ability to care for herself and her impaired spouse. In addition to the Family Support Group the worker recommended concrete services. The goal of work with the couple was to reduce the stress of caregiving by introducing relevant dementia-specific resources and by helping Mrs. N. re-assess her approach to caregiving.

A recommendation was made that Mrs. N. attend the once-a-week Family Support Group and that Mr. N. participate in the concurrent therapeutic recreation sessions. This provided Mr. N. with cognitive and social stimulation and was Mrs. N.'s first respite experience.

In the Family Support Group, Mrs. N. was exposed to other approaches to caregiving, received information about the disease process, obtained support and explored strategies for at-home management of her spouse. She had the opportunity to share her experiences in a safe, supportive environment. In the group, Mrs. N. developed relationships with other caregiving spouses that were continued during the week in-between group sessions. Mrs. N.'s pattern of help-rejecting complaining became evident and other caregivers kindly but firmly challenged her, giving her credit for her efforts and yet questioning her contribution in a self-defeating approach to caregiving. Mrs. N.'s participation in the Family Support Group opened an avenue for her to receive attention.

Staff worked with Mrs. N. to follow-up, on an individual basis, on issues raised in the group. During the three years of involvement in the project, the couple went from being isolated with no services to obtaining Meals-on-Wheels, Visiting Nurse Service, attending a twice-a-week social respite program, attending a local Senior Center and having a support network of peers. Recently, Mrs. N. worked through her reluctance to obtain medical attention for an urgent physical problem she was experiencing;

she placed her husband in a short-term residential respite and "took care of herself." Involvement with other caregivers and staff enabled her to look at what she has characteristically done with her own needs while she takes care of her husband who is so overtly in need of care.

The work done with this couple illustrates the efficacy of a multiple-intervention approach to service. Staff's in-depth assessment enabled the identification of a multi-faceted problem; this suggested the need for a comprehensive approach that included introducing the couple to relevant concrete services, dementia-specific services and addressing dynamic issues that were obstacles to the caregiver's effective utilization of services. Mrs. N. needed to be worked with in order to access and utilize services. Each move to accept a relevant service, be it meals-on-wheels a respite, was accompanied by extensive client preparation; it was necessary to address issues of separation, assertiveness, entitlement and other derivatives of low self-esteem that contributed to Mrs. N.'s neglect of her own health needs and her erratic approach to her husband's care.

Staff served several functions vis-à-vis this couple. Staff provided direct services such as the Family Support Group and social respite that were directly offered through the community-based project. Staff provided information and referral and helped the couple access other services that were relevant and not directly offered through the project. Staff provided case management, including an on-going assessment and evaluation of the couple's changing situation. As Mr. N.'s needs changed with the progress of the disease, staff were able to make relevant recommendations and help Mrs. N. access appropriate services. Staff provided information about the disease process and state-of-the-art strategies for at-home management. Staff counselled Mrs. N., working with her to remove obstacles to a realistic approach to caregiving.

This case illustrates that a worker can extend the caregiving capabilities of a couple by introducing services and simultaneously working with the caregiver on dynamic issues that interfere with effective coping strategies and effective utilization of health care resources. In the case of the N.s, the worker was able to reduce the burden of caregiving through the introduction of concrete services and to alleviate the caregiving spouses self-demand through the Family Support Group and individual counselling on an as-needed basis.

References

Caserta, M. S., Lund, D. A., Wright, S. D. & Redburn, D. E. (1987). Caregivers to dementia patients: The utilization of community services. *Gerontologist*, 27(2), p. 209-14.

Clayton, D. (1985). Community efforts help Alzheimer's victims. *Canadian Medical Association Journal*, 132(1), p. 68-69.

Held, M., Ransohoff, P. M. & Goehner, P. (1984). A comprehensive treatment program for severely impaired geriatric patients. *Hospital and Community Psychiatry*, 35(2), p. 156-160.

Endnotes

The following organizations worked collaboratively on the project:

Brookdale Center on Aging of Hunter College
Center of Geriatrics and Gerontology of Columbia University
Fort Washington Services for Elderly, Inc.
Isabella Geriatric Center
Memory Disorders Clinic of N.Y. State Psychiatric Institute and Columbia University
N.Y.C. Chapter of Alzheimer's Disease and Related Disorders (ADRD)
N.Y.C. Department for the Aging
The Presbyterian Hospital in the City of New York, Columbia Presbyterian Medical Center
Self Help
St. Elizabeth's Church Pastoral Care
S.T.A.R.
Washington Heights-Inwood Services and Transportation (WHIST)
YM-YWHA of Washington Heights and Inwood - Project Hopeé

Chapter 33

SOCIAL WORK PRACTICE IN A COMMUNITY-BASED SUBSTANCE ABUSE PROGRAM

Marvin D. Feit, PhD
Terence Mayes, MSW

Abstract

Social workers have provided treatment to substance abusers for many years. While treatment methods and services tend to be the same as in other facilities, local community-based substance abuse programs have several unique features for social work consideration. They provide services to populations living in the community, are independent treatment facilities, which tend to be more responsive to community and resident concerns, and their personnel are highly visible and accessible in the community. Social workers are likely to be employed at all levels in the agency and have direct responsibility in all aspects of outpatient care.

SOCIAL WORK PRACTICE IN A COMMUNITY-BASED SUBSTANCE ABUSE PROGRAM

Social workers have been serving substance abusers for many years. This chapter describes the activities of social workers in one aspect of the substance abuse field, a local community-based outpatient program. The substance abuse program is operated by the Community Services Board (CSB) of the City of Norfolk, Virginia. The members of its board of directors are appointed by the Norfolk City Council whose responsibility it is to see that it represents the residents of the city of Norfolk. The Board is chartered by the City of Norfolk and is legally established in the Commonwealth of Virginia.

The CSB established the Substance Abuse Outpatient Services Program to provide outpatient substance abuse services to the 279,000 residents living in Norfolk. It is estimated that the "at risk" population is substantial: 28,000 for alcohol; 5,000 for narcotics; and almost 15,000 for abusers of other drugs.

One distinguishing feature of the CSB is that since its board of directors are residents of the service area, it can better co-ordinate agency service with client and community need. In this regard, residents have the opportunity to be heard at board meetings and at public hearings, and they often interact with agency personnel by requesting information and services. Community persons usually perceive that they have a more direct impact on the agency, as demonstrated by the operation of several, smaller outreach or satellite centres.

Another distinct aspect of this community-based substance abuse outpatient program is that it operates independently of other health and medical care treatment facilities. The program maintains affiliations with selected treatment facilities and works co-operatively with a range of other community residents. It nevertheless is able to maintain its own identity and integrity.

The mission of the agency is to reduce the problems associated with substance abuse thereby decreasing social, economic and health problems through prevention, education, treatment, rehabilitation and research. The goal of the agency is to provide services to the substance abusing population and their families in the community. This goal often means working with employers, the

the courts, schools, probation and parole officers and other referral sources. Some of the services offered to clients include: prescreening evaluations and assessments; group, family and individual counselling; substance abuse and family education; discharge and aftercare planning and crisis intervention.

THE CLIENTELE

The Substance Abuse Outpatient Services (SAOS) provides services to a diverse population in the city of Norfolk. The SAOS has a central office, four satellite offices and a methadone clinic dispersed throughout the city, making the services accessible to the residents. Organizationally, the central office houses the administrative unit and also provides services. The four satellite offices have from one to three substance abuse counsellors each, depending on the size of the client population. Normal caseloads range from 35-40 clients per worker. There is one methadone clinic, which serves the entire city population.

Clients receiving services in the satellite or outreach offices represent various ethnic and racial groups. The location of each office often determines the characteristics of the treatment population, although clients may be served in any one of these five facilities. Because of uniqueness, methadone treatment is different and is discussed separately. Therefore, some social workers have clients who are predominately black or white, are employed or unemployed, and male or female. For example, one worker has a caseload which is all male, with 90% of them employed and about 60% are white and 40% are black.

In general, while many clients are employed full-time, there is a substantial portion of the treatment population who are unemployed, underemployed and/or receiving public assistance. Throughout the agency, about 80% of those treated are men, and the remaining 20% are women. Racial data are almost evenly split between black and white clients.

The agency makes a special effort to address the needs of different groups throughout the City of Norfolk, such as the poor and minorities. For example, it has developed a women's program, a program for black substance abusers, for adolescents and for clients with co-dependency problems. Typically, clients are walk-ins or are referred by other clients.

SAOS also operates a methadone program in one of its clinics. People admitted to the methadone program must prove continuous or episodic use of narcotic drug(s) for at least twelve months. Clients usually are experiencing social impairments related to narcotic drug use in their personal and/or occupational functioning. Such impairments typically involve loss of family and friends and missing work.

Admission to the methadone program involves a pathological pattern of abuse with one or more narcotic and other substances. This means using a narcotic substance daily for at least one month, increasing the intake of the drug to achieve the desired effect and experiencing a range of withdrawal effects such as rhinorrhea, pupillary dilation, piloerection, sweating, mild hypertension, tachycardia and others, as medically determined (Baum & Iber, 1988).

There are three types of clients exempted from the current physiological addiction requirements. One type is a person who has been released from a penal or chronic-care institution after being there at least one year. Such individuals may be admitted to the slow withdrawal phase of methadone treatment within fourteen days prior to, or within three months of being released or discharged from, such an institution without evidence to support findings of physiological dependence. Second, pregnant clients, regardless of age or prior addiction history, may be admitted to long-term withdrawal provided the Medical Director certifies that, in his or her judgment, such treatment is medically justified. Third, individuals who have been previously treated by the clinic are eligible for service when indicated.

PRACTICE ROLES AND RESPONSIBILITIES

The role of the social worker in the community-based substance abuse program is well defined. A social worker may be employed in every aspect of these programs and, for this chapter, only the direct service component is examined. In this capacity, a social worker has direct responsibility in the whole treatment process.

The treatment process normally involves an intake and assessment phase, acceptance into the program, the development of a contract and a treatment plan and a staffing contact with other members of the treatment team. At times, the social worker, after developing a discharge plan, may also work with the client in aftercare.

In the initial interview, the social worker is trying to assess many things. For example, questions such as why is the client seeking treatment at this time, how does the client define the presenting problem, how long has the client had the problem, has the client sought treatment before, what does the client think will be the outcome of treatment and do family members or others need to be involved in treatment are addressed. These are just a few key questions explored in the initial interview, but they help to obtain as clear a picture as possible of the client and the current situation. Where indicated, the social worker may co-ordinate the initial interview with the physician in order to obtain a more complete picture of the case and to assess whether a client needs hospitalization.

Upon completion of the intake/initial interview, identifying information is recorded on an intake form for each client. In this "pre-acceptance" phase a treatment plan is also developed, a medical and social history is obtained and a service agreement is completed. Only after all of this work is completed can a client be accepted, assigned a social worker and be "staffed," which means to be officially accepted for treatment in the agency. This pre-acceptance phase normally takes up to 30 days.

Once in treatment, methods of intervention may include: individual counselling, group therapy and family counselling, involving those members who have been affected by the client's substance abuse. It also involves referring clients to other community resources. When situations involve child abuse, child neglect, drinking and driving offences and employment problems, the worker must liaise with other agencies. Some of the typical duties and responsibilities include filing reports with protective service workers, preparing court reports for judges, attorneys and employers and, in rare instances, testifying in court.

In this program, clients accepted for treatment are assigned a primary worker, who is responsible for documenting the services received by the client and for monitoring the treatment plan. One task for the primary worker is to ensure that the services received by a client are congruent with those prescribed in the treatment plan. This entire process is monitored, in turn, by the program supervisor, who serves as a quality assurance monitor.

One of the most important tasks of a social worker is the development of the treatment plan. This plan is based on a needs assessment being done with the client, determined from the intake interview and other reports, and it reflects the major concerns identified by Louis, Dana and Blevins (1988). Thus, the client and worker negotiate a treatment contract, which becomes the mutually agreed upon treatment plan and forms the basis of the type and frequency of services offered as the client moves toward recovery. In this agency, becoming and remaining drug-free is the goal for each client, and this goal forms the basis of each contract.

Other goals are discussed with each client and may become part of the treatment plan. Such goals usually pertain to family life, or are related to work, or may involve the legal system. In any event, and as Brill (1981) stated, it is important that these goals be clear, achievable and provide direction to the client's purpose for being in treatment. Thus, each client has an individualized treatment plan.

Social workers are likely to be active in working directly with clients throughout the entire treatment process. Initially, contact is established through individual counselling. However, clients are encouraged to participate in substance abuse education and group treatment programs, which may be led by social workers, as clients have often benefited from them (Lewis, Dana, and Blevins, 1988).

POTENTIAL FOR ROLE DEVELOPMENT

Social workers have been serving substance abuse clients for many years and have served them in many capacities. For example, social workers have served as intake interviewers, individual, family, marital and group counsellors, referral specialists, supervisors, evaluators and administrators. The range of roles, responsibilities and tasks have been diverse and comprehensive.

There seems to be one primary area where role development could take place. Aftercare services have traditionally not been the most developed of the services provided to such clients. Much of the reason for this occurrence is that funds have generally not been provided for this service. In an effort to help clients maintain a drug-free state, case management services in aftercare programs have the greatest potential for utilizing community resources appropriately.

CONCLUDING REMARKS

There are several features that need to be taken into account when working in community-based substance abuse programs. While Lewis and Lewis (1983) identify important features of community counselling, some of the more prominent ones in this program are the impact an environment places on the lives of clients and their families, the visibility of the program and its staff in the community and the input from community residents.

It is important to note that much of what social workers do in community-based substance abuse programs is consistent with acceptable practice in other treatment settings (Lewis, Dana, & Blevins, 1988). This means that in many cases, they must deal with a client's denial system, use confrontation skills to hold clients to task, work with family members, make referrals when indicated and so forth.

However, the setting itself seems to affect the practice of social work in several ways. First, and most obvious, is that the client remains in the community and is connected to all of his or her community systems. Treatment must, therefore, take place in the context of this same environment, and usually the same conditions, which brought the client into the agency. However, it may be difficult to contend with an active and well-developed environmental support system in the context of treatment. For example, attending AA meetings on a daily basis often requires major shifts in the daily functioning of a client. One must make time to travel to and from the meetings, attend and respond to friends regarding the use of this time; i.e., where they went, what did they do, why are they avoiding them and so forth.

In another view, the visibility of the program and staff are higher in such settings than in other settings. For example, clients and their families are more likely to talk about their social workers because of their accessibility and the likelihood that they will be seen again in the community. Social workers can quickly gain a negative or positive reputation due to such high community visibility, which may in turn place a degree of stress on their performance.

There is a distinctly different feeling when one works in a community-based substance abuse program that can't always be captured by words. However, the treatment program is an integral part of the life of any community and its residents. At times, residents feel and act as if they can make a more direct impact upon the functioning of the agency. Further, clients may be quick to remind workers of their vulnerability by being accessible. Workers often wonder whether or not their intervention makes a difference in the context of clients living in these communities.

These are some of the features social workers must contend with when working with clients and their families in community-based substance abuse programs. Constant reminders in treatment, relative to the effect any treatment intervention has on a client's functioning in the community, is critical to effective counselling. Unlike other treatment settings, in community-based programs, treatment exists as an integral part of one's life and not as an abstract reality to be analysed and that one returns to at a later date.

CASE EXAMPLE

The following is a typical case served by social workers in a community-based program. All of the issues addressed in this chapter are evident, particularly the intervention strategy of the social worker. Some questions remain that may not be germane to community-based programs but need to be made explicit. For example, while this client is a self-referral, further discussion reveals that his recent work performance has suffered and his relationship with his wife and children has probably changed. Thus, his employer and/or his wife may have pressured him to seek treatment.

Mr. D. is a 46-year-old white male and a self-referral to Substance Abuse Outpatient Services for alcohol treatment. He is a native of Norfolk, Virginia and is the second oldest of five children. He describes his childhood as being normal with no developmental crises. He states that his relationship with his peers and siblings is good. Mr. D. is married and has two daughters aged 21 and 19. Mr. D. and his family are currently living in a mobile home. He completed the 12th grade of formal education and has been employed as a machinist for eight years. He had a good work record until he began missing work due to hangovers about a year prior to seeking treatment.

Mr. D. said, during the intake interview, that he had been drinking about a fifth of gin 2 or 3 days each a week. He also reported having experienced blackouts and withdrawal systems due to his excessive drinking behaviour.

His history revealed that he started drinking alcohol around age 20. He would have a few drinks (3 to 4 ounces per drink) to relax. His alcohol intake increased around age 39 when he began experiencing financial problems. However, after Mr. D. was able to reorganize his budget in order to meet his financial obligations, he continued with his abusive drinking pattern. This behaviour resulted in his experiencing blackouts and an increased alcohol tolerance level. At this time, he admitted to having interpersonal problems and employment problems. Interesting to note in his history was that he reported that neither of his parents had problems associated with alcoholism. However, while he said he felt good about himself, described himself as being out-going and well-adjusted, he stated that he drank alcohol to deal with life and was unable to cope with some very stressful situations. He came to the clinic because he wanted to stop drinking.

The social worker's impression was that Mr. D. admitted to having a problem with alcohol, which indicated some level of motivation. He also expressed serious problems with alcohol and has experienced several symptoms of alcoholism, such as

1) excessive drinking;
2) blackouts;
3) physical and psychological dependency and
4) withdrawal.

The prognosis in this case appears favourable, as a result of the client's awareness of his problem.

When Mr. D. came into the agency, he was unsure of the services offered by Substance Abuse Outpatient Services. The social worker explained to Mr. D. the services provided by the agency and explored the client situation during the intake and assessment phase. The client and social worker agreed on several "next steps" in developing an appropriate treatment plan.

The client agreed to attend individual counselling sessions to become involved in a growth group, to attend Alcoholics Anonymous meetings in the community and to attend a three-day social detoxification program. The social worker will be the one monitoring the clients' progress, doing the counselling, perhaps conducting the growth group and making referrals for participa-

participation in the social detoxification program and AA meetings. When indicated, the social worker is likely to work with the family, make contacts with other institutions on behalf of the client, (courts, health, employer) and work to help the client achieve his or her own objective.

References

Baum, R. A. and Iber, F. (1988). Initial treatment of the alcohol patient. In S. E. Gitlow & H. S. Peyser (Eds.), *Alcoholism: A Practical Treatment Guide* (2nd ed.) (pp. 54-66). Philadelphia: Grune & Stratton.

Brandsoma, J. M. & Welsh, R. J. (1982). Alcoholism outpatient treatment. In E. M. Patterson & E. Kaufman (Eds.), *Encyclopedia Handbook of Alcoholism* (pp. 885-893). New York: Gardner Press.

Brill, L. (1981). *The Clinical Treatment of Substance Abusers.* New York: Free Press.

Lewis, J. A., Dana, R. Q. & Blevins, G. A. (1988). *Substance Abuse Counselling.* Belmont, CA: Brooks/Cole.

Lewis, J. A. & Lewis, M. D. (1983). *Community Counselling: A Human Services Approach* (2nd ed.). New York: J. Wiley.

Chapter 34

SOCIAL WORK PRACTICE IN A THERAPEUTIC COMMUNITY CONTEXT

Neal Ruton, MSW, CSW
Tracey Foreman, BSW, MSW

Abstract

This chapter will examine the roles of social work practice in the unique setting of the therapeutic community (TC). A descriptive analysis of the TC milieu combines with an exploration of the drug addict's nature and treatment needs to yield an engaging vision of the potential for social work role development. Prompted by the conspicuous absence of our profession's involvement in the TC setting, this submission challenges the social work aspirant to pioneer new vistas of effective theory and practice to confront the darkening shadow of the escalating drug abuse crisis pervading contemporary times.

SOCIAL WORK PRACTICE IN A THERAPEUTIC COMMUNITY CONTEXT

THE CLIENTELE

I. The Settings

The Therapeutic Community (TC) is a unique and highly specialized approach to the treatment of substance abuse. In contrast to traditional settings of hospitals and prisons, the TC milieu establishes new levels of rehabilitative achievement in the field of drug addiction. The TC is a microcosm of the larger social environment, in which the client (generally referred to as resident, or member) undergoes two fundamental processes: drug-free lifestyle disruption followed by resocialization of a renewed, healthy self.

With regard to the "hard-core" drug addicts who are the TC's target population, the TC philosophy rejects modalities that focus short-term treatment endeavours on long-term problems, or interventive efforts that provide drugs to the drug abuser (e.g., methadone maintenance). The treatment stance of the TC is that the behaviourial abuse of drugs is an overt symptom of a covert problem; that addiction is a lifestyle. These fundamental premises of the TC demand expansive treatment goals related to self-examination and a restructuring of life, in all aspects, for the addict. Thus, it is not surprising that the TC treatment format and process is intensive and long-term.

The TC asserts that two central requirements are implicit in the resocialization process: a) exposure to responsible concern, coupled with b) firm behaviourial limits. Further, the structural components of the treatment process are linked to specific learning objectives. The catalystic elements of the TC include the concept of self-help; positive peer pressure; confrontation; structures to facilitate expression; role modelling; internalized constructive attitudes developed through achievement; living in a self-sufficient group; open communication and shared decision making; isolation from the outside community; pressures used to recruit and motivate clients; individual counselling; education and formalized

615

skill training; supervised contact with the outside community; organized recreation; public confession; ritual participation and the concept of uniqueness. Sugarman (1982) lists several learning objectives that correspond to the aforementioned elements, including: short-term behaviourial modification; impulse control; development of empathy and helping skills; expression and integration of feeling; sense of competence and pride; development of responsibility; encouragement of decision-making skills; growth of insight; development of socialization skill; healthy utilization of leisure time; development of specific employment related skills; and, finally, the integration of a "group solidarity" philosophy. While all of these treatment components can be found in all therapeutic communities, their specific application in the rehabilitative process is varied.

There are two distinct TC types, commonly referred to as the "European" and the "American" models. Essential differences between the models are summarized by the following chart:

	EUROPEAN	AMERICAN
1) Conception of client	More value placed on individual	Treat them like "emotional babies"
2) Staff roles	Facilitators Supportive Authoritative	Directive Judgmental Authoritarian
3) Role models	Be the good person you have the potential to be	Ex-addict: "Be more like me"

(Please refer to Halpern & Levine, 1979)

Therapeutic Communities based upon the European perspective view some types of "learning experiences" (i.e., wearing signs, shaving heads, humiliating task assignment) conducted by American model T.C.s as degrading and punitive. The controls, restrictions and value judgments imposed upon clients in some American Therapeutic Communities are considered to be of debatable clinical value (Sugarman, 1982).

The European TC model conceptualizes the client as an individual and utilizes staff members as facilitators and senior residents as role models. The ultimate goal of the European Therapeutic Community is to separate the rehabilitated drug addict from the intensive bonds of the family-like TC atmosphere and reintegrate him back into society as a healthy and contributing member. The American TC model, by contrast, uses ex-addicts as staff members and has a tendency to employ harsher methods of confrontation, and humiliating sanctions for unwanted behaviours. In many cases, the former addict graduates through the ranks of the American TC, yet remains within the TC framework in an ex-addict staff member role. In more recent years, it is apparent that both schools of thought are aware of the value of professional staff, together with the essential role of the ex-addict. Many American TCs have now hired professionally-trained staff, and the European TC, for its part, utilizes the value of the ex-addict as a role model.

Stonehenge Therapeutic Community (STC), founded upon the European model, is Canada's first TC. STC was created in 1971 by Dr. John M. Dougan, Director of the Community Psychiatric Hospital, Guelph, Ontario. At that time, drug-dependent individuals were being treated by the traditional forms of health service systems and a substantial number were being incarcerated as a result of the criminal/deviant lifestyle necessary to maintain an expensive drug habit. Addicts were afforded in-patient and out-patient treatment approaches, chemotherapy, occupational retraining, etc. These, collectively, resulted in duplications of service; wasted treatment endeavours and an accumulation of cost. Hospitalization or incarceration for the particular social problem of drug dependency, without treatment, was as unsuccessful then as it is now.

Since 1971, the Stonehenge Program has become nationally recognized as Canada's most viable treatment approach to drug addiction.[1] This is due to the fact that,

> Stonehenge views drug addiction as a symptom of a maladaptive mode of living rather than focusing treatment on the actual behaviourial abuse of drugs. The therapy deals with the alteration of a person's entire lifestyle and the discovery of a new set of values and goals. This process concludes in the successful rehabilitation of the ex-addict into society as whole. Rehabilitating the addict offender is a very long and complex process. (Ruton, 1982)

Indeed, as Ruton (1982) further states, "The program is distinguished from conventional modalities by its philosophy as well as its environment. Addiction is a lifestyle and therapeutic intervention focused solely on the behaviourial or physiological aspect of the non-medical usage of drugs is only temporarily effective at best."

Snyder's (1979) analysis of the success of Stonehenge focusses on the fact that,

> Stonehenge uses a theoretical approach of lifestyle disruption and resocialization. The professional staff actively and intensively engage in disrupting those aspects of the addict's lifestyle which predispose him or her to a drug dependent existence and, therefore, a life of crime. Addicts are carefully screened and only a small percentage of highly motivated individuals are admitted for treatment (p. 21).

The residents spend the majority of an average 12-month treatment term in isolation from the rest of the community. The setting of STC is pastoral, located just outside Guelph, Ontario, and provides the necessary geographical and social environment.

The Stonehenge Program produces a 75% curative outcome, as defined by lack of return to the behaviourial abuse of drugs, and stability within society (Holt, 1979). In addition to dramatically reduced recidivism rates, the Stonehenge Program provides significant savings to the taxpayers of Canada through cost effective treatment — as compared to the burden of expenses generated by addict offenders through the traditional processes of incarceration, or delivery of health care services.

Stonehenge is the only program of its kind to have been accredited by the Canadian Council on Hospital Accreditation. In recent years, its rehabilitative endeavours have been favourably recognized as an alternative to incarceration by Ontario Courts. Other countries are desirous of obtaining bedspaces for their citizens within the STC facility, as evidenced by ever-increasing referrals from international sources. At the present, Stonehenge Therapeutic Community provides 18 beds to the Ontario Provincial Ministry of Health; 12 beds for the Ontario Ministry of Correctional Services and approximately 5 beds for the Correctional Services of Canada. As an independent non-profit organization established by Letters Patent, and governed by a community-based Board of Directors, STC also receives funding as a registered charitable organization.

The highly structured daily and weekly program includes the following treatment modalities:

Group Therapy: Goal-oriented group therapy occurs 3 times per week, in sessions of 3 hour duration. Intensive levels of peer confrontation provide the impetus for self-reflection and change. As individual responsibility is promoted, and visible behaviourial change becomes apparent, the resident prepares to advance through the hierarchy of role responsibilities and privileges as determined appropriate by this peer group. Ultimately, however, the professionally trained group therapist is responsible for the nature of the corrective emotional experience shared by the group members.

Occupational Therapy: TC philosophy maintains that the survival of the community is based upon mutual interdependence. Thus, each individual plays an integral role in the maintenance of the environment (i.e., cooking, cleaning, gardening, etc.), recognizing and experiencing himself as a valued member of the total community. The occupational therapy program simulates the real job environment as closely as possible. Toward this end, residents prepare job applications, resumes, are interviewed, compete and proceed through a hierarchial structure as they demonstrate responsible work habits. This upward mobility is signified by earned increases in a weekly token salary and progressively higher levels of authority.

Activity Therapy: Physical fitness and awareness are promoted within the treatment structure, in sharp contrast to the addicts' former abuse of their own bodies. Progressively improving health, participation in sporting events and a developing sense of physical awareness and well-being serve to increase the client's somatic and mental awareness. This aspect of the program also stimulates and encourages the development of positive future leisure time activities.

Life Skills Program: The purpose of the Life Skills Program offered at STC is to provide clients with both educational opportunities and to enhance their skill capabilities. Emphasis focusses on the development of communication, relaxation and social skills.

Art Therapy: Art Therapy is offered on a weekly basis at STC and encourages intra-interpersonal insight through artistic expression. A variety of mediums (e.g., clay, paint, pastels, collage, etc.) are utilized. Each resident's representation is discussed in his art therapy group, which is comprised of different Community members from the resident's day therapy group. As opposed to the day group therapy sessions, the art therapy group is non-confrontational in nature.

Individual Therapy: Individual therapy sessions, also available at

STC, are confined to specific issues and are administered by a highly skilled multi-disciplinary staff team. Individual work may be undertaken in response to crisis, stagnation or in conjunction with the specialized expertise of a staff member in dealing with a particular client treatment dynamic (i.e., incest, parenting, guilt and shame issues, etc., not resolved in the group therapy format).

Discharge and Follow-Up: STC prepares its graduating residents for separation from the program by maintaining the same dual person/environment focus evidenced throughout the treatment stay. No member is allowed to leave the treatment setting without first having obtained a job or acceptance to an educational institution. Residents must also have prepared the necessary requirements for general societal membership (i.e., an apartment, source of income, etc.) Community resource networks are established and expanded (i.e., family relationships, non-drug-abusing friends, attendance at Narcotics Anonymous sessions and involvements with community organizations or groups). The agency recognizes graduation from the Program as a final rite of passage and the Community, as a unit, shares in the resident's success through his "consensus." (i.e., a graduation ceremony). To mark this occasion, members of the Community prepare a tribute to the graduating resident, usually in the form of a dinner, followed by comical theatrical skits, incorporating reflections of the past, testimonials of the present and well wishes for the future. Upon separation from the Program, the graduate resident attends follow-up care in the form of bi-weekly out-patient sessions with a professional therapist.

Special Treatment Focus Groups: Women's issues and parenting groups are conducted on weekends for selected residents to assist with specific areas of concern.

II. Descriptive Features of the Clients

Recent research at STC provides quantitative and qualitative data concerning types of drugs abused; frequency of use; length of drug abuse involvement; the method of self-administration of drugs; previous treatment contacts; nature of initiation into the drug abuse subculture; age; educational and socioeconomic backgrounds of clients in treatment and compounded or secondary problems (i.e., alcohol abuse). Assessment staff at the treatment facility also report individual resident commonalities/differences and distinctive medical and social histories of the clients. Agency statistics offer data regarding geographical residency of clients;

gender characteristics; incest involvement and criminal-judicial backgrounds, etc.

Client Features at STC

(a) **Descriptive data:**

primary type of drug consumed:
> 38.4% Opiates
> 17.4% Amphetamines
> 11.6% Cocaine
> 10.5% Sedatives
> 7.0% Hallucinogens (of Poly Substances)

frequency of drug use:
> 93.0% Daily
> 4.7% Weekly
> 1.2% Weekend only
> 1.2% Reported other

length of drug use:
> 34.9% Reported 6 - 11 years
> 27.9% Reported 11 - 15 years
> 24.4% Reported 1 - 5 years
> 10.5% Reported over 15 years
> 1.2% Reported 0 - 1 year

method of administration:
> 85.0% Self-administered by intravenous injection

previous treatment experience:
> 89.5% (Psychiatric, medical and/or
> community-based)

initiation of drug use:
> 16.7 Years (average age)

average length of active drug abuse:
> 7.75 Years

average age of clients in treatment:
> 23.88 Years

alcohol-related problems:
> 78.3% of population
> (Wilhelm, 1988, pp.44)

(b) **data collected by assessment staff:**

individual commonalities:

        limited community connection;
        previous criminal histories;
        suicide attempts;
        poor self-concept

    distinctive female characteristics:
        bulimia/anorexia;
        prostitution;
        incest/abuse;
        loss of child custody

(c) **ongoing program statistics:**

    addict commonly alienated from family and friends;
    addict commonly insular minority immersed in drug culture;
    addict commonly reluctant to seek formal medical treatment
      because of distrust and alienation from traditional health
      care system.

    geographical residency of clients:
            92.94% primarily Southern Ontario
            7.06% Guelph and Area

    gender characteristics:
            68.6% male
            31.4% female

    educational backgrounds:
            50% partial Secondary School
            29.1% Secondary School graduates
            10.5% any Post-Secondary School
            10.5% Elementary School only

Zastrow (1985) offers a general symptomalogical schema for substance abusers, which includes the following: denial; rationalization; projection; delusion; low self-worth and physical symptomalogy directly related to substance abuse. Interested readers should investigate the chapter of his book, which takes a process-oriented approach similar to that of STC with regard to the characteristics of clients.

The client entering treatment at Stonehenge is generally a youthful or adult addict, with a lengthy history of involvement with serious drugs (i.e., heroin, cocaine, prescription drugs, etc). These pre-selected, "hard-core" members of the overall drug-abusing population present for treatment with a previous lifestyle that is more dysfunctional than the actual drug abuse itself. These clients have been described as "highly motivated individuals," actively seeking admission to STC's self-help rehabilitative community. In fact they are, more aptly, individuals driven by desperation to participate in the very demanding process of rehabilitation.

While the majority of drug addicts on the street are very familiar with the rehabilitative opportunities at Stonehenge, it is usually only those who are facing crises in their drug dependent lifestyles who seek admission. The force of law may prompt an individual to apply to the agency. Drug-dependent prisoners seeking an early release to what they initially perceive as a more comforting setting than jail will often apply for a transfer to STC. Female addicts coerced by the removal of their children by social service agencies engage in the treatment program at Stonehenge to become drug-free, responsible mothers and regain custody of their offspring. Also, many individuals seek treatment at STC without judicial intervention. Some simply become exhausted from the vigorous demands of the street lifestyle. They have seen their friends or siblings overdose and die and reach a point where they are desperate to change. While the motivation of many entrants is less than sincere, the client who remains within the program eventually develops a genuine, internalized commitment to their process of self-change.

The agency recognizes, in addition to the aforementioned characteristics of the clientele, several factors related to entry into the TC as a treatment modality. The following list of commonly observed facts about new residents in TCs, accompanied by several cognitive and behaviourial practice suggestions for facilitation of the client into the treatment modality, will assist in an understanding and enabling of the client population:

1) The new resident is generally distrustful of everyone at the TC. The new resident frequently comes to treatment from the street, or a correctional institution. The client's modes of behaviour reflect the mistrust and suspicion that were functional for survival in their previous lifestyle. An effective therapeutic stance related to this issue begins with an expectation of initial distrust and/or an unconventional motivation for seeking treatment (i.e. hiding out, avoiding judicial repercussions, etc). Empathy, as opposed to sympathy, and the cognitive understanding of the client's present situation is essential.

2) The new resident is frequently physically weak and may have reactions associated with drug withdrawal and culture shock. Many new TC residents have been physically inactive for long

periods of time and find the immersion into a vigourous daily routine difficult. After entering the drug-free therapeutic environment, the new resident becomes more stable after approximately 4 weeks. During this initial time period, confrontation and expectation are held to a minimum to facilitate adjustment.

3) The new resident is a stranger to the setting and frequently feels alienated from the rest of the community. The client entering treatment will need time to make the cognitive shift from self-orientation to the Community-oriented philosophy and treatment atmosphere of the TC. As practitioners, we assist in this process by creating an atmosphere of trust and acceptance, while not condoning the previous dysfunctional lifestyle of harm to self and others. The professional therapist encourages hope in the new resident and facilitates his involved membership in the community as precursor to freedom from drugs and a functional, successful future in society.

4) The new resident, in most cases, is unskilled at direct, honest communication. New residents, unlike more experienced TC clients, are likely to find direct confrontative interpersonal exchanges unfamiliar and threatening. Their self-expression is typically reflective of their former lifestyles (i.e. deceitful and manipulative). They are often purposefully vague and defensive and avoid honest exchange. As professional practitioners, we assist in this area by providing explicit explanations of the TC treatment modality, including the jargon employed within the setting and modelling the direct interpersonal communication that is expected. Self-disclosure is encouraged, with an accompanying tolerance of the client's initial difficulties in relating emotion-laden material.

5) The new resident is unaware of the group-oriented philosophy and process of the TC. New residents may find the authority of the TC day group awkward and unpleasant, until they recognize the central necessity of this mechanism to the treatment modality. The TC staff facilitate understanding by providing explicit explanations and examples of group processes used in the TC, such as feedback, confrontation, openness, self-disclosure, isolation and phases of treatment achievement.

6) The new resident is unsure of the program and its effectiveness; hence, he may be suspicious of the goals and intent of the various interventions. New residents are initially concerned

with the potency of the treatment modality to impact upon their future lives. In many cases, this professed concern is a mechanism to avoid self-responsibility and represents a fear of becoming committed to a drug-free, successful life. The TC addresses this resistance through direct discussion and, more effectively, it provides visible role models. Senior and graduate residents provide personal, quantifiable, observable testimony to the program's efficacy.

7) The new resident may perceive senior residents and/or staff members as he would traditional authority figures. For many years previous to entering treatment, TC clients have been involved in a lifestyle segregating the addict from other members of various social strata. The "us/them" dichotomy (i.e., the "addict" versus "straight member of society," or the "addict offender" versus the "prison guard" figure) initially contaminates an objective perception of roles within the TC. It requires time and a developing basis of trust for the new resident to assimilate a full understanding of the hierarchial structure of the therapeutic community and his upward mobility within it. As effective practitioners, we facilitate the new resident's development of an accurate cognitive blueprint for his goals and objectives within the TC structure. The staff and residents assist the new client to understand the universal application of TC principles, gradually eroding traditional client/staff stereotypes.

8) The new resident experiences initial disorientation and new, confusing emotions. This phenomenon occurs because, for the first time in years, they are free of the mental and emotional "blocking effect" of intoxicating drugs. Former emotions related to guilt and shame are no longer vague and stifled. The resident may also experience levels of joy and exhilaration related to their first positive steps toward a retrieval of self. This signifies, for many, the first pleasurable experiences in years not synthetically induced by drugs.

9) The new resident often needs "time to breathe". Carefully considered flexibility in allowing time-limited periods of solitude affords the new resident an opportunity to regain perspective, and also relieve pressure attributable to the confrontative group process. However, over time, the resident will learn to assimilate the constructive criticism of others and,

in combination with their own self-reflection, actively participate in the group exchange format of the TC.

10) The new resident is frequently overwhelmed with the rigour and intensity of the TC program. Acknowledgment that immersion into the TC's unique treatment process can produce anxiety and pressure is essential. Nonetheless, when managed appropriately, this dynamic is precisely the type of functional stress that produces the impetus for change vital to ultimate rehabilitative recovery.

III. Presenting Problems and Needs

While the presenting problems of drug addicts fall into several distinguishable categories, from the obvious physical repercussions associated with self-abuse (eg., dirty needle sharing and drug overdose) to criminal, familial and marital issues, the most profound problems are related to the all-encompassing addicted lifestyle and accompanying distorted sense of self. The needs of the client are much more complex than would initially appear under traditional treatment format scrutiny. Several major categories of presenting needs and problems of drug addicted clients are delineated below

Physical Problems: The behaviourial act of ingesting an illicit drug automatically imposes a physical retribution. Simply stated, for every high there is a corresponding low — which can range from a mild depression after a drug experience, to the ultimate price, overdose. Drugs can be self-administered orally, rectally, inhaled or by intravenous injection (IV).

The majority of clients at Stonehenge are IV drug abusers. These individuals place themselves at risk of contracting many diseases through the sharing of syringes, thereby exchanging blood with other drug abusers. The two diseases of significance most common to needle-sharing addicts are serum hepatitis (hepatitis B) and AIDS. HIV+ (positive) drug addicts have now superseded members of the gay community in contracting AIDS and represent the gateway for the spread of HIV+ infection to the heterosexual population. Other physical problems manifested may include the inducement of epilepsy; the collapsing of veins after prolonged IV use; numerous psychosomatic maladies as a result of bodily and personal health neglect; liver damage and physical problems from former suicide attempts, accidents and drugs "cut" (mixed with a substance to increase the overall quantity of the drug) with other harmful chemicals. The authors wish to stress that the physical problems associated with needle-sharing have significantly increased over the previous years with the growing popularity of cocaine. Because the cocaine "high" is so much shorter than that of other drugs, such as heroin, the addict has to inject at a rate 7 to 10 times more frequently to achieve comparable effects when using cocaine. This accelerated use only increases the chances of contracting diseases and experiencing resultant physical problems.

Criminal/Judicial: While all drug addicts may not have a criminal record, they all participate in criminal acts. The possession or use of a restricted drug is, in itself, a crime. The majority of drug addicts, however, will become involved with the criminal-judicial system resultant of the lifestyle they undertake to maintain an expensive drug habit. The average cost of a cocaine or heroin habit for a resident receiving treatment at STC is $500 to $1,000 a day. The acquisition of this amount of income necessitates criminal involvement for the majority of our clients. The selling of drugs to other addicts, prostitution, theft, forgery and fraud, double doctoring and various other crimes eventually catch up with the addict. Consequently, they are often placed in settings (i.e., incarcerated, hospitalized) where drugs are still available to them, where rehabilitative opportunities are limited and where their anti-social attitudes are reinforced when they are eventually released back onto the street to continue with their drug abuse. Perpetuating the cycle, they commit further crimes to maintain their habits, again to be caught and incarcerated.

Family and Marital Relationships: It is inaccurate to assume that the majority of clients at STC turned to drug abuse because of abusive backgrounds or deprived childhoods. While their histories often present developmental traumas, it is also the case that the addict has been destructive to the stability of their family of origin and has caused his loved ones a great deal of anguish and pain. It is common practice for addicts to steal from their mothers' purses; forge cheques from their fathers' companies; squander their inheritances from deceased parents and display consistently disruptive behaviour within the family unit. In the marital dyad, the drug addict behaves as an irresponsible father/mother/spouse, and a great deal of therapeutic intervention must be directed towards a reunification of the family, if this is a mutually desirable therapeutic goal. During the course of the treatment term, aspects of guilt and shame, sexuality, parenting and role relationships within the family of origin and marriage are investigated and resolved.

The Self: Of greatest importance in the treatment of addicts within the therapeutic community context is the development of a new self. All other presenting problems related to physical disorders, criminal/judicial background and relationship to the family and/or marital dyad must be viewed as secondary to the problem of disordered character development and awareness of self. The four psychosocial elements below distinguish the drug addicted personality from general societal membership:

1) *Self-Orientation*

While "healthy" members of our society seek personal attainment and gain, the majority do not significantly harm others to do so. Drug addicts present as more self-centred individuals, who will harm people, steal from their loved ones, etc., and feel compelled to place their needs for immediate gratification ahead of the concerns of others. In treatment, addicts are taught to be creatively self-involved and selfish. Be selfish — look after your body; stop using drugs and needles. Be selfish — participate in the treatment, graduate from the program, get a job, be happy. Successful treatment intervention will refocus an addict's impulse toward self-gratification into productive and socially-acceptable channels.

2) *Poor Self-Concept*

While many of us may at times become constructively self-critical, a "healthy" person is not immersed in self-hatred. Addicts do not like what they are, and, after all, they have plenty of legitimate reasons to verify their poor self-image. Their self-destructive behaviourial use of drugs, the crimes necessary to finance the habit and the degrading acts that are part of their lifestyle reinforce an addict's negative self-concept. On the surface, many substance abusers are gregarious and possess the engaging interpersonal skills necessary for "hustling" the money to support a drug habit; but, when they are alone, when they are not under the influence of drugs, they do not like what they have become. An addict is caught in a vicious cycle. They dislike what they are, and therefore experience anxiety and depression. Consequently, they take drugs to alleviate this anxiety and sensation of worthlessness (i.e., get high to feel better). The problem is, the drugs wear off, and they again become depressed — resuming the pattern by seeking more drugs. This pattern is illustrated by the chart shown over.

In essence, then, drug addicts are self-medicating their own illness. In effective treatment, this cycle is broken, the drug addict faces who they are, and begins building a legitimate positive self-concept. The first step is their decision to invest in and commit to the arduous process of change.

3) *Perception of Time*

As we grow, we learn from our earlier mistakes and develop confidence from our past triumphs. Addicts, on the other hand, reject the reality of their pasts. This is understandable, when one considers that their pasts are filled with criminal activities, negative repercussions and a street lifestyle permeated by guilt and shame, which, if soberly reflected upon, would do nothing less than demand a cessation of drug abuse in the present.

The reluctance of drug addicts to make a commitment to denouncing the patterns of the past reflects their co-existing awareness of their lack of success in the present and dread of continued failure in the future. To protect himself from this experience, the addict injects drugs, which produce a relative lack of concern with what may happen within even minutes. It is possible to overdose and die from one injection. With this kind of immediate repercussion impotent as a deterrent, it is not difficult to conceive the addict's similar lack of concern for long-term consequences, such as contracting AIDS or hepatitis. The addict's perception of past, present and future consequence is altered in the TC process, demanding self-reflection without the escape of substance abuse.

4) *Manipulation*

Drug addicts find manipulation a functional necessity for maintaining expensive drug habits. They are "cons" not solely by nature of their previous criminal involvement, but owing to their addiction and resultant lifestyle. Most addicts have good interpersonal skills, which they have distorted into tools for their deceptions. In treatment, the client's former manipulations of others for their own gain is refocussed — toward a retention of their original interpersonal skills, while rejecting their use in service of fraudulent purposes. Post-treatment, these skills are applied to legitimate ends, such as employment roles, social support network advancement, etc.

For further information, Turner (1984, pp. 453) offers a social work perspective on the psychosocial treatment of drug addiction. The following chart summarizes his conceptualization of the process involved. Interested practitioners may elect to read his detailed chapter on this subject.

Table 1 *A Social Work Model for Treating Drug Abuse: Supportive Resources for Psychosocial Treatment*

PHASES OF PSYCHOSOCIAL TREATMENT

1. Preparation:	Knowledge Attitudes Supervision	4. Intervention:	Treatment Primary care Collaboration
2. Induction:	Relationship Motivational counselling Information	5. Evaluation:	Follow-up Relapse Prevention Corroboration
3. Negotiation:	Assessment Selection of treatment Consultation		

PRACTICE ROLES AND RESPONSIBILITIES

A fundamental role of social work in all settings is that of advocate. This role is particularly applicable to the field of drug addiction and even more critical in the specific area of residential treatment services provided to serious drug addicts. When one considers that there are only two therapeutic communities in the entire country, one based on the American model and the other (Stonehenge) based upon the European model, it is evident that there is a great need for social workers to advocate in this field. The situation is further intensified by the fact that Stonehenge is the only TC in Canada based upon a program directed by professionally-trained staff. To the authors' knowledge, there are only three professional social workers in our nation directly employed in a TC setting. These positions are all held at Stonehenge Therapeutic Community. In contrast to other nations, which are proud to have numerous therapeutic communities and social workers serving their drug-dependent populations, our country should be ashamed of the lack of development, foresight and response to the needs of Canadian addicts. As seen in the following delineation of social work roles in TC settings, advocacy on behalf of this target population is an underlying theme — indeed, a crying need.

I. Group Therapist

Professional social work roles undertaken in the context of the group therapy session are multifarious. Moreover, they are often developed in an *ad-hoc* fashion, as warranted by considerations such as

a) stage of individual progress/self-disclosure of each client;
b) stage of group life (i.e., pre-affiliation, power and control; intimacy; differentiation; termination) and
c) appropriateness with regard to timing, group purpose, group function, etc.

In general, as identified earlier, the underlying theme of all professional social work roles in the TC context is advocacy. Seen in this light, the professional social worker actually advocates on behalf of the client with his fellow group members, enabling them to fulfil the following roles:

1. *challenge* — group members are helped to bring to bear questions, consideration of consequences and reality testing on the output of their peers.
2. *confrontation* — group members are helped to make explicit faulty, self-serving and dysfunctional cognition and behaviour.
3. *support* — group members are helped to provide support for incremental and successive approximations of functional, healthy cognition and behaviour.

In terms of the professional social worker's exclusive responsibilities in the group, several other roles can be delineated, including

1. *facilitator* — aids the group members in processing challenge, confrontation and support in a fashion that promotes change and growth.
2. *executive* — the group leader retains the right to make final

decisions on issues; however, vetoing group decisions is considered a "last resort," as the focus of the therapy group in the TC is on enabling group decision making and problem solving.

3. *evaluator* — the group leader is responsible for the consistent monitoring of both individual and group processes and should be able to define these, together with pursuant plans of treatment, at all times.

4. *innovator* — the group leader, positioned between the agency administration and the group, is able to suggest and implement new and creative plans to enhance the group (e.g., group-exclusive outings, treatment processes, etc.)

II. Individual Therapist

Professional social work roles for individual therapy in the TC are similar to clinical roles in other progressive treatment settings and include: challenge; facilitation; enabling; support; innovation; confrontation; clarification; partialization; concretization and problem solving. The critical differences inherent in individual therapy in the TC is that the ultimate aim in closure of the individual therapy sessions is preparing the resident to process the issues discussed in his therapy group. To reiterate, group therapy is the primary method of treatment in the TC and one-to-one work is viewed as critical in certain cases (e.g., guilt and shame issues, etc.), yet supplemental to the group-oriented treatment focus.

III. Administrator

Stonehenge Therapeutic Community is a non-profit incorporated organization, with a budgetary base in excess of $1,000,000 per fiscal year, and a community-based Board of Directors. While it may be unpalatable in terms of the philosophical ideas held by certain social work practitioners, the therapeutic community is a business, with demands similar to profit-making businesses. While some companies manufacture and sell "widgits," the TC's product is people. If the company does not produce an exemplary product, it will not survive in either economic or social service marketplaces. Without the desired outcome, there would be no funding base and, therefore no production, or service. It is the administrator's role to ensure the viability of the company, or, in our profession's vernacular, "the good health of the agency."

The primary role of the administrator is to carry out agency policy and goals as determined by the Board of Directors. The social work practitioner, in the role of Chief Executive Officer, is a salaried employee of the Board and responds to the Board of Directors — directly and through a management sub-committee. All other job roles within the setting are responsible to the Chief Executive Officer as employees of the agency. The social work administrator is empowered to be involved in all aspects of the agency's functioning and reports, both verbally and in writing, to the Board of Directors.

The administrator is responsible for all fiscal aspects of the agency's function. In a sense, it is analogous to monitoring the heartbeat of a living organism. Both governmental funding sources and commonsense require the monitoring of dollar for value service. The administrator, in liaison with the financial officer and the agency's auditor, attend to the fiscal duties. These responsibilities can range from something as simple as signing an invoice for payment authorization to the preparation of annual budget forecasting. The Chief Executive Officer is required, through the financial officer, to invest any capital surpluses and is empowered to develop methodologies to avoid deficits. The administrator is also responsible for the agency's purchases. Individual staff responsible for specific program areas are allocated a spending ceiling applicable to each fiscal year and are monitored by the Chief Executive Officer. Unlike more traditional social work settings, such as institutions and government ministry organizations, the TC is not structured to include purchasing departments, as one might find in a hospital, for example. Therefore, the administrator, with the assistance of his staff, ensures proper fiscal functioning of the agency. The Chief Executive Officer is also responsible for salary administration; specifically, the implementation of competitive wage grids and the development of a progressive fringe benefit package to be approved by the Board of Directors. It is important that the TC be able to attract appropriately credentialed and skilled staff persons and, to do so, it must remain competitive with other agency settings. As the TC is generally a non-profit entity, the Chief Executive Officer is responsible for the encouragement of tax-deductible donations.

The social work administrator is responsible for all personnel matters, including the hiring, firing and supervision of staff. In the therapeutic community, staff team-building is a very important role of the agency's administrator. Developing a sense of personal commitment to the agency's philosophies and goals is an integral part of the achievement of high-quality treatment service delivery. The administrator is responsible in many ways for the team spirit, through staff development and leadership role style.

Finally, the administrator maintains the ultimate responsibility for the quality of resident care. Administrative staff are charged with the maintenance of patient's statistics and demographic information. Through both fiscal and personnel allocation, resident care is monitored and enhanced, from the physical setting to the attainment of treatment goals.

IV. Community Development and Social Policy

Undeniably, the role of advocate is the most visible when considered in terms of facilitating the process of social change. Prior to the introduction of a professional social work role, STC was relatively unknown and desperately underfunded. While it offered an exceptional quality of treatment service, its resources could only assist a few addicts. In 1975, the agency accommodated 10 drug abusers, with a staff of 6, maintained by a budgetary base slightly in excess of $100,000. The fiscal resources for the program's grant from the Federal Non-Medical Use Of Drugs Directorate had expired, and the treatment facility was facing extinction. The responsibility for funding the program fell mostly on the role of the professional social worker.

At the present time, the agency is funded by the Provincial Ministry of Health, the Provincial Ministry of Correctional Services, the Correctional Service of Canada, the Ministry of Community and Social Services (COMSOC) and by private donations. STC employs a staff of 25, serving the needs of 40 residents, and has recently developed educational and community awareness resources in the areas of drug abuse and HIV-AIDS Infection. STC enjoys an international reputation for expertise in the field of addiction, and has impacted significantly upon the fashion in which addict offenders are treated in the province of Ontario. The role of the practitioner as a catalyst for social change has been essential to the agency's initial survival and subsequent growth. Specific duties related to this role include the development of community-based support and the formulation of program proposals for application to various funding ministries. More often than not, "proper process" of funding application, by itself, will not ensure that the legitimate needs of the client group are met. Instead media involvement (in promotion of enhanced public awareness) and political lobbying represent the vehicles to effective change and support in response to our society's ever-growing problem with drug abuse.

V. Educator

Stonehenge Therapeutic Community is a teaching centre, and has a mandate to promote public awareness concerning substance abuse, HIV infection, the nature of the addict and addiction treatment modalities. As a placement setting for the graduate school of social work at Wilfrid Laurier University; the Conestoga College School of Social Work; the George Brown School of Addictions Studies, and as a resource to the University of Guelph, students from these educational institutions participate in various learning involvements at STC. They are supervised by the agency's social work practitioners. Inasmuch as one-to-one teaching/learning relationships benefit the students through exposure to a unique community health care setting, it also provides the agency with ongoing new perspectives, sometimes absent in settings devoid of student involvement. STC's social workers are actively engaged in educational responsibilities in the form of lectures, seminars and presentations to universities, schools, community groups and other social service agencies. Publications in various journals have been forthcoming from the agency's social workers. Whether at the lectern at an international conference, the front of a classroom, speaking at a community group's meeting or during a supervision session with a student, the role of educator is regularly evident in the practice roles and responsibilities of social workers at STC.

VI. Researcher

The role of the researcher has been minimal throughout the agency's history. While research studies have been completed, the majority were conducted by students on placement as requirements for their various degrees/certificates. It is the agency's philosophy to encourage research within its setting, but also to avoid bias by having research carried out by qualified persons outside the agency. Toward this end, research proposals have been developed by faculty members of the University of Guelph and are presently awaiting Governmental funding to commence. The role of the Stonehenge social worker is, therefore, to co-operate with the researching body through the provision of case studies, medical records, client statistics, etc.

VII. Private Practitioner

This chapter has mentioned the scant representation of professional social workers employed in this specific field. It is, therefore, not surprising that the role of "expert" applies to the agency's social workers. It is commonplace for the expertly qualified social worker to be hired to provide either assessment and/or testimony in court on behalf of drug addicts. Most commonly, the social worker is hired by a lawyer (usually the counsel for the defence) to interview an inmate and, in the form of a detailed psychosocial assessment report, provide an accurate personal history, including criminal involvement and background of addiction. Forthcoming sentencing recommendations are suggested for the court's consideration, and the social worker may be called upon to provide expert testimony during the court procedure.

To a very limited extent this agency allows its social workers to engage in private practice through the provision of individual treatment of an out-patient nature to drug-dependent persons and their families. The duties involved in all private practice matters require a contract for service, provision of the service and subsequent billing for the service.

VIII. Role Model

The "role of role model" permeates both inter-resident and intra-staff relationships. In many ways, the clients of the agency look to the staff member as a role model in terms of devising their lifestyle restructuring plan. It is natural for personnel trained in other disciplines to possess a curiosity concerning the skills developed through professional social work training. While the job responsibilities of the "role of role model" are difficult to define, the authors feel it is important to note that TC clients attempt to utilize the social worker's manifested interpersonal, communication and relationship skills as the blueprint for their own developing "healthy" personalities.

IX. The Role of the Self-Observer

The nature of our profession encourages the social worker to be an architect for his own personal growth and change. Self-observation not only assists us in job performance, but enhances skill development. The role of self-observer is promoted through the process of supervision, in which all the agency's social workers participate. Constructive, reflective feedback from one's supervisor and colleagues assists in the development of an observing self. While the job roles within the agency demand varying levels of authority, all members of the staff team endeavour to function within a "horizontal hierarchy." Specifically stated, a requirement of the job role is to remain open to other team members' constructive criticism. Therefore, differential levels of authority and responsibility within the functioning of the agency should not preclude an egalitarian "team" approach to the shared goals of client rehabilitation and overall agency philosophy.

POTENTIAL FOR ROLE DEVELOPMENT

If measured by sheer lack of numbers of professional social workers within the TC setting, the potential for role development and growth in this field is greater than in all other contexts of social work practice. Historically, there has been a dearth of professional social workers entering the TC modality. This phenomenon is based on three issues. First, as therapy in the TC is structured into days that are generally 15 hours in length, therapists work irregular shift hours, including evenings and weekends. Second, there is the intensity of work commonplace to a residential setting, which is devoid of the luxury of a private office, and often without time for isolation (i.e., for the therapist to "regroup" between client interactions). Finally, there is the recognition that the majority of the therapeutic processes occur in the group format, which, in the case of the TC, is confrontative, direct and intense. Some incompatible social worker may find this unpalatable to their style and to their ideals concerning the therapist-client relationship. The fact, however, remains that there are only a few social work job roles (at the MSW level) currently employed in Canada in this setting. As for residential treatment settings in general, a brief review of the Ontario College of Certified Social Workers Registry confirms the distinct lack of professional social work involvement in these settings. The majority of professional social workers remain in the relative comfort of governmental institutions and larger formalized settings.

CONCLUDING REMARKS

The TC treatment context is uniquely demanding. The call for skilled social work involvement in this field is a compelling mission fundamental to the essence of our profession's mandate. Historically, social work representation in TC settings has been sparse, but vital. Both new and experienced practitioners can embrace exciting opportunities to develop new horizons of theory and practice in the TC setting.

Recognizing that drug addiction is a pervasive and ever-increasing problem of epic proportion in contemporary society, the challenge for professional social work is indeed undeniable.

CASE EXAMPLE

The following case examples, which appeared in the *Kitchener-Waterloo Record* on Thursday September 1, 1988 are reflective of typical STC clientele.

Case #1

The decline of one addict from a young entrepreneur worth millions of dollars to a drug-crazed robber reads like a cliche, but his presence in the rehabilitation centre attests to its truth.

The former president of a Toronto air-conditioning company, Tony, 24, is part-way through a nine year sentence for 22 armed robberies. Under a special agreement with the centre and the federal corrections department he traded jail for Stonehenge.

Everybody he met during his year in jail had used cocaine. "That was their downfall," he said.

Before he was 20, Tony had smoked some hashish but wasn't seriously into drugs and didn't even drink alcohol. But then one day at a party he experimented with cocaine. "I tried that, and it was nothing like I ever tried before," he said. "I was addicted from that point on."

He bought $1,000 worth of cocaine that night. He loved cocaine so much he began a $600 a day habit that grew to $1,000 a day, then $1,500 a day. Within about eight months, he had spent his trust fund and his entire savings.

"It goes very fast when you smoke it," he said. "Spending $2,000 in 24 hours is very easy."

Because of his credit rating, he could buy $4,000 worth of cocaine from any dealer he knew. He tried to deal coke but because he was so addicted, ended up using it himself.

Tony, heavily in debt and owing $20,000 to a member of a motorcycle club, was given an ultimatum.

In order to pay the debt, Tony and his girlfriend embarked on a crime spree, holding up banks and gas stations with a toy gun. "I needed money or I was going to be shot," Tony said.

He and his girlfriend were eventually caught and convicted, making headlines as the "Bonnie and Clyde" of Toronto. Presently, Tony is successfully reintegrating into society. He has established a drug-free lifestyle and is maintaining gainful employment. Tony is a positive reflection of what an addict can do for himself when provided with the corrective resources proffered by STC. Tony will be on parole until 1990.

Case #2

A 21-year-old Cambridge woman has also opted for Stonehenge instead of jail where she was to spend two years for robbery, prostitution, theft, possession of a stolen vehicle, an indecent act and bail violations.

Donna's parents were alcoholics and very poor. She was beaten as a child, molested by a friend of the family when she was five and eventually placed in a foster home.

She left there at age 16 and immersed herself in a world of drugs and petty crime.

"I was really bad into cocaine. I needed it every second or just one after another. If I'd do one, I'd need another one," Donna said.

"I got into a lot of trouble with it. I felt like it followed me everywhere that I went. It's like it's your husband."

She would "do anything for this cocaine."

"I went out there and did the robberies to get the money or I'd go to the stores and steal. I used to be a thief just to get this cocaine. I was a prostitute," she said.

Her former boyfriend used to rob banks to have enough money for drugs.

"So the money would just come in. I don't know how much. From 16 to now, I must have spent billions on it. Every penny that I made, it would go towards the cocaine," Donna said. Drug use almost cost Donna her life.

"Doing cocaine, I'd find I've stabbed myself, I cut my wrists. If I didn't get it, I'd go and slash myself," she said.

Donna continues to progress through the program's phases of treatment, looking forward to her own consensus.

References

Halpern, S. & Levine, B. (Eds.) (1979). *Proceedings of the Fourth International Conference of Therapeutic Communities.* New York: U.S.A.

Holt, S. (1979). *A Follow-Up Study of Participants of a Residential Drug Related Treatment Program.* Unpublished manuscript.

Ruton, N. (1980). Cost effective rehabilitation for drug dependent persons. *Dimensions in Health Service.*

Ruton, N. (1982). Pre-trial perspectives for the addict offender. *Criminal Lawyers' Association Newsletter, 4(9).*

Ruton, N., & Vincent, S. (1986). *The Canadian T.C. — A Sentencing Option for the Addict Offender.* Paper presented to the Tenth World Conference of Therapeutic Communities, Eskilstuna, Sweden.

Snider, G. M. (1979). Developing rehabilitative factors in drug sentencing. *Criminal Lawyers' Association Newsletter, 1.*

Sugarman, B. (1982). Towards a new, common model of the therapeutic community: structural components, learning processes and outcomes. In *Third Generation of Therapeutic Communities: Proceedings of the First European Conference on Milieu Therapy.* Sweden: European Federation of Therapeutic Communities.

Turner, F. (Ed.) (1984). *Adult Psychopathology.* New York: The Free Press.

Wilhelm, J. (1988). *Clients of the Stonehenge Therapeutic Community: An Examination of the Relationship Between Selected Client Characteristics and Program Completion.* Unpublished manuscript.

Zastrow, C. (1985). *Social Work With Groups.* Chicago: Nelson-Hall.

Endnotes

1. "We have seen it emerge as one of the finest programs for youth with emotional and lifeskill problems in Ontario. Stonehenge's program skilfully combines warmth, love and kindness with discipline, self-reliance and self-independence." Communications from M. Rutte, Program Director, *The Non-Medical Use of Drugs Directorate*, Ottawa, Ontario, 1979.

   "This committee, in conducting an inquiry into drug abuse and possible solutions has found only one viable therapeutic community in the Province of Ontario — Stonehenge." Mayor Mel Lastman's Committee on Narcotic Addiction, Dr. J. Cooper and Edward L. Greenspan, Toronto, Ontario 1978.

   "It (Stonehenge) is considered the most viable treatment program in Canada." *Drug Alert*, Marilee Wiseman, Wiley Publishing Inc., Toronto, Ontario 1979.

   "The success of this treatment program is very impressive." News release, from the Chairman of the Management Board of Cabinet, the Honourable George McCague, April 14, 1980.

Chapter 35

COMMUNITY SOCIAL WORK PRACTICE: HEALTH PROMOTION IN ACTION

Judith Dunlop, MSW
Michael J. Holosko, PhD

Abstract

Current health care policy in North America reflects the political, economic and social realities of our culture. The crisis in health care that North America is presently experiencing has been brought about by forces that seek to change the priorities of health care funding from high technology institutional treatment to preventive programs with a community-based orientation. The profession of social work, through community social work practice, has a major role to play in empowering the community to strengthen itself and thus the community health and health of individual citizens.

COMMUNITY SOCIAL WORK PRACTICE: HEALTH PROMOTION IN ACTION

THE CLIENTELE

The desire to build a collaborative community to empower citizens to take control over a healthy, social economic and physical environment leads a social work practitioner into an exciting and challenging arena of political intrigue. The collaborative activities to be discussed in this chapter were carried out in three communities of Southwestern Ontario, when the first author (J. Dunlop) was a social worker in a public health unit. This concept of "community as client" is fundamental to the development of community social work practice. The community itself may be the clientele or user of service, and it is a distinct entity that requires indirect or direct intervention. At a macro level, this community practice intervention may take the form of helping all members of the community to take control over creating healthier communities, while at a micro level, the clientele may be defined as an "at risk" population with the intervention focussed on developing a network of informal relationships in a neighbourhood setting. Both of these definitions of community as client allow the integration of community social work practice models with recent health promotion policy documents to produce a de facto application of community social work skills in health promotion program implementation.

A common theme advocated in all recent health promotion policy documents is an identification of the need to go beyond specific health problems of individuals and to deal with the social, behaviourial and environmental determinants of health and illness in the population. Canada has created policies that provide universal access to health care, and the Canadian health care system seems to be on a much firmer foundation than the American system, whose current debate centres on the rationing of health care to curb expenditures. Conversely, the American health care system has in fact created two kinds of citizens in the health realm. Despite steady increases in health expenditures and the existence of sophisticated technology, for example, in 1987, 37 million Americans had neither private health insurance nor government health benefits (Hiatt, 1987). The success achieved by Canada in building an accessible health care system has provided the impetus to move forward looking for direction in addressing the realm of health promotion as advocated by the World Health Organization (WHO).

In *Targets for Health for All by the Year 2000*, it is agreed that the goal for all governments should be to ensure that everyone achieves a level of health that enables them to lead a socially and economically productive life (WHO, 1986). This goal has been adopted by the Canadian government in the recently released report *Achieving Health for All: A Framework for Health Promotion* (Epp, 1986). Affirming the World Health Organization report (1986), this document identifies three leading strategies of response to health challenges;= one of which is to co-ordinate policies between those sectors of the community that have a direct bearing on health. This focus on inter-sectoral action at the community level is reflected in three recently released provincial health reports from Ontario. *The Report of the Panel on Health Goals for Ontario* has identified that community development may contribute significantly to improvement in a community's health (Spasoff, 1987). Spasoff further identified the community development process as one whereby a community organizes itself to identify and solve its own problems using a consensus approach. Further, Dr. J. R. Evans, Chairman of the Ontario Health Review Panel in *Toward a Shared Direction for Health in Ontario* (1987) identified that new approaches to improve linkages among various levels of health services and related social services involved new organizational arrangements. For example, by re-organizing a community, a process could be developed whereby health could be an explicit consideration in all the policies, plans and programs of not only municipal governments but of other significant public and private organizations in the community whose actions may affect health.

The emphasis on the role of individuals and communities in determining their own health status is strengthened by the *Report of the Ministries Advisory Group on Health Promotion — Health Promotion Matters in Ontario* (Podborski, 1987). In its recommendations, it recognizes that public health units have an important role to play in creating community-based prevention programs. This chapter describes a social work role carried out within a public health unit in Ontario whose focus was community organization strategies to develop inter-sectoral planning and co-ordination of prevention in three communities of the region.

The massive problems of ill health cannot be addressed effectively without an understanding of the need to join together in the struggle to establish alternatives to the present high technology treatment system. This means not only joining with other health and social service professionals, but also with clients in order to gain a broad base of support and to make clients aware of their own oppression within the system. Thus, social work can examine the social and environmental causes for bad health and lobby for eliminating poverty, poor housing, poor nutrition and environmental pollution. Although change in the health care system is only part of a fundamental social change, the development of alternatives to the present sick-care system must be a goal of such social work practice. Community social work practice, whether the approach taken is community development, political action or social planning, offers an opportunity to move health promotion policy implementation from rhetoric to reality.

PRACTICE ROLES AND RESPONSIBILITIES

While there is no typical or "carved-in-stone" intervention technique that can be prescribed, to some degree all community workers are likely to adopt any one of three approaches: community development social action and, social planning. The selection of an approach is dependent upon the circumstances in which the community practitioner finds her/himself. Community organization approaches encompass

1) locality development with its focus on neighbourhood or rural community involvement;
2) social planning with its focus on inter-agency problem-solving and planning and
3) social action with its emphasis on social movements and political strategies seeking a redistribution of power, resources and community decision making (Rothman, 1979).

Inherent within all these approaches is the role of the community organizer, as one of the critical skills necessary for effective community interventions is the capacity to build relationships within it. This is based on the ability of the worker to use her/himself and use of relationship skills whether the group is a grassroots citizen's organization or inter-agency planning, and/or co-ordinating group. The focus on strategy development within an ever-changing environment involves a great deal of creativity, risk-taking, autonomy and competence. The "community as client" arena of community practice requires that for successful action the practitioner possesses skills of analysis, planning and organization together with the formidable interaction skills previously mentioned. It is without question, no small order being responsible for constant innovation in addition to managing many diverse and competitive interests.

This is not territory for the faint-hearted or for those who need immediate and/or concrete results. Perhaps one of the major responsibilities of the community practitioner is to cling to her/his faith in the educative process of community work while seeing no measurable achievement at either a structural or task-accomplishment level. How are we to convince social work students of the primacy of community organization given the results of the territory?

Karger (1983) posits that community organization skills taught in schools of social work need to be re-assessed. Practitioners need to be developed who have more precise, specialized skills and knowledge appropriate to the political economy of the 1980s and 1990s. The core areas of skills and knowledge suggested by Karger (1983) are as follows:

1) political and critical thinking;
2) analysis of relationships of power at different bureaucratic and government levels;
3) coalition building;
4) fundraising skills;
5) social action research skills and the ability to interpret the research to constituents;
6) administrative skills including; a) supervision and training, b) organizational development and c) budgeting and
7) technological skills a) information gathering and processing, b) knowledge and use of computers.

The skills and knowledge outlined by Karger (1983) represent a focus on community organization practice that has as its purpose the empowerment of the community and the redistribution of resources and power. It is in this arena of political and systems advocacy that we can once again return to the application of social work practice in health promotion. Community organization as an intervention seeks to facilitate collective action on the part of its clientele, be it a whole community or a collection of individuals linked by a neighbourhood. The participation of people in the decisions that influence their health, and the health of the community, affirms the commitment of the social work profession to social justice.

The principle of social justice fuels the community practitioner's motivation to effect change in the political and economic systems in the community. To suggest that inter-agency collaboration to plan and co-ordinate services arouses enthusiasm in the health, social service or education sectors would be ludicrous. It is possible, however, in some small measure to build a collaborative process at the community level by taking small, incremental, thoughtful steps toward building a structure for inter-organizational relations. As mentioned earlier, community practice is not the domain of the "quick fix" practitioner or for those who are afraid to go into the proverbial "lion's den" of community power structures.

For those who are willing to venture out of the easy shelter of the agency, work in isolation for a hundred masters and endure long and irregular working hours that take a toll on your private life, community practice offers a seductive lure for those with a vision of a better new world. The current climate of support for a movement to prevention/health promotion orientations is a heady climate for community social work indeed.

In examining community practice methods for implementing health promotion policy, Lappin's (1986) insights make a valuable contribution. Community practice is viewed as a two-level system:

1) embodying a direct form of work with community residents and

2) indirect community work carried out by representative bodies or community surrogates that function in the areas of social service planning, co-ordination of services and programs, setting priorities with respect to community needs and establishing standards of service among local social agencies.

It is in this second level of indirect community work or inter-group work where we must examine social work roles and their application in this chapter.

Before leaving the area of direct community work or community development, however, it is important to better understand this concept. Lappin (1986) described it as a one-level system of direct community work concerned with the total needs of residents whether in rural villages or urban neighbourhoods. We would be remiss in not directing the reader to the work of Paolo

Freire, who has had a profound impact on community development in the third world and whose practice of conscientization has influenced community organizers in direct practice in both South and North America.

The inter-group process carried out under the auspice of one public health unit in Southwestern Ontario resulted in the development of three local planning and co-ordinating coalitions whose purpose was to advocate for the prevention of developmental disabilities. The desire to become "systems advocates" for prevention within a tri-county geographic area led to the development of an advocacy planning role for the community practitioner. The role strain present in this particular intervention was based on the de-emphasis on community development that is currently present in health systems. While community representatives were becoming effective preventive advocates, the system they eventually challenged was the employer of the community worker. This experience illuminated the role of the community worker whose primary loyalty was to the community groups.

In an enabling role, the community worker must empower the community group to articulate their discontent and to develop the leadership skills necessary to work through expected conflict with the power brokers of the community who are resisting change. Grosser (1986) identified the roles of the political action organizer as educator, resource developer and agitator. As educator, the worker helps people to identify issues, to partialize the sources of their problems and to develop alternative solutions. The worker will work collaboratively to build the structure and teach leadership skills. The worker further acts as a resource developer by finding and linking resources to the organization.

Taylor (1986) discusses the community liaison model of practice as having three distinct functions:

1) inter-organizational relations, including referrals, inter-organizational exchange and joint agency action of behalf of its clients;
2) mobilization of community supports for the agency, its programs, financing and ideology and
3) change of community resources, including initiation, revision, elimination or combination of services needed on behalf of the agency's clients.

An examination of community practice methods, activities and roles illustrates once again the "person in environment" matrix that is the guiding unit of analysis in social work practice. While various conceptual models exist, there is considerable ambiguity present even within these models of practice. The rapidly changing environment requires the community worker to be constantly reflecting, analysing and manipulating the political environment to effectively advocate for change for the constituency s/he represents.

Along with a conceptual base for practice obtained through formal educational processes and well-supervised practice experiences, the personal attributes necessary for effective community practice cannot be understated. Some of these qualities that are crucial both to the task accomplishment and interactional process of community work are tact, diplomacy, maturity, resilience, political sensitivity, tolerance, self-confidence, drive, capacity for hard work, initiative, discipline and a degree of detachment and objectivity. The integration of the personal and the professional challenges enables the community organizer to develop a high level of conscious practice. The integration of knowledge and skills with these personal qualities creates the opportunity to ethically carry out the demands made of a social change agent.

POTENTIAL FOR ROLE DEVELOPMENT

It is in the area of coalition-building to improve a community's health that social work can provide a much-needed vision for the future. The cry for mandated inter-sectoral collaboration is faint at the community level. It is through the complex work of inter-organizational relations that social work provides a conceptual and experiential pathway. Thomas (1976) envisioned the social work roles necessary for coalition building as follows:

1) advocate — advocate for co-ordination and planning;
2) innovator-stimulator—collect data from services on their service provision and client;
3) advisor — advice and consultation to workers in voluntary and statutory agencies;
4) informant — collecting and disseminating information on local needs and
5) co-ordinator — a) bring agency staff together for discussions, b) bring agency staff and consumers into joint discussions.

The focus on inter-sectoral collaboration in health promotion

651

policy allows for the expertise of indirect community practice to be utilized in an effective way. The experience of the inter-sectoral collaborative planning coalitions carried out for planning prevention services has shown that the notion of a coalition can be nurtured at the community level. The ability of the community social work practitioner to respond flexibly and sensitively to each situation facilitates necessary collaborative relationships where each of the parties has skills and resources that it makes available to others for the benefit of the community. This specific role of enabler, which is the best approach to use to help a community define its own needs, belongs to community social work practice. The ability of the worker to engage the necessary representation in the community, to encourage the involvement of key representatives in inter-group work and the development of leadership skills among participants is based on the process intervention of community practice, which seeks to develop enabling relationships, mobilize citizen participation and build an organizational structure that will strengthen community involvement in managing local health challenges. Change can also be effected through direct interventions that seek to build collaborative networks for informal and formal social supports, self-help groups and the development of community participation in the voluntary sector.

Recent developments in health promotion policy areas have opened up a flood-gate of opportunity for social workers trained in community practice. For years, the community practitioner has been seen as a "somewhat amusing, somewhat confusing" aberration in North America, tolerated perhaps by their clinical peers but hardly considered an equal partner in the professional practice arena.

CONCLUDING REMARKS

The movement of the health care system away from high technology institutional treatment provides fertile ground for a lively and productive area of development for social work community practice. The training of community social workers needs to be undertaken by practitioners who have experienced what one could call the "art" of community practice; for it is the nuances of community work that allow the worker to achieve social action at the community level. Community groups need quick successes to effect commitment to collaboration and it is the worker's challenge to develop a learning environment where success is truly reinforced.

This "art" requires not only the functions for a procedural technician, but the type of inter-personal skills required of all leaders: the ability to motivate, negotiate, stimulate and resolve conflicts. No training in procedures and methods will compensate for lack of inter-personal skills.

Community practitioners must have the requisite professional training and attributes, and also the appropriate personal qualities to accept the limitations of the work while struggling to maintain the vision of a healthier community. In the words of Twelvetrees (1986), "you have to aspire to change the world to do community work, otherwise you will not find the motivation to do the job." In conclusion, there are a few caveats that are important to consider for those practitioners courageous enough to venture forth into the public arena of community practice. The choice of a professional practice in community social work needs to be examined through the following filters:

1) Social change is a continual phenomena — it is never finished!
2) The political action at the community level is dangerous — make sure you can take the heat if things go wrong.
3) Reflect upon and integrate the philosophy of social work into your practice; there will be many pushes and pulls by vested interest groups — you need an anchor!
4) Community work is a process that unfolds uniquely in each community and with each group and individual; don't expect surefire techniques to get you through — there aren't any!
5) Above all be honest in your dealings with community players — the role is one of perceived neutrality and the first self-serving intervention will destroy your credibility with the community.
6) Learn to live with isolation. Your client group needs you to be objective and detached — you are not in a collegial relationship with any of your fellow community members.

CASE EXAMPLE

The Prevention Project outlined in this case example was funded by the Ontario Ministry of Community and Social Services and administered through a local county public health unit. The goal of the project was to publicize what is known about the prevention of developmental disabilities and to promote a community response that would reduce the incidence of developmental disabilities throughout the three counties in the region. The community organizer (J. Dunlop) was hired as a Prevention Co-ordinator reporting to the Director of Infant Stimulation for the health unit. A model for program development had not been identified prior to the hiring of the staff position. This allowed the social work practitioner considerable autonomy in proceeding with a plan for locality development in each county.

In order to carry out the goals of the project, a Tri-County Advisory Committee and four local sub-committees were developed, which allowed for two levels of action to be operationalized in each community. These two levels, namely task accomplishment and structure building, allowed the project to work simultaneously toward its stated objectives of providing specific staff training and community education on the prevention of developmental disabilities and promoting inter-agency and inter-sectoral collaboration to improve services to populations at risk.

Participants in the project included the administrative and direct service levels of key service agencies, professional and community groups and parent advocates. Over sixty representatives from health, social service, education and voluntary organizations worked collaboratively for two years to carry out the stated objectives of the project.

The task accomplishment of the project's Sub-Committees was carried out utilizing a strategic planning process resulting in a set of action plans for each locality that included critical path dates for the activities to be carried out. The goal of the project had been to develop strong preventive networks in each community and while the project was successful in building these coalitions, it was in the realm of organizational structure that problems were encountered. The individuals and organizations of the three counties who were committed to the implementation of prevention programs in their respective areas sought to continue the networks that had been established by the project; however, they did not wish to continue under the current organizational structure. This development is a logical consequence of the particular community intervention techniques used by the organizer. The assessment of local needs and power structures allowed the organizer to mobilize coalitions with specific interests and specific definitions of at-risk populations that were relevant to that specific community.

Once these community groups were established as effective advocates for prevention, their desire or need to interact with an administrative body in another county, which in effect controlled the project and the co-ordinator, became a problem in continuing with the structure. These local groups consequently lobbied the Ontario Ministry of Community and Social Services for funding at the local level and were successful in accessing these funds. The co-ordinator worked individually with each community to strengthen their advocacy position and became an effective change agent to end this particular structure.

The inter-group process of building prevention coalitions was successfully implemented in this project. The role of the community social work practitioner was not well understood in this instance by the employing organization. The external limitations of time and travel were the most easily identified part of the process that had an impact on the co-ordinator's role. Along with this, the perception of the co-ordinator as an employee of the health unit was problematic in two counties outside the employing agency's territory. While there was successful engagement of the appropriate agency representatives, in two counties, the "out-of-community" position of the co-ordinator did not allow for the utilization of the informal power network in these communities as was possible in the local "home" area. This is a common problem in locality development and one that contributed to the decision not to continue on a Tri-County basis. There was, further, a lack of clarity about the co-ordinator's role being one of consultant on loan to respective community groups and some lack of understanding of the organizational accountability, which is necessary when the sponsoring organization gives auspice to this kind of inter-sectoral project.

This project was very successful in building community coalitions to advocate for prevention. The autonomy afforded to the practitioners allowed the project to develop a clear response to community needs that was eventually in direct conflict with the needs of the employing agency. The model for intervention in three communities was discussed with health unit administration at the inception of the project. However, due to lack of training and experience with the community social work practice and the relative unimportance of the project to the organization's functioning, the development of the project as a strong advocacy body for prevention services caused the sponsoring organization to experience both internal and external conflicts.

This case example points out the need for community social work practitioners to have a clear sense of the constituency s/he purports to represent. Inevitably, there will be a conflict between the service provider agency employing the community worker and the constituency developed by the organizer to whom s/he owes her/his primary loyalty.

References

Epp, J. (1986). *Achieving Health for All: A Framework for Health Promotion*. Ottawa: Health and Welfare Canada.

Evans, R. (1987). *Toward a Shared Direction for Health in Ontario: Report of the Ontario Health Review Panel* (p. 16). Toronto: Government of Ontario.

Friere, P. (1985). The Politics of Education, Culture, Power and Liberation. London: MacMillan Ltd.

Grosser, C. E. & Mondras, J. (1986). In S. H. Taylor & R. W. Roberts (Eds.), *Theory and Practice of Community Social Work* (p. 161). New York: Columbia University Press.

Hiatt, H. J. (1987). *America's Health in the Balance — Choice or Chance*. Toronto: Fitzhenry and Whitehead.

Karger, H. J. & Reitman, R. (1983). Community organization for the 1980's: Toward developing a new skill base within a political framework. *Social Development Issues, 7*(2), 50-62.

Lappin, B. (1986). In S. H. Taylor & R. W. Roberts (Eds.), *Theory and Practice of Community Social Work*. New York: Columbia University Press.

Podborski, S. (1997). *Report of the Ministries Advisory Group on Health Promotion Matters in Ontario*. Toronto: Ministry of Health.

Spasoff, R. A. (1987). *Health for All: Ontario Report of the Panel on Health Goals for Ontario* (p. 100). Toronto: Government of Ontario.

Taylor, S. H. (1986). In S. H. Taylor & R. W. Roberts (Eds.), *Theory and Practice of Community Social Work* (p. 184). New York: Columbia University Press.

Twelvetrees, A. (1986). *Community Work* (p. 128). London: MacMillan Education Ltd.

Thomas, D. M. (1976). *Organizing for Social Change: A Study in the Theory and Practice of Community Work* (p. 131). Great Britain: Biddus Ltd.

World Health Organization (1986). *Targets for Health for All* (p. 1). Copenhagen: World Health Organization.

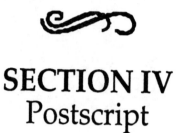

SECTION IV
Postscript

Chapter 36

NEW WAVE SOCIAL WORK: PRACTICE ROLES FOR THE 1990s AND BEYOND

Patricia A. Taylor, MSW

NEW WAVE SOCIAL WORK: PRACTICE ROLES FOR THE 1990s AND BEYOND

As we approach the 21st century, the primary thrust of the delivery of health care is embodied in the concept of "prevention." Not only does this approach respond to the problems of cost containment and the demands for service, but it furthers the goal of making the best possible use of limited health care dollars.

Critical to the concept of prevention is research that will contribute to the present body of health care knowledge in new and unusual ways. The increasing demand for social work research is putting the entire profession on notice that the direction of health care delivery is changing and consequently the profession must come up with both creative and practical solutions to its problems. The general trend to community-based health care is a clear example of a new direction for social work.

The concept of prevention is far broader in scope than rehabilitation alone. Jesse Williams, as quoted in Kenneth R. Pelletier's book, *Holistic Medicine,* stated that "Health as freedom from disease is a standard of mediocrity; health as a quality of life is a standard of inspiration and increasing achievement" (p. 16). Today's emphasis on living a healthy social, emotional and physical lifestyle as embodied in the general concept of holistic medicine certainly predicts a change in health care delivery from the disease/cure model to a broader based, more adaptable health care system. As Pelletier (1979) points out, "It is more evident that health never has been and never will be the sole responsibility of doctors but increasingly that of the consumer working in concert with medical, psychological and environmental counsellors" (p. 16).

An important construct in the new trend in health care delivery is that of the patient as consumer. The challenge to the power base of the traditional system is obvious. At the same time, the patient cannot control the system. Consequently, the patient as consumer needs an advocate from within the health care system, someone to make the patient aware of the services available and to assist the patient in making the best possible choice among these services. While many health care professions such as medicine and nursing assume this function, the role of patient advocate would be better if left in the hands of social work. The generalist theoretical background of social workers together with the special skills in mediating the system that they have developed through practice are solid justification for social workers to assume this advocacy. As Kane (1979) in her editorial in *Health and Social Work* stated:

> The social worker assists the individual patient in clarifying priorities and weathering whatever unavoidable stress is associated with the choices. On an organizational level the social worker is alert to institutional policies (such as visiting rules in a hospital or routines of a nursing home) that are antithetical to other social values (such as family cohesiveness or individual autonomy). Indeed in the future this is where social work is going to have a great impact (p.3).

EMPOWERING THE PATIENT

Historically, the doctor-patient relationship was founded on trust and expertise. Based on a particular background of knowledge and the results of empirically based tests, the doctor had the obligation to form a professional judgment and the right to prescribe treatment. It was improper for a patient to question a diagnosis or seek a second opinion. As Parsons (1957) observed, the "good" patient was supposed to surrender himself to the care of the professionals.

More recent literature has highlighted a change in the role of the patient. Patients and their families are challenged to question the doctor's dominance (Freidson, 1970) and more actively negotiate and participate in their own care (Hayes-Bautista, 1976) by changing physicians if they feel it is necessary (Ugalde, 1984) or by seeking out the most competent doctor (Williams et al., 1960). Certainly the direction of the medical relationship suggests a more active role for the patient. The role of social work in helping patients make choices for themselves is clear. Not only is the basic tenet of social work embodied in the directive of "helping the patient to help himself" but the expressed values of the profession support this approach. Self determination, acceptance and a non-judgmental attitude lend themselves to an approach that supports the patients' right to be included in the decision making about their care. Empowering patients to maintain a level of control over their treatment without alienating themselves from medical services is critical. The role of social work in advocating for this empowerment within the health care team is equally important.

NEGOTIATING THE SYSTEM

A primary goal of social work practice in health care is to ensure that the system meets the needs of the patient. Negotiating health care treatment in the political and administrative context of fiscal restraints, the professional context of advancing medical technology and the personal context of increasing ethical dilemmas and choices is the new wave of social work practice. Balancing the financial costs to the system with the psychosocial costs to the patient defines a clear role for social work. Negotiating, however, is a complex process. It calls for the social worker to acquire a knowledge of what services are needed, where the services exist and how to access them. In addition, a social worker who works well in tandem with other health team members will be more effective in securing special services. The social worker is frequently called upon not only to advocate for the patient, but, in a very positive way, to educate other health care professionals and services about the rights and values that are directing either the patient's or the institution's choice of services. Networking with families, friends and involved others on behalf of the patient is often a part of the negotiation.

Finally, the provision of health care is a legitimate concern of a democracy. The governmental threats of future privatization of segments of the health care system for motives of profit put a serious stress on the individual patient. Under such a system social workers will have an increasing responsibility to negotiate the best possible solutions for the patient's needs within the system.

CREATING A CARING COMMUNITY

The effect of the patient/consumer model has many serious implications for the direction of the delivery of health care services. Consumers classically define services by how they use them and what they want them to offer. In examining the trends in community-based health care over the last fifteen years the increase in self help groups, and also disease-oriented organizations and special patient group clinics, reflects consumer needs that were previously neglected. The early discharge of patients from overburdened hospital facilities is only successful if the community is equipped to receive them. From The Cancer Foundation to The Hospice, to Friends and Families of Schizophrenics, the community trend is to develop specialized services that can assist in both the treatment and the management of patients with both chronic and critical diseases outside of the hospital. The success of these organizations is acknowledged by patients and institutions alike. The role of social work in this trend is defined by the profession's global perspective that has traditionally followed the patient from the hospital to the community and home. Indeed, the work involved in preparing the patient to return to the community is frequently pivotal in achieving successful rehabilitation. As both demand for and cost of in-patient hospital beds increase, that role will continue to expand.

Another feature of the community-based, consumer-oriented system is the increase in services offered for special patient populations. Women's Health Care, Teen Health Care and Geriatric Health Care function so successfully at present that one can only predict an on-going growth in the community of health care centres based on the demands of special interest groups. The implication of this trend for social work education and research is obvious. Informed intervention that reflects specialized knowledge, values and skills will be required in both community- and hospital-based delivery systems where controversial issues around quality of life, abortion and costs of services are debated. Schools of Social Work have a new incentive to develop courses involving medical, legal and ethical issues as they impinge upon social work knowledge if future health care social workers are going to be adequately equipped to meet the challenges of a changing health delivery system.

While the role of social work in counselling families, supporting patients, discharge planning and co-ordinating resources will continue into the next century, they will be refined by a more educated and pro-active consumer and directed by a more creative and responsive community. The new frontier in health care delivery will require the increased intervention of social workers to fully realize its mandate to promote and support the health of the nation. As Schwaber-Kerson (1985) suggests:

> Although the goal of making the system more responsive to need has been clear since the inception of social work in health, the imperative has never been more in the profession's focus. More than ever, the interests of social work's clients and the specialty of social work in health will depend on the

profession's ability to influence the delivery of health care (p. 350).

Social work as a profession has a rich history and tradition steeped in a human response to a human need. The particular features of helping clients when they become patients has been addressed in both philosophical and practical ways in this text.

The variety of specialized services and the creative responses of practitioners to these services are a blueprint for practice today, but more importantly they highlight the direction of social work practice in health care in the 21st century.

References

Freidson, E. (1970a). *Professional Dominance*. New York: Atherton.

Hayes-Bautista, D. E. (1976). Termination of the patient-practitioner relationship: Divorce, patient style. *Journal of Health and Social Behaviour, 17*(1), 12-21.

Kane, R. A. (1979). Social work, social values and health. *Health and Social Work, 4*(3), 3-7.

Parsons, T. & Fox, R. (1952). Illness, therapy and the modern urban American family. *Journal of Social Issues, 8*, 31.

Pelletier, K. R. (1979). *Holistic Medicine*. New York: Dell Publishing.

Schwaber-Kerson, T. (1985). Responsiveness to need: Social worker's impact on health care. *Health and Social Work, 10*(4).

Williams, J. F. (1979). Personal hygiene applied (Philadelphia: W. B. Saunders, 1934), as quoted in Kenneth R. Pelletier, *Holistic Medicine*. New York: Dell Publishing.

Williams, T. F., White, K. L., Andrews, L. P., Diamond, E., Greenberg, B. G., Hamrick, A. A. & Hunter, E. A. (1960). Patient referral to a university clinic: Patterns in a rural state. *American Journal of Public Health, 50*(10), 1493-1507.

Ugalde, A. (1984). Where there is a doctor: Strategies to increase productivity at lower costs. The economics of rural health care in the Dominican Republic. *Social Science Medicine, 19*(4), 441-450.